SOCIETY OF GENERAL PHYSIOLOGISTS SERIES

Synaptic Transmission and Neuronal Interaction

Volume 28
SOCIETY OF GENERAL PHYSIOLOGISTS SERIES

Synaptic Transmission
and
Neuronal Interaction

Editor:

M. V. L. Bennett, D.Phil.

*The Rose F. Kennedy Center for Research in Mental Retardation and Human Development
and the Department of Anatomy, Albert Einstein College of Medicine, New York City*

Raven Press, Publishers ▪ New York

The publication of this volume was supported by a grant from the National Institutes of Health (NS–10438).

Made in the United States of America

International Standard Book Number 0–911216–56–1
Library of Congress Catalog Card Number 73–83886

D
612·81
S4N

Preface

Since Sherrington's *Integrative Action of the Nervous System*, it has become a truism of neurobiology that the synapse is the primary locus of neuronal information processing. To be sure, the neuron's impulse initiating site encodes synaptic potentials into impulse activity, but, to a good approximation, the axon merely represents a reliable conductor of these impulses. It is integrative action that leads the synaptologist to regard the synapse as the most important element of the nervous system, even if he recognizes that axons are as essential to neuronal function as are hearts and lungs. Furthermore, he must acknowledge that much of our understanding of membrane properties comes from axonology, and that the paradigm for the study of elementary electrical events remains the space and voltage clamped axon. Admittedly then, the synaptologist is in the difficult position of regarding one link of a causal chain as more important, but this is not so much a logical blunder as an esthetic judgment, based primarily on the original assertion that the synapse is the site of neuronal information processing.

Our knowledge of the synapse is expanding rapidly, and this volume brings together a number of recent developments in electrophysiological, structural, molecular, developmental and behavioral aspects. It is intended to provide an overview of current concepts and a representative sampling of new technical approaches. The following is the editor's highly condensed summary of the contents.

Grundfest's introductory chapter surveys the diversity of neural membranes and their influence on form and function. In the section on conventional synapses,* Quastel proposes an unconventional model for the role of calcium ions in transmitter release at the neuromuscular junction. Calcium ions and other activators are presumed to act independently to reduce an energy barrier for release, a mechanism which predicts quite different results from the usual model of a release site that becomes effective when it binds a fixed number of calcium ions. Stevens' presentation modifies the conventional view of electrical linearity of subsynaptic membrane. He shows that the postsynaptic conductance increase at the neuromuscular junction is, after all, affected by the membrane potential. The degree of

---

*The editor admits that a division of synapses into conventional and unconventional types is difficult, and in this case it refers primarily to the amount they have been studied. Some ambiguity arose because conventional has two meanings: that which is agreed upon and that which is commonplace. What is conventional in the former sense can change for it is a matter of convention; what is conventional in the latter sense can also change as the distribution of observations changes. For all their faults these terms are retained because references to them are found in several contributions and it would be difficult to edit them out and confusing to leave them unexplained.

alteration, though small, is consistent with the action of an applied field on a conformational change in a membrane-bound receptor molecule.

One of the more exciting elaborations of the conventional view of transmission is the concept of membrane recycling. While the equivalence of vesicles and quanta was hypothesized almost from their discovery, the evidence has been weak. Heuser and Reese have now correlated stimulation and depletion of vesicles which for some reason was never convincingly demonstrated before. More important, by their inventory of membrane and pulse labeling with peroxidase they have obtained convincing evidence that membrane cycles from vesicles to surface by way of exocytosis to coated vesicles by way of endocytosis to cysternae from fusion of coated vesicles to new vesicles which bud off from the cysternae.

Kuno discusses factors affecting the magnitude of postsynaptic potentials at central synapses, sites from which it is much difficult to obtain data than from peripheral synapses.

The unconventional synapses considered include both peripheral and central ones. The retina, which quite recently appeared a can of worms, now seems to be comprehensible, at least in broad outline; much of this advance comes from the correlated morphological and physiological studies of Dowling and his collaborators. The curious hyperpolarizing responses to light become conventional when viewed as responses to dark, the absence of impulses in the outer layers is reasonable for cells where the input and output parts of the cells are close together in terms of electrical space constants. And, having given up impulses, why not have continuous transmitter release that is modulated up and down by appropriate stimuli? Furthermore, demonstrated connectivity patterns of the retina begin to explain the different kinds of responses observed in the retinal output elements, the ganglion cells.

Steinbach assembles available morphological and physiological data on synapses between nonphotic receptor cells and afferent fibers, and presents new physiological results on an acoustico-lateralis receptor. At least some of these synapses are proving to be conventional in terms of the action of calcium ions and quantal release, but they may also have tonic transmitter release that is modulated oppositely by appropriate stimuli. Again, the short length of the receptor cell allows an electrogenic action at one region of the receptor cell surface to act directly upon transmitter release at presynaptic regions elsewhere on the cell.

It would seem that synapses involving decreased rather than increased conductance, as discussed by Weight, will remain unconventionally rare, for their speed of action must always be limited by a time constant at least as great as that of the resting membrane. Still, the mechanisms demonstrated here clearly support similar but less compelling findings in certain central neurons. An as yet largely unexplored question is whether the conductance decreases involve membrane distant from the actual synapse and are mediated by an intracellular, second messenger, as has been widely demonstrated for hormonal actions.

Bennett (the Editor) describes new data on electrically coupled systems. Although electrotonic synapses are undoubtedly many fewer in number than chemically transmitting synapses, they now comprise a respected minority. Mechanisms are shown here by which the degree of electrical coupling can be under physiological or synaptic control, thus allowing neurons to act synchronously or asynchronously under appropriate conditions and extending the number of sites where electrotonic coupling could be of functional significance.

Although the temporal resolution of electrophysiological techniques has allowed one to make inferences about fast chemical changes such as transmitter release, the direct demonstration of the underlying chemical events, including those which are electrically silent, remains a primary if somewhat reductionist goal. The papers by Klett, Fulpius, Cooper, and Reich and by Lindstrom and Patrick concern their pursuit of the subsynaptic receptor molecule for acetylcholine using the recently developed technique involving very tight and specific binding with a particular toxin from a snake venom. While the concept of a synaptic channel has had an obvious appeal, strengthened, one might add, by the demonstration of channel formation in bimolecular lipid membranes, the evidence has been quite inferential. The potentiality for isolation of the receptor molecule suggests that direct demonstration of the channel and of its gaiting mechanism may not be too far off.

A weak point in the skein of evidence for transmitter release from vesicles has been the somewhat varied population of vesicles isolated from central nervous tissue. The successful application of subcellular fractionation techniques to *Torpedo* electric organs is described by Whittaker and Zimmermann. These organs contain a vast and pure population of cholinergic synapses, and extraordinarily homogenous vesicle preparations can be obtained. Now direct measurements of their acetylcholine content are becoming consistent with electrophysiological and morphological estimates. Furthermore, there is new information suggesting mechanisms of storage in high concentrations. Schwartz explores cholinergic mechanisms using the single neuron techniques that are so beautifully applicable to the large and identifiable neurons of many molluscs. Although the predominant synthesis of acetylcholine must be in the terminals, the cell body clearly plays a role in providing the packaging machinery (as well as a minor amount of packaged acetylcholine).

Tissue culture provides an important technique for analysis of development, and three contributions concern the formation of neuromuscular junctions *in vitro*. Fischbach and his collaborators describe their results with dissociated embryonic cells. Of particular interest are the local hot spots of sensitivity to acetylcholine that are found in perinuclear regions and the possibility of tracing their origin by electron microscopic observation of labeled receptor molecules. Fambrough and colleagues focus on the molecular biology of acetylcholine receptors, their synthesis, and their appearance in the membrane. Harris uses continuously dividing lines of cultured cells that have the advantage of genetic uniformity if they are not entirely normal. The point of his presentation is that neuroblasts that do not make acetylcholine attach to myoblasts and that these sites have an increased sensitivity to acetylcholine. If, indeed, the sensitivity appears after contact is made, there is a strong case for trophic influence at the neuromuscular junction that is not mediated by acetylcholine.

The final paper by Carew and Kandel presents their analysis of habituation of a withdrawal response. They have found much of the underlying neural circuitry and are very close to defining the cellular events involved in this primitive but almost universal form of learning.

The papers thus range from the molecular characterization of excitability to the cellular analysis of a simple form of behavioral plasticity. Obviously the stories here are not complete, yet they provide an indication of the directions in which cellular neurobiology will be going for some time to come.

M. V. L. Bennett

Contents

Contributors

M. V. L. Bennett
Rose F. Kennedy Center for Research in
  Mental Retardation and Human Develop-
  ment
Department of Anatomy
Albert Einstein College of Medicine
New York, New York 10461
and
Marine Biological Laboratory
Woods Hole, Massachusetts 02543

A. C. Breuer
Behavioral Biology Branch
National Institute of Child Health and Hu-
  man Development
National Institutes of Health
Bethesda, Maryland 20014

Thomas J. Carew
Department of Neurobiology and Behavior
The Public Health Research Institute of the
  City of New York
and
Department of Physiology and Psychiatry
New York University Medical School
New York, New York 10016

S. A. Cohen
Department of Pharmacology
Harvard Medical School
25 Shattuck Street
Boston, Massachusetts 02115

D. Cooper
Rockefeller University
New York, New York 10021

John E. Dowling
The Biological Laboratories
Harvard University
Cambridge, Massachusetts 02138

Douglas M. Fambrough
Department of Embryology
The Carnegie Institution of Washington
115 W. University Parkway
Baltimore, Maryland 21210

G. D. Fischbach
Department of Pharmacology
Harvard Medical School
25 Shattuck Street
Boston, Massachusetts 02115

B. W. Fulpius
Rockefeller University
New York, New York 10021

Harry Grundfest
Department of Neurology
Columbia University
College of Physicians and Surgeons
New York, New York 10032

A. John Harris
Department of Physiology
University of Otago Medical School
Dunedin, New Zealand

H. Criss Hartzell
Department of Embryology
The Carnegie Institution of Washington
115 W. University Parkway
Baltimore, Maryland 21210

M. P. Henkart
Behavioral Biology Branch
National Institute of Child Health and Hu-
  man Development
National Institutes of Health
Bethesda, Maryland 20014

J. E. Heuser
Department of Biophysics
University College
London, England

Nancy Joseph
Department of Embryology
The Carnegie Institution of Washington
115 W. University Parkway
Baltimore, Maryland 21210

Eric R. Kandel
Department of Neurobiology and Behavior
Public Health Research Institute of the City
  of New York
and
Department of Physiology and Psychiatry
New York University Medical School
New York, New York 10016

R. P. Klett
Rockefeller University
New York, New York 10021

Motoy Kuno
Department of Physiology

University of North Carolina
School of Medicine
Chapel Hill, North Carolina 27514

Jon Lindstrom
Salk Institute for Biological Studies
P.O. Box 1809
San Diego, California 92112

F. M. Neal
Behavioral Biology Branch
National Institute of Child Health and Human Development
National Institutes of Health
Bethesda, Maryland 20014

Jim Patrick
Salk Institute for Biological Studies
P.O. Box 1809
San Diego, California 92112

Jeanne A. Powell
Division of Biological Sciences
Smith College
Northampton, Massachusetts 01060

David M. J. Quastel
Department of Pharmacology
Faculty of Medicine
University of British Columbia
Vancouver, British Columbia, Canada

John E. Rash
Department of Molecular, Cellular, and Developmental Biology
University of Colorado
Boulder, Colorado 80302

Thomas S. Reese
Laboratory of Neuropathology and Neuroanatomical Sciences
National Institute of Neurological Diseases and Stroke
National Institutes of Health
Bethesda, Maryland 20014

E. Reich
Rockefeller University
New York, New York 10021

James H. Schwartz
Department of Microbiology
New York University Medical Center
and
Department of Neurobiology and Behavior
Public Health Research Institute of the City of New York
New York, New York 10016

Alan B. Steinbach
Marine Biological Laboratory
Woods Hole, Massachusetts 02543

Charles F. Stevens
Department of Physiology and Biophysics
University of Washington
School of Medicine
Seattle, Washington 98195

Forrest F. Weight
Laboratory of Neuropharmacology
National Institute of Mental Health
St. Elizabeths Hospital
Washington, D.C. 20032

V. P. Whittaker
Department of Biochemistry
University of Cambridge
Cambridge CB2 1QW, England

J. Whysner
Behavioral Biology Branch
National Institute of Child Health and Human Development
National Institutes of Health
Bethesda, Maryland 20014

H. Zimmermann
Department of Biochemistry
University of Cambridge
Cambridge CB2 1QW, England

Synaptic Transmission and Neuronal Interaction
Raven Press, New York 1974

On the How and Why of Synapses

Harry Grundfest

Laboratory of Neurophysiology, Department of Neurology, College of Physicians and
Surgeons, Columbia University, New York, New York 10032

Some 20 years ago Altamirano and I observed that the postsynaptic potentials (PSP's) of eel electroplaques could not be evoked directly by
electrical stimuli but were responses to electrical stimulation of the nerve
fibers (Altamirano and Grundfest, 1954; Altamirano, Coates, and Grundfest, 1955). The special geometry and properties of the cells permitted the
conclusion that the membrane component that generates the PSP is electrically inexcitable in contrast to the electrically excitable component that
generates the spike of the same cell. A theoretical analysis led to the
generalization that the input membrane both of neurons and muscle fibers is
electrically inexcitable (Grundfest, 1957a). Some of the properties associated with electrical inexcitability are also exhibited by sensory receptor
cells (see Grundfest, 1971). Thus, a relationship was formulated between
the various types of input membrane, which clarified the adaptations involved in the functioning of the neuron as a system of communication. I
shall survey briefly here some of the characteristics of input electrogenesis
which have particular bearing on the knowledge of the general physiology
of excitable membranes.

I. TERMINOLOGY

The organizer of this volume has classified as "conventional" what I
prefer to designate simply as "synapses." This is not entirely because
conventional has somewhat pejorative connotations for a superannuated
bohemian as well as to members of the now generation. The "unconventional" synapses discussed here are either the synaptic junctions of various
specialized receptor cells with sensory neurons (Grundfest, 1971) and thus
are "conventional" or they are low-resistance ephaptic (or electrotonic)
junctions (Grundfest, 1959) which have been studied so effectively by
Bennett and his colleagues (Bennett, 1966; Auerbach and Bennett, 1969).
Terming these junctions as "synapses" (albeit electrical or unconventional)
implies an equivalence between the rather simple dynamics of electrical
transmission (Watanabe and Grundfest, 1961) and the far richer possibilities that are embodied in the complex interactions among three functionally

distinct components of the neuron and between the presynaptic and post-synaptic elements of synaptic junctions (Grundfest, 1957a, 1961a, 1967). Electrical transmission can play a role in mobilizing a population of cells for better synchronization of their activity (Bennett, 1966). However, the complexities and subtleties which arise from the relationships of synaptic transmission give the nervous system very different dimensions, even more, perhaps, than Sherrington (1906) appreciated in his pioneering work.

II. THE NEURON AS A SYSTEM

The classical concept (Sherrington, 1906) of the two neuron reflex arc as the simplest element of communication in the nervous system, with separate receptor and effector sides connected by excitatory and inhibitory synapses, does injustice to the functional complexity of a single neuron. In actuality, each neuron is a complete independent system for communication with other cells. It is at the same time an electrical power source, signal detector, signal generator and encoder, an insulated conductor and a relay. These various functions may or may not be delimited geographically, but they are very effectively separated by their different physiological properties (Fig. 1). The input section of the cell receives specific information which may be chemical, mechanical, photic, or thermal in the case of the primary sensory neuron, but must be chemical in all other neurons, since the input membrane is electrically inexcitable (Grundfest, 1957a). The information received at the input is transformed into an electrical signal, the graded generator or postsynaptic potential which can induce a frequency-number coded message of spikes in the electrically excitable, conductile, axonal component. This transformation from the graded electrogenesis of the input is necessary because only spikes can propagate to the output without decrement in the long-line electrical cable which is the axon. Since the input membrane is electrically inexcitable, the interface between input electrogenesis and that of the axon is polarized, being coupled only in the forward direction. Thus, the large changes in membrane potential that are associated with spike electrogenesis do not appreciably affect the response of the input.

The transfer of information from the terminals of a neuron or receptor cell to the input of the next cell (another neuron or effector) must be by a chemical signal, since the second input is also electrically inexcitable. Thus, the electrical message carried by the spikes in the axon of the first neuron must effect release of a transmitter agent that is recognized by the input of the following cell. The obligatory change to a secretory function at the output justifies the term "chemical synapses" even though direct evidence for chemical action at the synapse is often hard to come by.

Axons can also respond to chemical, mechanical, photic, or thermal stimuli, but this responsiveness has little if any functional validity. To

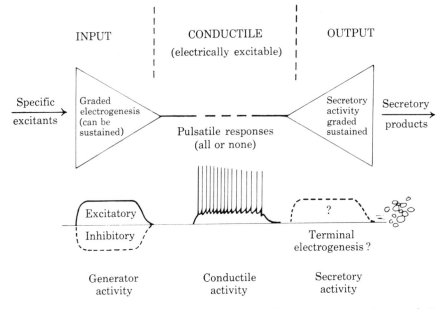

FIG. 1. The neuron as a system for communication. The input component responds to specific stimuli which may result in excitatory and/or inhibitory electrogenesis that cannot be evoked by electrical stimuli. The depolarizing generator potential or excitatory postsynaptic potential (EPSP) acts upon a conductile, electrically excitable component, generating spikes. The latter command the secretory activity of the output component. Although the coupling between spikes and secretion is electrical, secretory activity need not be associated with an electrical activity or the latter, if present, may be of either sign.

perform its function as an undecremented conductor, the axonal membrane must be electrically excitable. Electrical inexcitability, on the other hand, endows the neuron with the capability of functional diversity, since the input membrane is isolated from the conductile in a beautifully simple way. The input electrogenesis is then also a fairly linear response to stimuli that may be graded both in amplitude and duration.[1]

III. FUNCTIONAL AND STRUCTURAL DIVERSITY AMONG NEURONS

The properties of the three components of a neuron may vary independently, and different assortments of the components can, therefore,

---

[1] Hubbard, Llinas, and Quastel (1969) view electrical inexcitability as merely a "christening" (i.e., renaming) of "chemical synapses" (p. 59). Recognition of electrical inexcitability predicts that synaptic transmission is obligatorily a neurosecretory, chemical process. The converse, that chemically excitable membrane is electrically inexcitable, is not true. Electrical inexcitability of synaptic membranes was neither predicted nor recognized by proponents of chemical transmission during the prolonged controversy regarding electrical versus chemical transmission (see Grundfest, 1957b), although some evidence was available (Bernard, 1859; Rosenblueth and Cannon, 1934), which was ignored or rejected (see Grundfest, 1966a).

give rise to many types of neurons. Only one such example will suffice here, the striking difference between slowly and rapidly adapting crayfish stretch receptors (Fig. 2). Electrically inexcitable membrane is insensitive to saxitoxin (STX) or tetrodotoxin (TTX) (Reuben and Grundfest, 1960*a;* Grundfest, 1961*a*) in contrast with that of the Na-spike generators (Narahashi, Moore, and Scott, 1964; Nakamura, Nakajima, and Grundfest, 1965*a,b*). When the spikes of the receptor neurons are eliminated by TTX both the "slow" and the "fast" cells generate similar graded sustained potentials in response to various degrees of stretch (Fig. 2, right). On the left of Fig. 2 is a demonstration that the slowly adapting cell continues to generate spikes for a long time when it is stimulated by intracellularly applied currents. The rapidly adapting cell, on the other hand, responds only for a brief time (Nakajima, 1964). Thus, the difference between the "tonic" and "phasic" receptor neurons resides in a specialization of the electrically excitable membrane (Nakajima and Onodera, 1969) at or close to the region of the trigger zone (Edwards and Ottoson, 1958) of the axon.

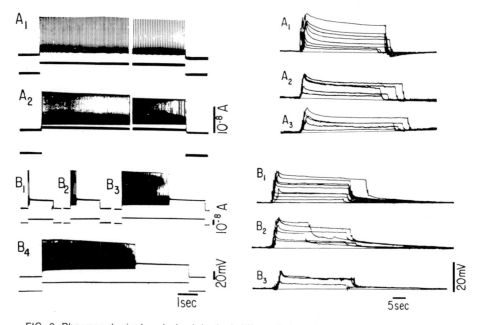

FIG. 2. Pharmacological and physiological differentiation of input and conductile membrane in slowly adapting *(A)* and rapidly adapting *(B)* crayfish stretch receptors. *Right:* Spikes were abolished after exposure of the cells to TTX. Generator potentials were still elicited in response to stretch. They were similar in both cells, graded and sustained in accordance with the stimuli. *Left:* These two cells were depolarized with intracellularly applied currents, monitored in the lower of each pair of traces. The frequency of the spikes induced by the depolarization increased with increasing currents, but the durations of the discharges were brief in the rapidly adapting cell. In the slowly adapting receptor the discharge continued throughout the applied current (140 sec in A_1; 26 sec in A_2) (modified from Nakajima, 1964).

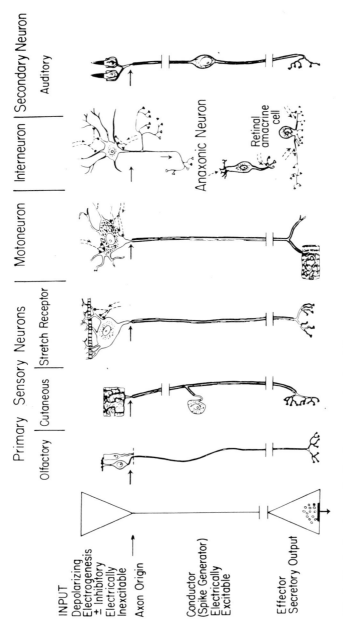

FIG. 3. Similarity of organization in neurons having different structures and functions. The diagram on the left represents the generalized neuron of Fig. 1. Further description in text (modified from Bodian, 1967).

The tripartite functional organization is a general characteristic independent of the geometry of the cells (Fig. 3). In some neurons the cell body lies between the receptive and conductile components; in others it is athwart the axon; and in still others it is located on a side branch of the axon. The spike arises in the axon and in many cases the soma lacks the capacity for spike electrogenesis, or the soma spikes may not require the presence of a Na gradient (Koketsu, Cerf, and Nishi, 1958; Koketsu and Nishi, 1969). Synaptic contacts between most invertebrate neurons are made at fine branches of the axon which proliferate into the neuropil.

The conductile capability of a neuron may be dispensed with if the distance between input and output is small. Anaxonic neurons or receptor cells then behave essentially as neurosecretory elements (Fig. 4). Contrariwise, neurons with axons may be frankly neurosecretory (Bennett and Fox, 1962), the conductile activity linking commands from the input to secretion at a distant site.

The input to a postsynaptic neuron being electrically inexcitable transmission across the synapse may be independent of the presence or absence of electrogenesis in an anaxonic neuron or receptor cell, or of the sign of the electrogenesis, if it is present. This accounts (Grundfest, 1958, 1971)

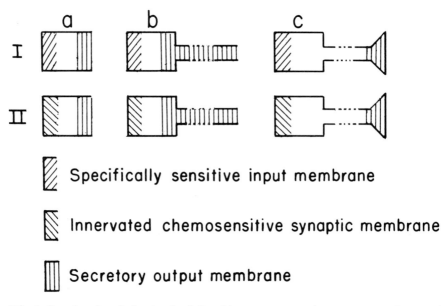

FIG. 4. Functional and structural relationships among secretory, neurosecretory, and receptor cells and neurons. I. Cells that receive commands from external or internal specific stimuli. II. Cells that are excited via their innervation. (a) Gland, neurosecretory, or receptor cells. (b) Neurosecretory or receptor cells. (c) Neurons. The input and output are far apart and their coupling requires an intermediate activity, the electrically excitable spike generator (from Grundfest, 1961b).

for the fact that puzzled its discoverer (Svaetichin, 1956), that light-induced hyperpolarization in cells of the vertebrate retina nevertheless results in an excitatory action upon ganglion cells.

A. Synaptic Electrogenesis

Although the dynamics are vastly different, the basic principles of electrogenesis in electrically excitable and electrically inexcitable components are similar (Fig. 5). The electrical driving forces are concentration cells,

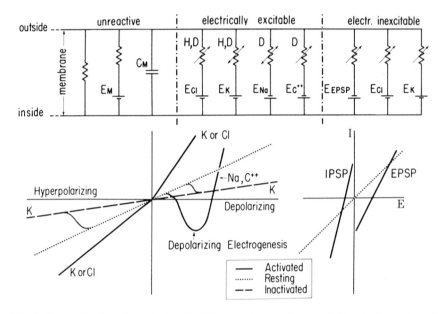

FIG. 5. Generalized equivalent circuit of the membrane of an excitable electrogenic cell *(top)* and the current-voltage (I–E) characteristics of its various components. Unreactive elements are the fixed-leak resistances and the capacity (C_M). Electrically excitable components are shown as ion-selective channels, each with a specific ionic battery and a resistance which can vary in response to depolarizing (D) or hyperpolarizing (H) stimuli. The opening of usually closed gates (activation ↗) or the closing of open gates (inactivation ↙) is controlled by the membrane potential and results in the change in conductance for the channel. Electrically inexcitable channels are opened only by specific stimuli. Depolarizing electrogenesis (generator potential or EPSP) develops when the channels for a mixed ionic battery (E_{EPSP}) are opened. Inhibitory electrogenesis involves only the channels driven by E_{Cl} or E_K.

The nonlinear characteristics of the electrically excitable components are shown in lower left. For description see Grundfest (1966a). The electrically inexcitable components retain their linear I–E relationship when activated by specific stimuli but the slope changes, in correspondence with the higher conductance. The origin of the high conductance characteristic is translated on the voltage axis toward depolarization for the EPSP or generator potential. In the diagram the characteristic for the inhibitory component is translated to hyperpolarization. The resting and active characteristics of the membrane components intersect at the "reversal" or "equilibrium" potential which indicates the net driving force for the electrogenesis.

ionic batteries for specific ions. Specific membrane sites act as gates, diagrammed as resistances in Fig. 5, that can open or close to alter the permeability (or conductance) for a given ion or several ions. The electrical response thus is a function of the driving force and of the degree of change in
the conductance.

The depolarizing electrogenesis of EPSP's or generator potentials is
usually due to more or less simultaneous increase in the permeability to
Na and K, so that the maximum emf for this response lies somewhere
between the inside negative E_K and the inside positive E_{Na}. Where E_{Na} is
very large (e.g., eel electroplaques, Ruiz-Manresa and Grundfest, 1971),
E_{EPSP} is correspondingly inside positive. Inhibitory electrogenesis involves
increased conductance for K or Cl. The change in potential is small even
when these synapses are fully activated and the electrogenesis may be of
either sign, or absent, depending on how close E_K or E_{Cl} is to the resting
potential. As the membrane potential is changed by an applied voltage or
current, the amplitude of the electrically inexcitable potentials varies
(Fig. 5). The I–E characteristic remains linear but the slope changes to
correspond with the change in conductance and the origin is translated
along the voltage axis by the amplitude of the response measured from
the resting potential. The ohmic behavior of the active as well as the resting
membrane is in marked contrast to the nonlinear characteristics of electrically excitable components (Grundfest, 1961c).

The inhibitory effect of a conductance increase for K or Cl is out of
proportion to the small change in potential during the IPSP. The strong
inside negativity of the respective ionic batteries tends to "clamp" the
membrane at or close to the resting potential. However, if E_K or E_{Cl} is made
considerably less negative than the resting potential, the increased conductance can induce large depolarization, which can in turn lead to excitation of the spike generating membrane. This effect has been achieved experimentally in cells where the IPSP is due to Cl activation (Fig. 6). In cat
spinal motoneurons E_{Cl} was changed by injecting Cl (I). In the crayfish
stretch receptor (II) and snail neurons (III) E_{Cl} was changed by removing Cl
from the bathing solution. In each case a depolarization resulted when the
"inhibitory" membrane was excited and it was large enough to evoke spikes
in the electrically excitable component.

The existence of anion permselective channels at inhibitory synapses
reenforces the view (Grundfest, 1966b) that the membrane is a hetero-
geneous electrochemical system. Cation permselectivity is predominant and
indicates that the membrane has mainly negatively charged selectivity sites,
but the existence at the same time of anion permselectivity indicates some
specialized positively charged sites. Thus the membrane does not obey the
requirement for microscopic electroneutrality which is assumed in the
Nernst-Planck relationships (see MacInnes, 1961).

Permselectivity of membrane sites is dependent upon the energetics of

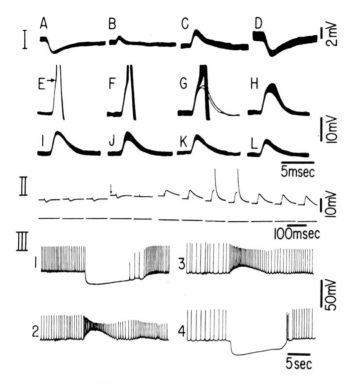

FIG. 6. Conversion of an inhibitory synaptic electrogenesis into excitatory.

I. Cat spinal motoneuron. The inhibitory hyperpolarizing electrogenesis (A) was reversed (B) by injecting Cl into the cell. More depolarization resulted from increasing the injection (C) and the potential reversed in sign when depolarized sufficiently (D). More Cl was then injected (E) and the "IPSP" became so strongly depolarizing that it evoked spikes (E-G). The depolarization then decreased progressively (G-L) as the Cl inside the cell leaked out.

II. Crayfish stretch receptor. Each trace shows the response to stimulating the inhibitor axon. This was a hyperpolarizing IPSP initially. At the arrow, external Cl was replaced with glutamate. The response now became depolarizing and could generate a spike in the axon. Redistribution of Cl across the cell membrane led to subsidence of the depolarization.

III. Spontaneously discharging snail neurons. Application of acetylcholine induced inhibitory activation (1). External Cl was then replaced with an impermeable anion. The response to acetylcholine now became depolarizing and excitatory (2, 3). The effect was reversed on restoring Cl (4) (from Grundfest, 1964b, where original references are given).

interaction between the ions and the charged sites in the membrane structure relative to the interactions of the ions with water (see Eisenman, 1962; Diamond and Wright, 1969) and upon the net charge and dimensions of the walls of aqueous channels through the membrane (see Hille, 1972). The pattern of permselectivity for cations or anions differs in various membranes and this indicates some degree of structural difference in different membranes. For example, the inhibitory synaptic membrane of lobster, but not of crayfish, is slightly permeable to propionate, which is a rather large and generally impermeable anion (Motokizawa, Reuben, and Grundfest, 1969).

The membrane conductance might conceivably decrease in response to a stimulus, in symmetry with the behavior of electrically excitable components in which inactivation processes are often observed (Grundfest, 1966a). A light-induced increase in resistance is associated with the hyperpolarization generated in vertebrate cones (Witkovsky, 1971). A change in potential could result if the resting membrane has a high conductance for Na and the resting potential is consequently closer to E_{Na} and farther from E_K. If the Na conductance is decreased, the contribution of E_{Na} is diminished. This type of change also occurs in the secondary receptor cells of the skate retina and is the basis of the hyperpolarization (S potential) of these cells (Dowling and Ripps, 1972). At rest the cones apparently release a transmitter which increases the conductance of horizontal cells for Na. The secretory activity is blocked not only by light but also by Mg. A decreased conductance is induced in rat taste buds by quinine (Ozeki, 1971) but the response of the receptor cell is a depolarization. The taste bud exhibits an additional complexity in that depolarizing receptor potentials also develop in response to salt, sugar, and acid, but these depolarizations are associated with an increase in membrane conductance.

IV. RESPONSES OF SYNAPTIC MEMBRANE TO DRUGS

Because the postsynaptic membrane responds only to chemical stimuli, and because synthetic chemistry has made available a wealth of chemical agents, pharmacological tools have yielded particularly rewarding data on synapses. The concept that ionic selectivity and gating[2] can assort independently (Grundfest, 1957c) has been confirmed by such data (Fig. 7). The D cells of *Aplysia* (I) respond with depolarization (excitation) to acetylcholine and with hyperpolarization (inhibition) to noradrenaline. The H cells, on the other hand, are inhibited by acetylcholine and excited by noradrenaline. Thus, these two agents are both "excitatory" and "inhibitory" in pharmacological parlance. They are both *synapse activators* (Grundfest, 1957c), increasing the conductance for different ions in different cells. Thus, the chemically reactive gates and the ion permselective sites

---

[2] The ion "gate" is the equivalent of the "receptor" of biochemists and pharmacologists. The former term is more general since it applies also to membrane sites that react to stimuli other than chemical, and, furthermore, describes more specifically the type of change that results in the electrogenesis. Under the stress of appropriate stimuli the molecular structures of gates are assumed to undergo conformational changes which lead to a change in the permeability of the permselective site or channel with which the gate is associated. In most cases the different gates are normally closed and are opened (activated) by the stimuli. However, gates may be open in the resting membrane, e.g., the electrically excitable K conductance system of eel electroplaques (Nakamura et al., 1965a), and are closed (inactivated) by an electrical stimulus.

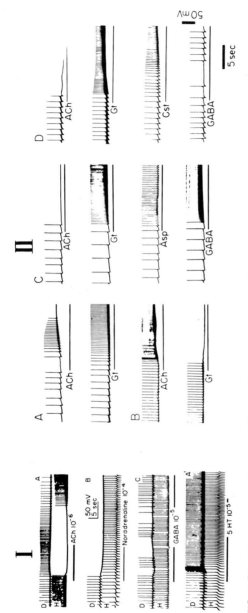

FIG. 7. Pharmacological evidence for different chemical structures of electrically inexcitable gates. I. Simultaneous recording from two *Aplysia* neurons, labeled D and H, respectively. Acetylcholine (*A*) caused depolarization and increased discharge in D cell, but the H cell hyperpolarized and its discharge was inhibited. *B*. The responses to noradrenaline are inverse in the two cells. *C*, *A′*. Responses of four cells (*A-D*) to applications of acetylcholine (ACh), glutamate (Gt), asparate (Asp), cysteine (Cst), and GABA. Modified (I) from Tauc and Gerschenfeld (1961) and (II) from Gerschenfeld and Lasansky (1964).

TABLE 1. *Electrophysiological and pharmacological characterization of five gates in synaptic membrane of an Aplysia neuron*

Electrogenesis	Ionic battery	Reversal pot. (mV)	Response blocked by
A. Cholinergic			
1. Depolarizing	E_{EPSP}	—	d-tubocurarine (dTC) hexamethonium (C_6)
2. Hyperpolarizing (rapid)	E_{Cl}	−60	dTC, not C_6
3. Hyperpolarizing (slow)	E_K	−80	neither
B. Dopaminergic			
1. Depolarizing	—	—	dTC
2. Hyperpolarizing	E_K	−80	ergot derivatives, not dTC

(Data from Kehoe, 1972*a*, and Ascher, 1972.)

which they control can assort independently, thereby giving rise to numerous possibilities for permutations and combinations of these components.

The chemical structures of the cholinoceptive and adrenoceptive gates in different cells must vary to some degree, as is shown by the different patterns of response to other agents. The D cells of *Aplysia* are somewhat inhibited by GABA, which has perhaps a small excitatory effect on the H cells, whereas both cell types are excited in the presence of 5HT. The different patterns of response of four *Helix* neurons to various amino acids (Fig. 7 II) reenforce this conclusion.

More precise evidence for the different assortment of gates and channels has been recently obtained by Kehoe (1972*a,b,c*) and Ascher (1972). Certain neurons of *Aplysia* generate three PSP's in response to acetylcholine and to neural stimuli (Table 1). The EPSP is an early, relatively brief depolarization. An early IPSP, also brief, is due to Cl activation. Another, later and much more prolonged hyperpolarization results from K activation (Kehoe, 1972*a*). In addition to the cholinergic gates for these three responses the neurons may have dopaminergic gates. One is for an early excitatory depolarization, the other is for a later and longer lasting hyperpolarization (Ascher, 1972).[3] All five gates have rather distinctive pharmacology, being blocked differently by different synaptic inactivator agents, indicating that their macromolecular structures differ to a degree.

---

[3] The various cholinergic and dopaminergic responses of the *Aplysia* neurons appear to be monosynaptic. Thus, the same transmitter can evoke early and brief or later and longer lasting electrogenesis. Does this signify that the gates for the briefer responses close before the transmitter is destroyed or diffuses away from the synaptic region? Alternatively, may it be that once the gates for the slow inhibitory electrogenesis are opened by the transmitter their subsequent kinetics are independent of "drug receptor" interactions? If would be also important to know whether the neurally evoked dopaminergic and cholinergic EPSP's have the same or different time courses.

The reactivity of a particular synaptic membrane to continued application of a synapse activator may decrease with time (desensitization, see Katz and Thesleff, 1957). The degree and rate of desensitization differ widely. Some crab neuromuscular junctions desensitize so rapidly to GABA (Epstein and Grundfest, 1970) that this activator may appear to have no effect on the conductance of the membrane (Florey and Hoyle, 1961), although inhibition occurs and persists because of a presynaptic inhibitory action of GABA, which is particularly prominent in crab, but also occurs in other crustacean systems (Grundfest, 1972). There is little if any desensitization to GABA in neuromuscular synapses of lobster (Grundfest, Reuben, and Rickles, 1959), crayfish (Ozeki, Freeman, and Grundfest, 1966), and insect (Usherwood and Grundfest, 1965). Considerable difference is also observed in vertebrate cholinergic synapses. Desensitization is evident in frog and mammalian neuromuscular synapses (Katz and Thesleff, 1957) and in the electroplaques of marine electric fishes (see Grundfest and Bennett, 1961). There is little or no desensitization in eel electroplaques (Ruiz-Manresa and Grundfest, 1971). If the synapse activators act to open gates, the degree and kinetics of desensitization may provide additional parameters for characterizing the chemical structure of gates.

V. IONIC CHANNELS

Kehoe (1972a,b,c) and Ascher (1972) have also obtained data that bear upon the nature of the ion-selective channels of the synaptic membrane.[4] Injection of TEA blocks the slow (K-activated) hyperpolarization and prolongs the spike, but does not affect the EPSP. Thus, the K channels of the inhibitory membrane may have a configuration similar to that which is postulated for the K channels in squid axons (Armstrong, 1971). Since the EPSP does not appear to be affected, the efflux of K during the EPSP must then occur in a different type of K channel, perhaps one that also permits inward Na movement.

A conductance increase for K in the absence of Na has been observed in frog neuromuscular synapses (Del Castillo and Katz, 1956; Katz and Thesleff, 1957). The experimental condition did not permit a decision as to whether the K and Na channels of the synaptic membrane behaved as one system or as two independent systems. In crustacean muscle, however, an activation of the synaptic membrane by glutamic acid requires the presence

---

[4] Further evidence that is available for the distinction between gates and channels will not be discussed here. It should be noted, however, that such a distinction may be absent in lipid bilayer artificial membranes. Cation selective channels may be formed randomly by transition of gramicidin molecules from an "inactive" to an "active" state (Hladky and Haydon, 1972). The transition is dependent on the concentration of gramicidin and temperature, but not upon electrical stimuli.

of Na (Ozeki and Grundfest, 1967). There is no conductance increase when the crayfish muscle fiber is bathed in Na-free saline (Fig. 8).

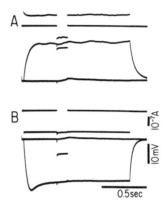

FIG. 8. Absence of depolarizing electrogenesis of EPSP's in crayfish muscle fiber in the absence of Na.

A. The resting potential is registered on the lowest trace. A brief pulse (monitored on second trace) delivered an ionophoretic jet of glutamate which causes maximal depolarization when Na is present. Only a small artifact is seen on the voltage trace. The cell was then depolarized with an intracellularly applied current and the chemical stimulus was again applied. Both currents are monitored on the upper trace. The absence of a conductance increase is shown by the absence of a change in the membrane potential.

B. Similar data except that the fiber was hyperpolarized (lowest trace) while glutamate was applied. Both currents are monitored on the second trace. The uppermost trace monitors the ionophoretic current applied to the resting cell (resting potential on third trace). As in *A*, the membrane potential did not change in response to glutamate (from Ozeki and Grundfest, 1967).

VI. HOW DO GATES REACT TO STIMULI?

It is generally supposed that the gating structure, which is presumably a macromolecular complex, undergoes conformational changes which cause a change in the ion-specific channel associated with its opening (activating) or closing (inactivating) the latter. Karlin (1969) has suggested that the acetylcholine "receptor" which gates the depolarizing electrogenesis of eel electroplaques has an S–S site and an anionic site, the two being located some 12 Å apart in the resting condition (Fig. 9*A*). Acetylcholine combines with both sites, drawing them together to approximately 9 Å *(B)*. Decamethonium, although a larger molecule, can fold *(C)* so as to combine with both sites and is also an activator of the synapse. Hexamethonium (C_6) is also too long but does combine with the anionic site, thereby blocking the access of synapse activators *(D)*. Thus C_6 is a competitive antagonist of the activators. More recently Karlin and his colleagues (Reiter, Cowburn, Prives, and Karlin, 1972) have isolated an affinity labeled fraction of

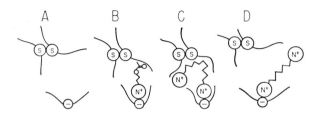

FIG. 9. Diagrammatic representation of the cholinergic gate for the EPSP of eel electro-plaques. *A.* The gate is closed in the resting state with the S–S site approximately 12 Å from an anionic site. *B.* Acetylcholine binds to both sites, bringing them to within 9 Å and opens the gate for depolarizing electrogenesis. *C.* Although decamethonium is a long molecule, it folds to combine with both sites, also activating the synapse. *D.* Hexame-thonium is also too long, but cannot fold. Not only does the gate remain closed but the anionic site is occupied by one quaternary nitrogen. This prevents access of a synapse activator agents and hexamethonium acts as a competitive inhibitor (modified from Karlin, 1969).

molecular weight (ca. 42,000), which they believe is the receptor protein of synapses in eel electroplaques. Karlin, Cowburn, and Reiter (1973) suggest that it exists as a dimer in the membrane.

VII. ELECTRICAL EXCITABILITY OF SYNAPTIC MEMBRANE

One class of receptors — the electroreceptors of fish — is, of course, sensitive to electrical fields and therefore may be considered electrically excitable (Grundfest, 1964a; Bennett, 1967). Although synaptic electro-genesis is not initiated by electrical stimuli, the kinetics of ion movements in the activated synaptic membrane may be affected by an electric field. Thus, once the frog end plate is activated by a neural or chemical stimulus, the kinetics of the conductance change is dependent on the membrane potential (Kordăs, 1969, 1972; Magleby and Stevens, 1972). This type of electrical excitability also occurs in the synaptic membrane of eel electro-plaques (Ruiz-Manresa and Grundfest, 1971) except that large depolariza-tions induce a decrease in conductance (Fig. 10) just as in the electrically excitable membrane. The activated synaptic membrane of the electroplaque also appears to be somewhat permeable to Ca and Mg.

VIII. THE INTERFACE BETWEEN CONDUCTILE AND SECRETORY ACTIVITY

The interaction between the message contained in the spikes and the secretory activity which it engenders is less well known than are the prop-erties of the input and conductile components and their interfacial behavior. The postsynaptic activity evoked by a nerve impulse or by an intracellular depolarization after TTX is applied to block the spikes is dependent upon

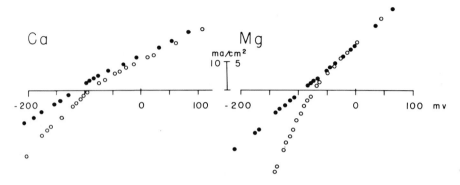

FIG. 10. I–E characteristics of synaptic electrogenesis in eel electroplaques. All Na and K were replaced with Ca *(left)* and Mg *(right)* and some Ba was added so that the electrically excitable membrane became essentially ohmic *(filled circles)*. Open circles show the change in conductance and membrane potential when the synaptic membrane was activated by carbamylcholine. The depolarization indicates that the activated synaptic membrane is somewhat permeable to both divalent cations. The conductance increase induced by the activator was reduced and abolished as the membrane was depolarized by the applied current, indicating a degree of electrical excitability (from Ruiz-Manresa and Grundfest, 1971).

the presence of Ca in the bathing medium and is blocked by Mg or Mn (see Katz, 1969). The "spontaneous" miniature EPSP's and IPSP's (Fig. 11) which persist after the spike of the axon is blocked are, however, independent of the presence or absence of Ca, Mg, or Mn (April and Reuben, 1971; April, 1972). There is also some question as to the randomness of the events (Bittner and Harrison, 1970; Van der Kloot, Cohen, and Kita, 1973).

Thus, for the present at least, one might distinguish between "spontaneous" and evoked secretory activity at synapses. Supporting this conclusion is the finding that the marked increase induced by Cs in the neurally evoked PSP's (Reuben and Grundfest, 1960*b;* Gainer, Reuben, and Grundfest, 1967; Ginsborg and Hamilton, 1968) does not affect the dis-

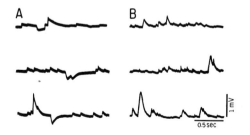

FIG. 11. Miniature PSP's occurring spontaneously in lobster muscle fiber. *A.* Both depolarizing and hyperpolarizing miniatures are observed but the latter are abolished *(B)* in the presence of picrotoxin. These responses occur in the presence of TTX or STX, which abolishes spike electrogenesis in the axon (from Grundfest, 1961*a*, and from unpublished data by Reuben and Grundfest, 1960*a*).

tribution of miniature potentials (Gainer et al., 1967; Lang and Atwood, 1972). The neurotoxin of black widow spider venom (BWSV) also affects the evoked potentials differently than it does the miniature potentials (Longenecker, Hurlbut, Mauro, and Clark, 1970; Kawai, Mauro, and Grundfest, 1972). The neurally evoked PSP's, both excitatory and inhibitory, are rapidly blocked, while the frequency of miniature PSP's increases markedly. The similarity of the effects of BWSV on vertebrate and invertebrate neurons indicates that the action is independent of the nature of the transmitters and thus of the synthesizing apparatus. After a time, which is correlated with the estimated content of vesicles in vertebrate synapses, the high-frequency spontaneous miniature activity stops and the nerve terminals are then seen to be empty of vesicles (Longenecker et al., 1970; Clark, Hurlbut, and Mauro, 1972). In crustacean junctions, random "giant" PSP's appear after the output of miniature PSP's stops (Kawai et al., 1972).

The function (if any) of the spontaneous activity is unknown. It might be a signal from the presynaptic to the postsynaptic cell, playing a part in modulating or determining the phenomenon associated with denervation sensitization of neurons and effectors. Noteworthy in this connection is the finding that the sensitivity of crayfish muscle to GABA is not altered appreciably for as long as 7 weeks after the nerve is interrupted (Fig. 12).

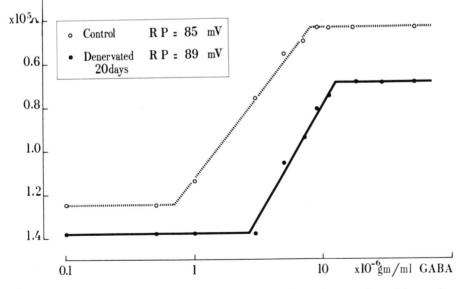

FIG. 12. Dose-response curves for the effect of GABA on the resistance of crayfish muscle fibers. An innervated fiber was more sensitive to GABA than a fiber in a preparation whose nerve had been severed for nearly 3 weeks. Although termed "denervated" the axons continued to function (from Grundfest, 1964b, after unpublished data by Girardier et al., 1962).

The severed axon remains excitable throughout this time (Girardier, Reuben, and Grundfest, 1962). Denervation does occur in insects and brings with it a variety of morphological and physiological changes (Usherwood and Wood, 1973).

Facilitation, the increase in successive PSP's on repetitive stimulation of the presynaptic nerve, and its inverse, defacilitation, arise from changes in the transmitter output. Different degrees of facilitation and defacilitation that occur in different pathways to a given neuron may have profound behavioral effects. The mechanisms of the changes are still unclear and they deserve further study. Crustacean neuromuscular junctions and the electroplaques of marine electric fishes would seem to be particularly useful objects for such studies. Different degrees of change may be observed on stimulating different excitatory or inhibitory axons in a multiply innervated fiber and some agents such as BWSV (Kawai et al., 1972) affect the degree of facilitation. A striking difference in the degree of facilitation is observed in electroplaques of the main and accessory organs of *Narcine* (Bennett and Grundfest, 1961). Those of the main organ, like the electroplaques of *Torpedo* and *Astroscopus* (see Grundfest and Bennett, 1961), respond with a maximal or nearly maximal PSP to every neural volley. Repetitive stimulation induces little or no growth in the depolarization, only a sustained summated response. A single volley to the accessory organ, however, produces only a small PSP in the cells, but successive volleys show marked facilitation so that a brief, high-frequency train of impulses results in a depolarization as large as that of the sustained depolarization in the electroplaques of the main organ.

ACKNOWLEDGMENTS

Work in the author's laboratory is supported in part by grants from MDAA, by USPHS research grant 03728 and training grant 05328 from the National Institute of Neurological Diseases and Stroke, and from the National Science Foundation (GB 31807X).

REFERENCES

Altamirano, M., Coates, C. W., and Grundfest, H. (1955): Mechanisms of direct and neural excitability in electroplaques of electric eel. *J. Gen. Physiol.*, 38:319.

Altamirano, M., and Grundfest, H. (1954): Three excitable systems of the synaptic unit in the innervated electroplaque preparation. *Trans. A.N.A.*, 79:79.

April, S. P. (1972): The effect of divalent cations on spontaneous and neurally evoked transmitter release at the crustacean neuromuscular junction. Ph.D. Thesis, Columbia University, New York.

April, S. P., and Reuben, J. P. (1971): The effect of divalent cations upon the evoked and spontaneous release of excitatory transmitter at the crustacean neuromuscular junction. *Fed. Proc.*, 30:557.

Armstrong, C. M. (1971): Interaction of tetraethylammonium ion derivatives with potassium channels of giant axons. *J. Gen. Physiol.*, 58:413.

Ascher, P. (1972): Inhibitory and excitatory effects of Dopamine on *Aplysia* neurones. *J. Physiol.*, 255:173.

Auerbach, A. A., and Bennett, M. V. L. (1969): A rectifying electrotonic synapse in the central nervous system of a vertebrate. *J. Gen. Physiol.*, 53:211.

Bennett, M. V. L. (1966): Physiology of electrotonic junctions. *Ann. N.Y. Acad. Sci.*, 137:509.

Bennett, M. V. L. (1967): Mechanisms of electroreception. In: *Lateral Line Detectors*, edited by P. H. Cahn, p. 313. Indiana University Press, Bloomington.

Bennett, M. V. L., and Fox, S. (1962): Electrophysiology of caudal neurosecretory cells in the skate and fluke. *J. Comp. Endocrin.*, 2:77.

Bennett, M. V. L., and Grundfest, H. (1961): The electrophysiology of electric organs of marine electric fishes. II. The electroplaques of the main and accessory organ of *Narcine brasiliensis*. *J. Gen. Physiol.*, 44:805.

Bernard, C. (1859): *Lecons sur les propriétés physiologiques et les altérations pathologiques des liquides de l'òrganisme*, Vol. 2. Paris, Baillière.

Bittner, G. D., and Harrison, J. (1970): A reconsideration of the Poisson hypothesis for transmitter release at the crayfish neuromuscular junction. *J. Physiol.*, 206:1.

Bodian, D. (1967): Neurons, circuits, and neuroglia. In: *The Neurosciences. A Study Program*, edited by G. C. Quarton, T. Melnechuk, and F. O. Schmitt, p. 6. The Rockefeller University Press, New York.

Clark, A. W., Hurlbut, W. P., and Mauro, A. (1972): Changes in the fine structure of the neuromuscular junction of the frog caused by black widow spider venom. *J. Cell Biol.*, 52:1.

Del Castillo, J., and Katz, B. (1956): Biophysical aspects of neuromuscular transmission. *Prog. Biophys.*, 6:121.

Diamond, J. M., and Wright, E. M. (1969): Biological membranes: The physical basis of ion and nonelectrolyte selectivity. *Ann. Rev. Physiol.*, 31:581.

Dowling, J. E., and Ripps, H. (1972): Effects of Mg^{2+} on skate horizontal cells; evidence for release of transmitter from receptors in darkness. *Biol. Bull.*, 143:458.

Edwards, C., and Ottoson, D. (1958): The site of impulse initiation in a nerve cell of a crustacean stretch receptor. *J. Physiol.*, 143:138.

Eisenman, G. (1962): Cation selective glass electrodes and their mode of operation. *Biophys. J.*, 2 (2, Pt. 2):259.

Epstein, R., and Grundfest, H. (1970): Desensitization of gamma aminobutyric acid (GABA) receptors in muscle fibers of the crab *Cancer borealis*. *J. Gen. Physiol.*, 56:33.

Florey, E., and Hoyle, G. (1961): Neuromuscular synaptic activity in crabs. In: *Nervous Inhibition*, edited by E. Florey, p. 105. Pergamon Press, London.

Gainer, H., Reuben, J. P., and Grundfest, H. (1967): The augmentation of postsynaptic potentials in crustacean muscle fibers by cesium. A presynaptic mechanism. *Comp. Biochem. Physiol.*, 20:877.

Gerschenfeld, H. M., and Lasansky, A. (1964): Action of glutamic acid and other naturally occurring amino-acids on snail central neurons. *Int. J. Neuropharmacol.*, 3:301.

Ginsborg, B. L., and Hamilton, J. T. (1968): The effect of cesium ions on neuromuscular transmission in the frog. *Quart. J. Exp. Physiol.*, 53:162.

Girardier, L., Reuben, J. P., and Grundfest, H. (1962): Changes in membrane properties of crayfish muscle fibers caused by denervation. *Fed. Proc.*, 21:357.

Grundfest, H. (1957a): Electrical inexcitability of synapses and some of its consequences in the central nervous system. *Physiol. Revs.*, 37:337.

Grundfest, H. (1957b): Excitation at synapses. *J. Neurophysiol.*, 20:316.

Grundfest, H. (1957c): General problems of drug action on bioelectric phenomena. *Ann. N.Y. Acad. Sci.*, 66:537.

Grundfest, H. (1958): An electrophysiological basis for cone vision in fish. *Arch. Ital. Biol.*, 96:135.

Grundfest, H. (1959): Synaptic and ephaptic transmission. In: *Handbook of Physiology, Section I, Neurophysiology I*, edited by J. Field, p. 147. American Physiological Society, Washington, D.C.

Grundfest, H. (1961a): General physiology and pharmacology of junctional transmission. In: *Biophysics of Physiological and Pharmacological Action*, edited by A. M. Shanes, p. 329. AAAS, Washington, D.C.

Grundfest, H. (1961b): Excitation by hyperpolarizing potentials. A general theory of receptor activities. In: *Nervous Inhibition*, edited by E. Florey, p. 326. Pergamon Press, London.

Grundfest, H. (1961c): Ionic mechanisms in electrogenesis. *Ann. N.Y. Acad. Sci.*, 94:405.

Grundfest, H. (1964a): Evolution of electrophysiological varieties among sensory receptor systems. In: *Physiological Evolution,* edited by J. W. S. Pringle, p. 107. Pergamon Press, London.

Grundfest, H. (1964b): Chemical determinants of behavior: The chemical mediators. In: *Unfinished Tasks in the Behavioral Sciences,* edited by A. Abrams, H. H. Garner, and J. E. P. Toman, p. 67. Williams and Wilkins Co., Baltimore.

Grundfest, H. (1966a): Comparative electrobiology of excitable membranes. In: *Advances in Comparative Physiology and Biochemistry,* Vol. 2, edited by O. E. Lowenstein, p. 1. Academic Press, New York.

Grundfest, H. (1966b): Heterogeneity of excitable membrane: Electrophysiological and pharmacological evidence and some consequences. *Ann. N.Y. Acad. Sci.,* 137:901.

Grundfest, H. (1967): Synaptic and ephaptic transmission. In: *The Neurosciences. A Study Program,* edited by G. C. Quarton, T. Melnechuck, and F. O. Schmitt, p. 353. The Rockefeller University Press, New York.

Grundfest, H. (1971): The general electrophysiology of input membrane in electrogenic excitable cells. In: *Handbook of Sensory Physiology, I. Principles of Receptor Physiology,* edited by W. R. Loewenstein, p. 135. Springer-Verlag, Berlin.

Grundfest, H. (1972): Neuromuscular transmission in arthropods. In: *International Encyclopedia of Pharmacology and Therapeutics,* Sec. 14, Vol. 2, edited by J. Cheymol, p. 621. Pergamon Press, London.

Grundfest, H., and Bennett, M. V. L. (1961): Studies on morphology and electrophysiology of electric organs. I. Electrophysiology of marine electric fishes. In: *Bioelectrogenesis,* edited by C. Chagas and A. Paes de Carvalho, p. 57. Elsevier Publ., Amsterdam.

Grundfest, H., Reuben, J. P., and Rickles, W. H., Jr. (1959): The electrophysiology and pharmacology of lobster neuromuscular synapses. *J. Gen. Physiol.,* 42:1301.

Hille, B. (1972): The permeability of the sodium channel to metal cations in myelinated nerve. *J. Gen. Physiol.,* 59:637.

Hladky, S. B., and Haydon, D. A. (1972): Ion transfer across lipid membrane in the presence of gramicidin A. I. Studies of the unit conductance channel. *Biochim. Biophys. Acta,* 274:294.

Hubbard, J. I., Llinas, R., and Quastel, D. M. J. (1969): *Electrophysiological Analysis of Synaptic Transmission.* Edward Arnold, London.

Karlin, A. (1969): Chemical modification of the active site of the acetylcholine receptor. *J. Gen. Physiol.,* 54:245s.

Karlin, A., Cowburn, D. A., and Reiter, M. J. (1973): Molecular properties of the acetylcholine receptor. In: *Drug Receptors. Biological Council Symposium on Drug Action.* Macmillan, London, *in press.*

Katz, B. (1969): *The Release of Neural Transmitter Substances.* University Press, Liverpool.

Katz, B., and Thesleff, S. (1957): A study of the "desensitization" produced by acetylcholine at the motor end-plate. *J. Physiol.,* 138:63.

Kawai, N., Mauro, A., and Grundfest, H. (1972): Effect of black widow spider venom on the lobster neuromuscular junctions. *J. Gen. Physiol.,* 60:650.

Kehoe, J. (1972a): Ionic mechanisms of a two-component cholinergic inhibition in *Aplysia* neurones. *J. Physiol.,* 225:85.

Kehoe, J. (1972b): Three acetylcholine receptors in *Aplysia* neurones. *J. Physiol.,* 225:115.

Kehoe, J. (1972c): The physiological role of three acetylcholine receptors in synaptic transmission in *Aplysia. J. Physiol.,* 255:147.

Koketsu, K., Cerf, J. A., and Nishi, S. (1958): Action of quarternary ammonium compounds on the neuron cell body. *Fed. Proc.,* 17:89.

Koketsu, K., and Nishi, S. (1969): Calcium and action potentials of bullfrog sympathetic ganglion cells. *J. Gen. Physiol.,* 53:608.

Kordaš, M. (1969): The effect of membrane polarization on the time course of the end-plate current in frog sartorius muscle. *J. Physiol.,* 204:493.

Kordaš, M. (1972): An attempt at an analysis of the factors determining the time course of the end-plate current. *J. Physiol.,* 224:317.

Lang, F., and Atwood, H. L. (1972): Cesium ion: Differential effect on crustacean neuromuscular synapses. *Fed. Proc.,* 31:334.

Longenecker, H. E., Hurlbut, W. P., Mauro, A., and Clark, A. W. (1970): Effects of black widow spider venom on the frog neuromuscular junction. *Nature,* 225:701.

MacInnes, D. A. (1961): *The Principles of Electrochemistry*. Dover, New York.

Magleby, K. L., and Stevens, C. F. (1972): The effect of voltage on the time course of end-plate currents. *J. Physiol.*, 223:151.

Motokizawa, F., Reuben, J. P., and Grundfest, H. (1969): Ionic permeability of the inhibitory postsynaptic membrane of lobster muscle fibers. *J. Gen. Physiol.*, 54:437.

Nakajima, S. (1964): Adaptation in stretch receptor neurons of crayfish. *Science*, 146:1168.

Nakajima, S., and Onodera, K. (1969): Membrane properties of stretch receptor neurones of crayfish with particular reference to mechanisms of sensory adaptation. *J. Physiol.*, 220:161.

Nakamura, Y., Nakajima, S., and Grundfest, H. (1965a): Analysis of spike electrogenesis and depolarizing K-inactivation in electroplaques of *Electrophorus electricus*, L. *J. Gen. Physiol.*, 49:321.

Nakamura, Y., Nakajima, S., and Grundfest, H., (1965b): The action of tetrodotoxin on electrogenic components of squid giant axons. *J. Gen. Physiol.*, 48:985.

Narahashi, T., Moore, J. W., and Scott, W. R. (1964): Tetrodotoxin blockage of sodium conductance increase in lobster giant axons. *J. Gen. Physiol.*, 47:965.

Ozeki, M. (1971): Conductance change associated with receptor potentials of gustatory cells in rat. *J. Gen. Physiol.*, 58:688.

Ozeki, M., Freeman, A. R., and Grundfest, H. (1966). The membrane components of crustacean neuromuscular systems. I. Immunity of different electrogenic components to tetrodotoxin and saxitoxin. *J. Gen. Physiol.*, 49:1319.

Ozeki, M., and Grundfest, H. (1967): Crayfish muscle fibers: Ionic requirements for depolarizing synaptic electrogenesis. *Science*, 155:478.

Reiter, M. J., Cowburn, D. A., Prives, J. M., and Karlin, A. (1972): Affinity labelling of acetylcholine receptor in the electroplax; electrophoretic separation in sodium dodecyl sulfate. *Proc. Nat. Acad. Sci.*, 569:1168.

Reuben, J. P., and Grundfest, H. (1960a): Inhibitory and excitatory miniature postsynaptic potentials in lobster muscle fibers. *Biol. Bull.*, 119:335.

Reuben, J. P., and Grundfest, H. (1960b): The action of cesium ions on neuromuscular transmission in lobster. *Biol. Bull.*, 119:336.

Rosenblueth, A., and Cannon, W. B. (1934): Direct electrical stimulation of denervated autonomic effectors. *Am. J. Physiol.*, 108:384.

Ruiz-Manresa, F., and Grundfest, H. (1971): Synaptic electrogenesis in eel electroplaques. *J. Gen. Physiol.*, 57:71.

Sherrington, C. S. (1906): *The Integrative Action of the Nervous System*. Cambridge University Press, Cambridge.

Svaetichin, G. (1956): Spectral response curves from single cones. *Acta Physiol. Scand.* 39: Suppl. 134, 17.

Tauc, L., and Gerschenfeld, H. M. (1961): Cholinergic transmission mechanisms for both excitation and inhibition in molluscan central synapses. *Nature*, 192:366.

Usherwood, P. N. R., and Grundfest, H. (1965): Peripheral inhibition in skeletal muscle of insect. *J. Neurophysiol.*, 28:497.

Usherwood, P. N. R., and Wood, M. R. (1973): Structure and physiology of denervated and re-innervated cockroach muscle. *J. Physiol. Proc.*, 230:1.

Van der Kloot, W., Cohen, I., and Kita, H. (1973): Miniature end-plate potentials are unlikely to be generated by a Poisson process. *J. Gen. Physiol., in press*.

Watanabe, A., and Grundfest, H. (1961): Impulse propagation at the septal and commissural junctions of crayfish lateral giant axons. *J. Gen. Physiol.*, 45:267.

Witkovsky, P. (1971): Peripheral mechanisms of vision. *Ann. Rev. Physiol.*, 33:257.

Synaptic Transmission and Neuronal Interaction
Raven Press, New York 1974

Excitation-Secretion Coupling at the Mammalian Neuromuscular Junction

David M. J. Quastel

Department of Pharmacology, Faculty of Medicine, University of British Columbia,
Vancouver, British Columbia

I. THE CALCIUM HYPOTHESIS

It is now well established that the quantal release of transmitter by verte-brate neuromuscular junctions that is evoked by motor nerve stimulation is dependent upon and graded with the ambient concentration of calcium ions (Feng, 1936; del Castillo and Stark, 1952; del Castillo and Engbaek, 1954; Liley, 1956; Jenkinson, 1957; reviewed by Rubin, 1970). As at the giant synapse of *Loligo*, this Ca^{2+} dependence is not secondary to any effect of Ca^{2+} on the presynaptic action potential (Katz and Miledi, 1965a,b; Miledi and Slater, 1966; Katz and Miledi, 1970). Similar Ca^{2+} dependence has been demonstrated for a variety of secretory processes, and in tissues (e.g., adrenal medulla and neurohypophysis) where measurement of Ca fluxes has been possible, excitation of secretion has been shown to be associated with influx of Ca into the secretory cells (reviewed by Douglas, 1968). Since the presynaptic action potential can be effectively mimicked by a passive depolarization in the squid nerve terminal (Bloedel, Gage, Llinas, and Quastel, 1966; Katz and Miledi, 1967; Kusano, Livengood, and Werman, 1967) and the same is likely to be true at the vertebrate junction (see Katz, 1969), as was suggested by Liley (1956), it has been proposed that the excitation-secretion coupling mechanism consists of (1) a system whereby depolarization of the nerve terminal causes influx of Ca^{2+} or a Ca complex (Ca^*), and (2) a system whereby intracellular Ca^{2+} or Ca^* stimulates release of transmitter quanta. This "calcium hypothesis" (Katz and Miledi, 1967, 1968, 1969a,b, 1970) gains some support from observation of a tetrodotoxin and tetraethylammonium-insensitive inward current, that may be carried by Ca^{2+} or Ca^*, in depolarized squid nerve terminals (Katz and Miledi, 1969a,b). However, it has yet to be demonstrated that Ca inside the nerve terminal can evoke transmitter release (Miledi and Slater, 1966).

II. QUANTITATIVE DIFFICULTIES

Quantitative studies of the relationship between transmitter release and [Ca] have not provided evidence in favor of the calcium hypothesis. Jenkinson (1957) found the actions of Ca and Mg on end-plate potential (epp) amplitude in the frog to be compatible with competition of Mg^{2+} for a Ca receptor (X), the facilitatory action of Ca^{2+} being secondary to formation of a complex, CaX (del Castillo and Katz, 1954). Epp amplitude was proportional to approximately the fourth power of [Ca] when [Ca] was low and/or [Mg] raised. These results were confirmed by Dodge and Rahamimoff (1967), who proposed that the power relationship indicated a constant stoichiometric relationship between transmitter release and calcium, because four Ca atoms were required for release of each quantum of transmitter. However, at the rat neuromuscular junction (Hubbard, Jones, and Landau, 1968*b*), as at the squid giant synapse (Katz and Miledi, 1970), the limiting slope of log transmitter release versus log [Ca] was approximately 2.7, rather than 4. Spontaneous frequency of miniature end-plate potentials (mepp's) has always been found to be much less steeply graded with [Ca] (frog: del Castillo and Katz, 1954; rat: Hubbard, 1961; Elmqvist and Feldman, 1965; Hubbard, Jones, and Landau, 1968*a*), indicating that, for spontaneous release, some quanta require no Ca at all for release whereas the liberation of others requires only one Ca atom per quantum (Hubbard et al., 1968*a*). At rat nerve terminals depolarized by 15 mM K^+, the relationship between transmitter release (mepp frequency) and [Ca] lies between that found for nondepolarized terminals and that for epp's (Gage and Quastel, 1966). Thus, it would appear that there are a variety of release systems (or quantal populations) distinguishable on the basis of a requirement for Ca varying between zero and four Ca atoms per quantum released. The effect of presynaptic depolarization would seem to be to increase the effectiveness of the high-order Ca complex(es) or the quantal population susceptible to these complexes (Hubbard et al., 1968*b*). The same conclusions could be drawn (Miledi and Thies, 1971) from data on the ionic dependence of the facilitation of mepp frequency and epp's during and after tetanization of the motor nerve, on the assumption that facilitation reflects persistence of intracellular Ca.

III. A SIMPLE ACTION OF ETHANOL AND ITS IMPLICATIONS

Whereas analysis of the Ca dependence of transmitter release, under various conditions, indicates a variety of release systems, other evidence suggests the reverse. In Table 1 are shown some conditions under which a given concentration of ethanol acts to produce the same multiplication of transmitter release. Gage (1965) found that ethanol (and related alcohols)

TABLE 1. *Conditions under which ethanol produces transmitter release*

Type of release	ETOH etc.	Facilitation — PTP
Spontaneous	√ Gage (1965)	√ e.g., Hubbard (1963)
epp	√ "	√ "
epp high Mg^{2+}	√ "	√ "
low Ca^{2+} spontaneous	√ Quastel et al. (1971)	√ Miledi and Thies (1971)
Ca-free spontaneous	√	—
"Anodal bursts"	√	√
Release evoked by same agent, i.e., log release rate proportional to dose or stimulation frequency	√ "	√ Maeno and Edwards (1969)

√ indicates *multiplication* of release rate.

gave equal multiplication of epp quantal content and spontaneous mepp frequency in rat diaphragm. Since the multiplication of release was unaffected by raised [Mg] and lowered [Ca], it was evidently not mediated by nerve terminal depolarization or by an effect on the nerve terminal membrane similar to that caused by presynaptic depolarization. These observations were extended by Quastel, Hackett, and Cooke (1971), who found that the multiplication of transmitter release by ethanol was exerted equally on release that was evoked by presynaptic depolarization, and on the release that persisted after strenuous removal of Ca from the bathing medium, and even on the peculiar "bursty" release evoked by nerve terminal hyperpolarization (Katz and Miledi, 1965a; Cooke and Quastel, 1973a). Moreover, release evoked by ethanol itself was multiplied by ethanol, i.e., transmitter release rate (mepp frequency) rose exponentially with ethanol concentration (Quastel et al., 1971). Similar action could be found with a variety of central depressant drugs, although for some, as with raised osmotic pressure, multiplication of depolarization-calcium evoked release was less than that of Ca-independent release, i.e., there appeared a combination of ethanol-like action with an action to inhibit depolarization-secretion coupling (Quastel, Hackett, and Okamoto, 1972). Whether the effects of ethanol and similarly acting agents are direct or mediated by a common "activator" (perhaps involving intracellular Ca, although this seems unlikely, in view of the apparent Ca-independence of the effects), these results clearly undermined the notion of a variety of release systems, or populations of quanta, since all these apparent release systems must be equally susceptible to acceleration by ethanol and other agents.

Moreover, action like that of ethanol is demonstrated by one form of depolarization-secretion coupling, that is, so-called "facilitation" or "post-tetanic potentiation" (Hughes, 1958), in other words, the enhancement of release that persists for seconds and even minutes after a nerve impulse or presynaptic depolarization. Thus (Table 1), if this persistent and cumulative response to depolarization is measured in terms of multiplication of transmitter release rate, it appears to be about equally exerted on release evoked by large depolarizations (i.e., on epp's) and on spontaneous release, and is not depressed by low Ca/raised Mg (Hubbard, 1963; Miledi and Thies, 1971), although it is absent after strenuous removal of calcium (Katz and Miledi, 1968; Cooke and Quastel, 1973*b*). When generated by focal depolarization of rat or mouse nerve terminals (Weinreich, 1970; Cooke and Quastel, 1973*a,b*), it can be seen also to multiply frequency of mepp's in "anodal bursts." Hurlbut, Longenecker, and Mauro (1971) have recently found that during repetitive nerve stimulation in Ca-depleted preparations mepp frequency grows exponentially in time; this relationship would follow if each presynaptic action potential in a series incremented to the same extent the amount of a "facilitation activator" to the concentration of which release rate were exponentially related. By this hypothesis one could also expect that net facilitation of epp quantal content would be exponentially related to stimulus frequency: such a relation has indeed been observed (Maeno and Edwards, 1969).

IV. AN UNCONVENTIONAL MODEL

The exponential response-dose curve for transmitter release versus concentration of an activator (e.g., ethanol) is not difficult to explain in terms of a model. Indeed, this relationship follows directly from basic principles, if an energy barrier normally limiting release of each releasable quantum of transmitter is reduced linearly with ethanol concentration. Moreover, with a scheme such as indicated in Fig. 1, the relationship can be derived on a stochastic basis, with only a few assumptions: (1) each particle of strategically located activator causes (on average) the same reduction of the energy barrier, independent of how many other particles are present, so that probability of release, in any arbitrarily small time unit,

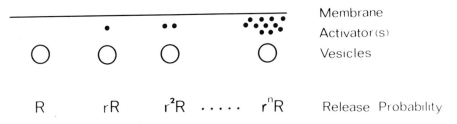

FIG. 1. Diagrammatic representation of model by which quantal release probability is continuously graded with local number of activator particles. This model predicts exponential relation between transmitter release rate and concentration of activator *(see text).*

is increased from R to $r^n R$ where n particles are present, and (2) number of particles is randomly, i.e., Poisson, distributed. Summing over all possibilities one obtains:

$$F = c \sum_{n-0}^{\infty} R r^n \; \lambda^n \; e^{-\lambda} (n!)^{-1} = cRe^{\lambda(r-1)}$$

where F is mepp frequency, c is a constant (depending upon the number of quanta available for release), and λ is the mean number of activator particles. If several different activators act independently, one obtains:

$$F = cRe^{\lambda_1 \; (r_1-1) \; + \; \lambda_2 \; (r_2-1) \; + \; \lambda_3 \; (r_3-1) \; + \; \ldots}$$

where each λ and r refers to one kind of activator. Since each r is a constant and each λ proportional to activator concentration, one can write:

$$\text{Log } F = a_0 + a_1[A_1] + a_2[A_2] + a_3[A_3] + \ldots \tag{1}$$

where each a is a constant and each $[A]$ the concentration of a specific activator. This equation is, of course, in the correct form to account for the multiplying action of ethanol and other agents on release rate, independent of how else release is stimulated, i.e., additive effects on the logarithm of release rate (Quastel et al., 1971). It should be noted that it is not necessary to suppose that any of these agents acts directly as an activator; if the concentration of an activator increases linearly with concentration of the agent, one would expect the exponential relationship to be maintained between transmitter release rate and concentration of the agent.

Now, it becomes of interest to examine what would be expected if a Ca-complex, namely $Ca_\theta X$, were to act on quantal release probability in the same way as ethanol appears to act, i.e., if $Ca_\theta X$ were an activator working in a continuously graded rather than all-or-nothing fashion. Grouping together (as α) all Ca-independent terms in equation (1), and using the usual kinetic equations to express $[Ca_\theta X]$ in terms of X_t (total X) and $[Ca]$ one obtains:

$$\text{Log } F = \alpha + a[Ca_\theta X] = \alpha + aX_t\{1 + K_1[Ca]^{-1} + \ldots K_1 \ldots K_\theta[Ca]^{-\theta}\}^{-1} \tag{2}$$

where K's are dissociation constants. If intermediate species of X, other than free X and $Ca_\theta X$, are always negligible in quantity:

$$\text{Log } F = \alpha + \beta\left\{1 + \left(\frac{\gamma}{[Ca]^\theta}\right)\right\}^{-1} \tag{3}$$

where $\beta = aX_t$ and γ is a constant. Differentiating equation (3) with respect to log $[Ca]$:

$$\frac{d \log F}{d \log [Ca]} = \beta\theta\left\{1 + \left(\frac{\gamma}{[Ca]}\right)^\theta\right\}^{-1} \left\{+ \left(\frac{[Ca]^\theta}{\gamma}\right)^{-1}\right\}; \left(\frac{d \log F}{d \log [Ca]}\right) \max = \frac{\beta\theta}{4}$$

Thus, according to this model, the maximum value of the slope, $d \log F / d \log [\text{Ca}]$ does *not* give the number of Ca atoms that "cooperate" in release of each quantum of transmitter. Moreover, the maximum slope could be expected to vary continuously with presynaptic depolarization if β alters with membrane potential. This would occur, for example, if presynaptic depolarization acted to increase influx of the activator, $\text{Ca}_\theta X$, into the nerve terminal. On the other hand, if influx of free Ca was altered by depolarization and the activator $(\text{Ca}_\theta X)$ was formed intracellulary, only γ would be expected to change, becoming smaller with increasing depolarization. A more complicated case would be Ca entry governed by the amount of a Ca complex on the membrane, as well as by presynaptic polarization: both β and γ would then alter with presynaptic potential.

V. THE CA-DEPENDENCE OF TRANSMITTER RELEASE FITS THE UNCONVENTIONAL MODEL

In order to test whether this model could indeed account for observed relationships between F and $[\text{Ca}]$ under various conditions, experiments were done (Cooke, Okamoto, and Quastel, 1973) in which the mepp frequency (F) versus $[\text{Ca}]$ relationship was studied (a) at various $[\text{K}^+]$, both by multiple sampling of end plates in each solution (Gage and Quastel, 1966) or by following F at individual end plates as $[\text{Ca}]$ was varied; (b) using focal polarization of whole end plates with large tipped electrodes (Quastel et al., 1971); and (c) with epp's. In each case, curves of $\log F$ versus $\log [\text{Ca}]$ were fitted to equation (3), by the standard nonlinear least squares method, to determine (a) whether data were indeed consistent with the equation, and, if so (b) whether θ was indeed constant, independent of presynaptic transmembrane potential, and (c) how parameters α, β, and γ altered with presynaptic membrane potential. For comparison, data series were also fitted to the equation corresponding to all-or-nothing increase of quantal release probability by a Ca-complex, namely:

$$F = \alpha + \beta \left\{ 1 + \left(\frac{\gamma}{[\text{Ca}]} \right)^{\theta} \right\}^{-1} \qquad (4)$$

With $\alpha = 0$ and $\theta = 4$, this equation becomes the same as one of those of Dodge and Rahamimoff (1967). With addition of terms in $[\text{Ca}]^{(\theta-1)}$, $[\text{Ca}]^{(\theta-2)}$, etc., and with $\theta = 3$, it becomes the equation used by Hubbard et al. (1968b). That is, the equations that were used by these investigators rest on the assumption that no quantum may have its release probability affected by more than one Ca-complex at the same time. It should be noted that the form of curve specified by equation (4) is sufficiently flexible that a series of points generated by equation (3) with any fixed θ can always be fitted fairly closely by equation (4) provided θ, as well as α, β, and γ, is free to vary.

A. Raised [K$^+$]

Figure 2 and Table 2 show some of the results of this investigation. Invariably, the relationship between log F and log [Ca] was sigmoid, with a Ca-dependent range of log F that increased with [K$^+$] at least up to 20 mM and a center of symmetry that moved to the left on the abscissa with increasing [K$^+$]. The curves drawn in Fig. 2 are from experiments using multiple sampling and were drawn to fit the equation:

$$\text{Log } F = \alpha + \beta\{1 + \gamma^2([Ca]^{-2} + \epsilon[Ca]^{-1})\}^{-1} \tag{5}$$

in each case with $\epsilon = 1$. This is the same as equation (2) with $\theta = 2$, and the term in [Ca]$^{-1}$ kept equal to the term of [Ca]$^{-2}$. In terms of the parameters in this equation, increasing [K$^+$] appears to increase β, for [K$^+$] $\leq$ 20 mM and to reduce γ. In addition, α appears to rise with [K$^+$]. However, other experiments show that α values tend to vary substantially from diaphragm to diaphragm, and these series were not all from the same diaphragm.

Although these data did show that the Ca-dependence of transmitter release could fit the new model, with a constant θ equal to 2, the multiple sampling method did not provide sufficient accuracy for establishing that θ was in fact independent of [K$^+$]. The derived data in Table 2 are from a number of experiments in which the relationship between transmitter release and [Ca] was determined at individual end plates. For each series of points θ was found by least squares to fit equations (4) and (3). Evidently, in each [K$^+$], θ by the new (log) model was not significantly different from 2, and there was no suggestion of alteration of θ with [K$^+$]. Moreover, for no individual end plate was the fit of data to equation (3) significantly better with θ free to vary than with θ fixed at 2. In contrast, with fitting to the "linear" model (equation 4), it was generally impossible to choose any fixed θ even at any one [K], which did not make the best fits obtainable appreciably worse than with θ free to vary. It may be remarked that adjustment of data for the inhibitory effect of high [Ca] on release evoked by raised

TABLE 2. *Estimates of θ and γ obtained by least squares fitting of F versus [Ca] curves to equations corresponding to linear and log models*

[K$^+$]	n	θ linear	θ log	γ linear	γ log
5	*	0.95	—	6.43	0.95 ± 0.23
10	*	1.51 ± 0.50	—	2.21 ± 0.24	0.68 ± 0.18
15	7	2.60 ± 0.21	1.94 ± 0.27	1.07 ± 0.16	0.45 ± 0.02
20	19	3.03 ± 0.12	1.99 ± 0.12	0.64 ± 0.05	0.28 ± 0.01
25	6	2.94 ± 0.17	1.74 ± 0.32	0.49 ± 0.07	0.19 ± 0.01
30	6	3.44 ± 0.21	1.96 ± 0.19	0.30 ± 0.02	0.13 ± 0.01
50	3	3.23 ± 0.19	1.8 ± 0.5	0.39 ± 0.21	0.10 ± 0.01

* Data from experiments using multiple sampling; one series each.

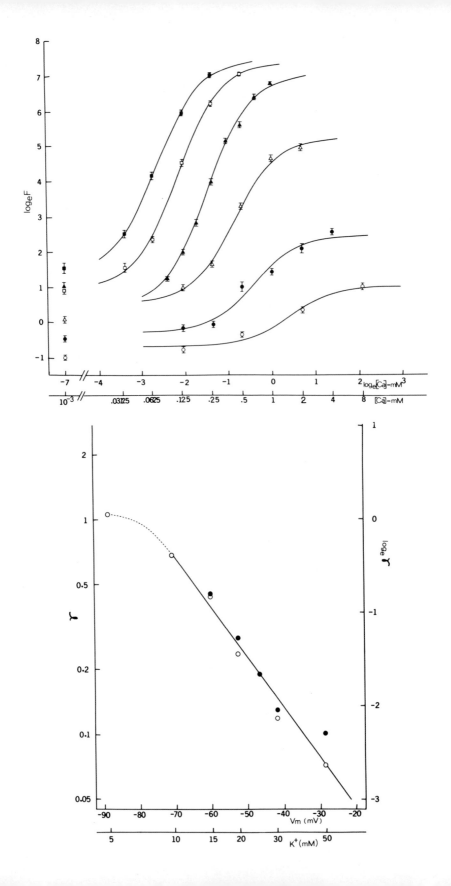

[K$^+$] (Cooke and Quastel, 1969, 1973a,b,c) did not alter derived values of θ appreciably, but improved fits to equation (5) relative to equation (3), with $\epsilon = 1$ when [Mg] $= 1$. In experiments using raised [Mg], fits were improved by raising ϵ (to 4, for [Mg] $= 5$ mM); ϵ did not appear to change with [K$^+$].

Thus, by the "log" model the data were compatible with the notion of the same Ca complex always mediating release, independent of the degree of nerve terminal depolarization. By the linear model, however, it would appear that depolarization acts to make transmitter release dependent upon progressively higher order Ca complexes.

It has already been pointed out that, if depolarization were to act to increase influx of free Ca or Ca from a complex into the nerve terminal, one would expect γ to become reduced with increasing depolarization. As shown in Fig. 2 (right), γ did indeed go down with increasing [K$^+$] and nominal transmembrane potential. Apparently, for membrane potential less negative than approximately -70 mV, γ^{-1} increases e-fold for every 18.9 mV increment of membrane potential ($r = .978$ for log γ versus nominal membrane potential). That β also rises with depolarization is inconsistent with the hypothesis that depolarization acts solely to increase influx of free Ca^{2+}, and implies either that Ca entry is also governed by the amount of a Ca complex on the membrane, or that intracellular Ca "receptor" increases with depolarization.

B. Focal Depolarization of Nerve Terminals

In Fig. 3 are shown results obtained using current pulses, applied focally to an end plate, of up to several seconds duration, to evoke enhanced mepp frequency, with [Ca] varied between .0625 and 8 mM. Evidently (Fig. 3 left) the maximum slope of log F (during pulses) versus applied current tended to be increased in low [Ca] (Landau, 1969). However, corresponding plots of log F versus log [Ca] (Fig. 3 right) are very similar to what was obtained with raised [K$^+$], i.e., the Ca-dependence of transmitter release evoked by focal depolarization fits equation (5). (Lines drawn are with α, β, γ, found by least squares fitting.) As previously, β is seen to increase with depolarization, but become reduced with very large depolarization. Again, log γ goes down linearly with depolarization. Indeed, from other data (see Cooke and Quastel, 1972a), it was possible to estimate the

---

←

FIG. 2. *(Top):* Graphs of log F versus log [Ca] obtained by multiple sampling from three diaphragms: (○) 5mM K$^+$, (●) 10mM K$^+$, (△) 15 mM K$^+$, (▲) 20 mM K$^+$, (□) 30 mM K$^+$, (■) 50mM K$^+$. Series in 5 and 10 mM K$^+$ from one diaphragm, 20 mM K$^+$ from another, and others from the third. All points except those for 5 and 10 mM K$^+$ have been raised to adjust for variation of α between diaphragms. Lines are theoretical curves fitting equation (5), with $\epsilon = 1$. *(Bottom):* Graph of log γ (found by fitting to equation 5, with $\epsilon = 1$) versus nominal membrane potential (Nernst equation): (○) γ's from multiple sampling experiments, (●) mean γ's from individual end-plate experiments. The solid line is linear regression line, point for 5mM K$^+$ omitted.

presynaptic polarization corresponding to each current applied, and, on this basis, the slope of log γ versus membrane potential was between $-.04$ and $-.055/mV$, (cf. $-.053/mV$ for the data from experiments using $[K^+]$).

What is also striking, of course, is the apparent increase of α, the Ca^{2+}-independent fraction of mepp frequency (as defined by fitting to equation 5), with presynaptic depolarization.

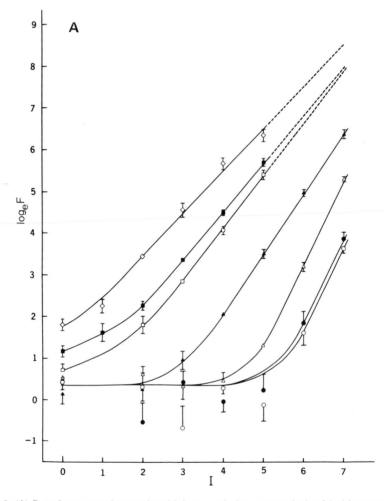

FIG. 3. (A) Data from experiments in which an end plate was polarized (arbitrary current unit $= -.24\,\mu A$) in 0.0625, .125, .25, .5, 1, 2, 8 mm Ca^{2+} (curves shift upward with increasing [Ca]). Lines drawn by eye. (B) Same data as (A), plotted as log F versus log [Ca], for $1 = 0$, 2, 3, . . . 7 arbitrary current unit. Curves drawn are theoretical curves fitting equation (5) with $\epsilon = 1$.
(C) Derived data from data in (A). Graph of log γ versus I (arbitrary units), γ found by least squares fitting of curves to equation (5).

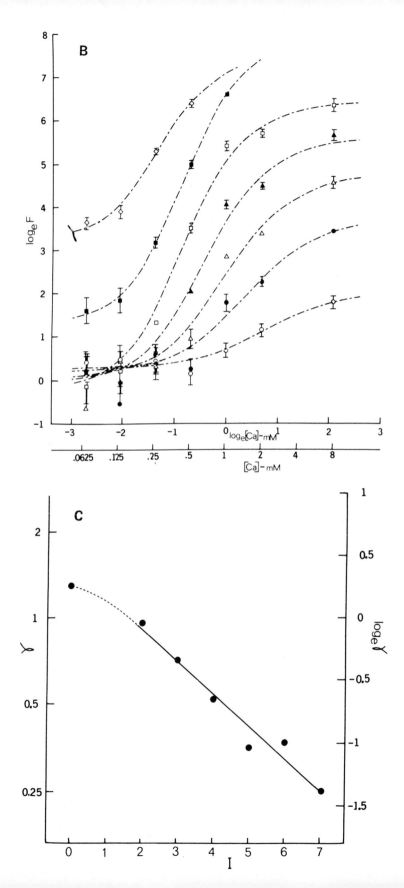

C. End-Plate Potentials

Figure 4 shows examples of the Ca-independence of end-plate potentials elicited by 30-sec stimulation, as [Ca] was varied. In all cases, as in those presented, the relationship between log quantal content and log [Ca] was sigmoid, with maximum slopes sometimes significantly more than 4 and sometimes less. Because muscle twitching occurred with exposure to low Ca^{2+}, unless [Mg^{2+}] were raised, [Mg] was raised to 5 mm for these experiments. The lines drawn are best fits to equation (5), with $\epsilon = 4$, as with 5 mm Mg^{2+} in raised K^+. As with previous data, the best fits obtained with this equation left residual mean squares no larger than expected from the accuracy of the data points. Of course, about equally good fits could also be

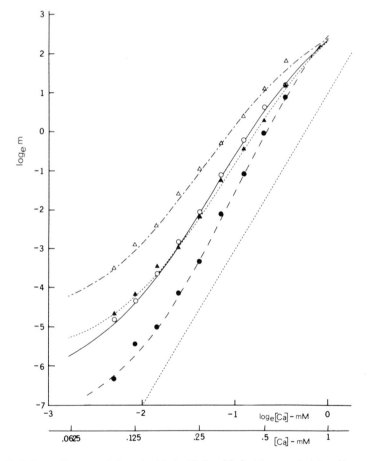

FIG. 4. Variation of log quantal content (m) with log [Ca] at four end plates. Nerve stimulated at 30.5 sec. [Mg] = 5 mm. Dashed straight line drawn with slope of 4. Each curve represents best fit of data points to equation (5) with $\epsilon = 4$.

obtained with the equation for the linear model, but with θ, the number of Ca atoms that "cooperate" approaching 5 (cf. Table 2).

VI. A MODEL THAT ACCOUNTS FOR Ca-DEPENDENCE OF DEPOLARIZATION-EVOKED TRANSMITTER RELEASE

Equation (5) is sufficiently complex that there are a number of physical models that would be compatible with it. However, if, as it appears, the term ϵ alters only with [Mg], and not with depolarization and hence γ, choice of possible models becomes greatly restricted. The simplest that fits the equation is the following:

(a) Transmitter release rate is exponentially related to the amount of a Ca complex, CaX, inside the nerve terminal $\text{Log } F = \alpha + a[\text{CaX}]$

(b) The amount of CaX is governed by the total amount of X (X_t) and local [Ca] available $[\text{CaX}] = X_t\{1 + K_c[\text{Ca}]_i^{-1}\}^{-1}$

(c) $[\text{Ca}]_i$, inside the terminal, is governed by presynaptic membrane potential (V) and the amount of a Ca complex involving two Ca atoms (Ca_2Y) on the membrane, i.e., $[\text{Ca}]_i = f(V)[\text{Ca}_2\text{Y}] = f(V)Y_t\{1 + K_2[\text{Ca}]^{-1} + K_1K_2[\text{Ca}]^{-2}\}^{-1}$ where $f(V)$ is a function of membrane potential, K's are dissociation constants.

Combining these equations one obtains equation (5) with $\alpha = \alpha$; $\beta = aX_t\{1 + K_cf(V)^{-1}Y_t^{-1}\}^{-1}$; $\gamma^2 = K_1K_2K_c\{K_c + f(V)Y_t\}^{-1}$; $\epsilon = K_1^{-1}$. The action of Mg is accommodated by competition at the various Ca-binding sites. In particular, Mg competition leading to formation of MgCaY will lead to linear increase of ϵ with [Mg]. It may be noted that the experiments with raised Mg also show increase of γ^2 with [Mg]: this is most readily explained in terms of competition of Mg with Ca on the intracellular binding side X. It may be recalled that Douglas and Poisner (1964) found that Mg inhibited secretion of vasopressia by the neurohypophysis to a greater extent than to be expected from the inhibition of calcium entry. Using this model, $f(V)$ is almost proportional to γ^{-2}. Thus, the slope of $\log f(V)$ versus V is between .08 and .11/mV.

The above equations make a specific prediction with regard to the relationship between β and γ^2, namely, these should be linearly related, with $\beta = aX_t$ when $\gamma^2 = 0$ and $\gamma^2 = K_1K_2$ when $\beta = 0$. However, graphs of β versus γ^2, (e.g., Fig. 5) from observed data (either raised K^+ or focal polarization) show a larger increase of β with low γ^2 (i.e., with depolarization) than that predicted by the model. It is necessary to postulate that X_t (or a) increases with presynaptic depolarization, perhaps to double or even triple its initial value, to account for the β of at least 13 which obtains for epp's. This could arise, for example, if the internal binding site for Ca^{2+} (i.e., X) were located on the inner surface of the nerve terminal membrane and depolarization caused a configurational change that increased the number of sites available for combination with Ca²⁺. Of course, once it is postulated that X_t is increased by depolarization, then this increase could be invoked to account entirely for increase of β with depolarization. On this basis the data is qualitatively compatible with a model in which Ca²⁺ entry requires no external binding of Ca, and it is a Ca_2X inside the terminal that mediates release. However, it becomes difficult to account for an ϵ that does not increase greatly with depolarization.

VII. NONINDEPENDENCE OF a AND β

The above models fail to account for the rise with depolarization of α (i.e., apparent Ca-independent portion of log F) and fall of β at higher levels of depolarization. The rise of α can, of course, be identified with the Ca-insensitive cumulative and persistent response to depolarization, already briefly discussed. In the experiments illustrated in Fig. 4, it can be seen that extrapolated quantal contents in very low [Ca], i.e., α (which in each case corresponded to 10^{-3} times observed mepp frequency in solution

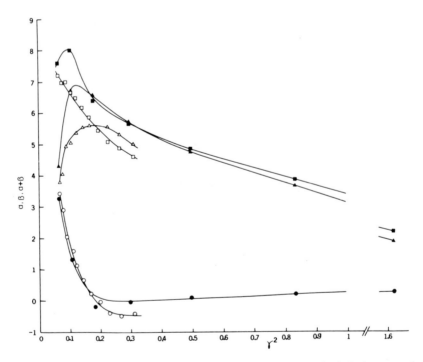

FIG. 5. Graphs of α (circles), β (triangles) and $(\alpha + \beta)$ (squares) plotted versus γ^2, for experiments using focal polarization of end plates. Open symbols = 20 mM K⁺, filled symbols = 5 mM K⁺ in bathing solution. Note β (or $\alpha + \beta$) is not linear with γ^2, as predicted by model.

containing EDTA and Ca, to give a [Ca] of $\sim 10^{-3}$ mM), varied considerably from one end plate to another, and tended to be negatively correlated with β. That is, a large Ca-independent fraction of log F was associated with a low Ca-sensitive fraction. When data from other such experiments were also considered, the negative correlation between β and α for end-plate potentials became insignificant. However, data from the experiments using raised [K$^+$] showed for each group a negative correlation between these parameters that was significant (at the 5% level) for most series. Figure 6 shows plots of β versus α (by least squares fitting to equation (5)) for the data series using 15 and 20 mM K$^+$ and for the epp data. Evidently, the observed relationship between β and α is compatible with a linear relationship between the two; by extrapolation β would be zero at $\alpha \simeq 7$, i.e., at Ca-independent F at approximately 10^3 sec. A simple explanation for this phenomenon would be the following: with depolarization there occurs not only an increase of the Ca receptor, X, but a transformation of X to a new form X', which needs no Ca attached to it in order to constitute an activator of transmitter release.

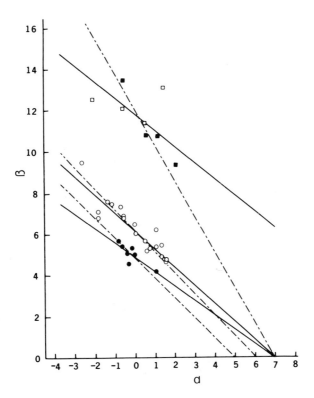

FIG. 6. Graphs of β versus α showing correlations from experiments in 15 m M K$^+$ (●), 20 m M K$^+$ (○) and end-plate potentials [with 6.8 added to α to make it equivalent to basal log mepp frequency, (■), 30.5 sec, (□), 5 sec]. In each case solid line is regression line for β versus α and interrupted line for α versus β.

To the extent that the rate and eventual degree of X → X' transformation varied from one end plate to another it would account for the wide variation of α at tetanized or depolarized junctions.

VIII. INACTIVATION OF DEPOLARIZATION-SECRETION COUPLING

If, indeed, the above hypothesis is correct, that raised α corresponds to the cumulative and persistent response to depolarization and consists of an alteration of the Ca receptor (X) to a form needing no attached Ca for activation of quantal liberation, it implies that concomitant with development of this response there should be a corresponding decline of X, and therefore of the degree to which nerve terminal depolarization can evoke transmitter release, i.e., an inactivation of coupling. Such is indeed the case. As illustrated in Figs. 7 to 9, the slow response to depolarization can readily be produced by focal depolarization of nerve terminals in the presence of tetrodotoxin (Cooke and Quastel, 1972*b*) and can appear as a large afterdischarge (Fig. 7), a slow phase of increased F during and persisting after a square pulse depolarization (Fig. 8), or, in very low [Ca] (added 1 mM-MgEDTA, no Ca^{2+}: estimated free [Ca] 10^{-4} mM), as a very slow rise of F during a depolarization, with relatively little aftereffect (Fig. 9). The asymmetry in Fig. 9 presumably reflects a permissive role of a small amount of

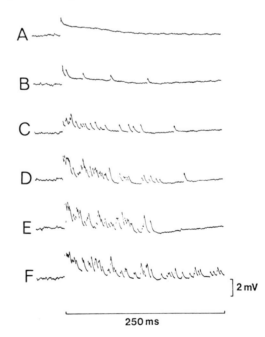

FIG. 7. Afterdischarges of mepp's following focal depolarization of an end plate for increasing periods, from .23 sec to 1.6 sec. Standard solution. Transmembrane depolarization during current application estimated ~ 45 mV.

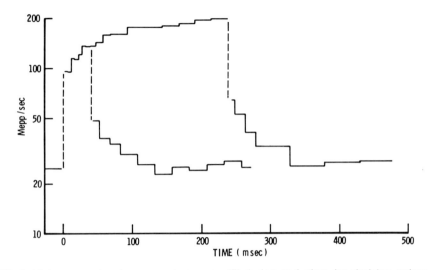

FIG. 8. Histograms showing mepp frequency *(F)* during and after depolarizing pulses (250 iterations of three 40-msec and one 250-msec pulse) applied focally to end plate in 20 mM K⁺, .25 mM Ca²⁺, 2 mM Mg²⁺. Note total response compounded of "square" response and exponentially rising and falling component of log *F*.

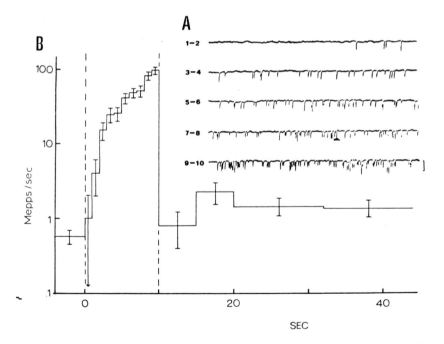

FIG. 9. Acceleration of mepp's during a focal depolarizing pulse, in solution containing ~ 10^{-7} M free Ca²⁺ (5 mM MgEDTA, 5 mM MgCl₂, no Ca²⁺). (A) Alternate seconds of pulse application. There was 1 mepp in first second. Voltage scale 1 mV. Each trace 1 sec. Note inversion of mepp's by local extracellular negativity. (B) Log *F* versus time. Pulse applied between dashed lines.

Ca^{2+} for development of the response, with enough present only during the depolarization, when some enters the terminal. It is noticeable in Fig. 8 that the fast response to depolarization was somewhat greater for the start of the depolarizing pulse than for its end; this was a consistent finding and is consistent with a small degree of inactivation. Figure 10 shows inactivation much more clearly. Here, pulses were virtually ineffective in raising F immediately following a large depolarization; the response returned to control level roughly in parallel with the decline of the afterdischarge. The tests with raised $[K^+]$ indicate that the apparent inactivation could not have been secondary to persistent increase of K^+ conductance or of local $[K^+]$ following the large depolarizing pulse (Cooke and Quastel, 1972*b*).

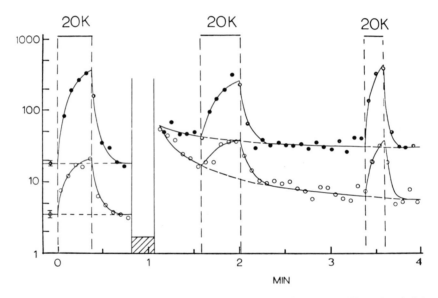

FIG. 10. Inactivation of coupling. The response of mepp frequency *(F)* to depolarizing pulses (1-sec duration, filled circles) was reduced during afterdischarge caused by large prolonged depolarization (cross hatch). Responses of *F* to raised [K] (20 mM) were reduced in parallel with responses to depolarization.

IX. EFFECTS OF DRUGS ON DEPOLARIZATION-SECRETION COUPLING

It was mentioned previously that with raised osmotic pressure and some central depressant drugs (the notable exception being ethanol) there occurs, in addition to the direct action to increase F, an inhibition of depolarization-secretion coupling (Fig. 11). Chlorpromazine (Fig. 11 left) caused a rise in spontaneous F, but a reduction of the extent to which depolarizing pulses multiplied F, i.e., a flattening of the presynaptic transfer function. Figure

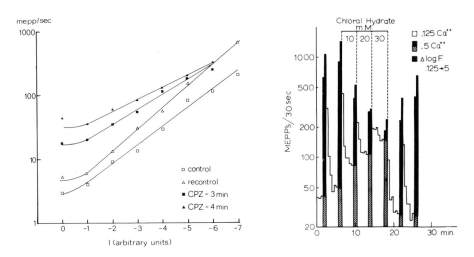

FIG. 11 *(Left):* Depression of slope of log F versus applied depolarizing current, by chlorpromazine. *(Right):* Depression, by chloral hydrate (10, 20, 30 mм) of response of F to increase of [Ca] from 0.125 to 0.5 mм, [K$^+$] constant at 20 mм.

9 left shows the converse phenomenon. At constant depolarization (20 mм K$^+$), the response to increase of [Ca] from .125 to .5 mм was attenuated by chloral hydrate (10, 20, 30 mм). Similar effects have been obtained with raised osmotic pressure, pentobarbital, and chloroform (Quastel et al., 1972). Presently under investigation is the mechanism(s) by which these agents work in terms of the model which has been put forward.

X. SUMMARY

Quantitative evaluation of the Ca-dependence of transmitter release (mepp frequency: F) by depolarized mouse nerve terminals has shown that the relation between log F and log [Ca] is always sigmoid. There occurs a progressive rise of maximum $\Delta \log F / \Delta \log$ [Ca] with increasing depolarization. The data are compatible with a model by which an energy barrier-limiting release of a quantum of transmitter is continuously graded with the number of particles of a Ca complex (CaX) located strategically, so that quantal release rate is exponentially related to the amount of CaX inside the nerve terminal. The action of presynaptic depolarization increases entry of Ca, to an extent also governed by a complex (Ca_2Y) on or in the membrane: Ca entry increases e-fold per between 9 and 13 mV. In addition, depolarization causes increase of the amount of the Ca receptor (X) available for combination with Ca. To explain the observation that with large prolonged depolarization there is increase of Ca-independent release (at [Ca] $>$ 10^{-4} м) with reduction of Ca-dependent release, it is proposed also that depolarization causes alteration of X, to a form, X', that can activate release (also in graded fashion) in the virtual absence of extracellular Ca. This last phenomenon also appears as "inactivation" of depolarization-secretion coupling.

ACKNOWLEDGMENT

The research reported in this chapter is supported by grants from the Muscular Dystrophy Association of Canada and Medical Research Council of Canada.

REFERENCES

Bloedel, J., Gage, P. W., Llinas, R., and Quastel, D. M. J. (1966): Transmitter release at the squid giant synapse in the presence of tetrodotoxin. *Nature*, 212:49–50.

Cooke, J. D., Okamoto, K., and Quastel, D. M. J. (1973): The role of calcium in depolarization-secretion coupling at the motor nerve terminal. *J. Physiol.*, 228:459–497.

Cooke, J. D., and Quastel, D. M. J. (1969): Mechanism of potassium action on transmitter release at the neuromuscular junction. *Abstracts, Third Int. Biophysics Congress*, p. 99.

Cooke, J. D., and Quastel, D. M. J. (1973a): Transmitter release by mammalian motor nerve terminals in response to focal polarization. *J. Physiol.*, 228:377–405.

Cooke, J. D., and Quastel, D. M. J. (1973b): Cumulative and persistent effects of nerve terminal depolarization on transmitter release. *J. Physiol.*, 228:407–434.

Cooke, J. D., and Quastel, D. M. J. (1973c): The specific effect of potassium on transmitter release by rat motor nerve terminals, and its inhibition by calcium. *J. Physiol.*, 228:435–458.

Del Castillo, J., and Engbaek, L. (1954): The nature of the neuromuscular block produced by magnesium. *J. Physiol.*, 124:370–384.

Del Castillo, J., and Katz, B. (1954): The effect of magnesium on the activity of motor nerve endings. *J. Physiol.*, 124:553–559.

Del Castillo, J., and Stark, L. (1952): The effect of calcium ions on the motor end-plate potentials. *J. Physiol.*, 116:507–515.

Dodge, F. A., Jr., and Rahamimoff, R. (1967): Cooperative action of calcium ions in transmitter release at the neuromuscular junction. *J. Physiol.*, 193:419–433.

Douglas, W. W. (1968): Stimulus-secretion coupling: The concept and clues from chromaffin and other cells. The First Gaddum Memorial Lecture. *Brit. J. Pharmac.*, 34:451–474.

Douglas, W. W., and Poisner, A. M. (1964): Calcium movement in the neurohypophysis of the rat and its relation to the release of vasopressin. *J. Physiol.*, 172:19–30.

Elmqvist, D., and Feldman, D. S. (1965): Calcium dependence of spontaneous acetylcholine release at mammalian motor nerve terminals. *J. Physiol.*, 181:487–497.

Feng, T. P. (1936): Studies on the neuromuscular junction. II. The universal antagonism between calcium and curarising agencies. *Chin. J. Physiol.*, 10:513–528.

Gage, P. W. (1965): The effect of methyl, ethyl, and n-propyl alcohol on neuromuscular transmission in the rat. *J. Pharm. Exp. Ther.*, 150:236–243.

Gage, P. W., and Quastel, D. M. J. (1966). Competition between sodium and calcium ions in transmitter release at a mammalian neuromuscular junction. *J. Physiol.*, 185:95–123.

Hubbard, J. I. (1961). The effect of calcium and magnesium on the spontaneous release of transmitter from mammalian motor nerve endings. *J. Physiol.*, 159:507–517.

Hubbard, J. I. (1963). Repetitive stimulation at the mammalian neuromuscular junction and the mobilization of transmitter. *J. Physiol.*, 169:641–662.

Hubbard, J. I., Jones, S. F., and Landau, E. M. (1968a): On the mechanism by which calcium and magnesium affect the spontaneous release of transmitter from mammalian motor nerve terminals. *J. Physiol.*, 194:355–380.

Hubbard, J. I., Jones, S. F., and Landau, E. M. (1968b): On the mechanism by which calcium and magnesium affect the release of transmitter by nerve impulses. *J. Physiol.*, 196:75–86.

Hughes, J. R. (1958): Post-tetanic potentiation. *Physiol. Rev.*, 38:91–113.

Hurlbut, W. P., Longenecker, H. B., Jr., and Mauro, H. (1971): Effects of calcium and magnesium on the frequency of miniature end-plate potentials during prolonged tetanization. *J. Physiol.*, 219:17–38.

Jenkinson, D. H. (1957): The nature of the antagonism between calcium and sodium ions at the neuromuscular junction. *J. Physiol.*, 138:438–444.

Katz, B. (1969): *The Release of Neural Transmitter Substances*. Liverpool University Press, Liverpool.

Katz, B., and Miledi, R. (1965a): Propagation of electric activity in motor nerve terminals. *Proc. Roy. Soc. B*, 161:453–481.

Katz, B., and Miledi, R. (1965b): The effect of calcium on acetylcholine release from motor nerve endings. *Proc. Roy. Soc. B*, 161:496–503.

Katz, B., and Miledi, R. (1967): A study of synaptic transmission in the absence of nerve impulses. *J. Physiol.*, 192:407–436.

Katz, B., and Miledi, R. (1968): The role of calcium in neuromuscular facilitation. *J. Physiol.*, 195:481–492.

Katz, B., and Miledi, R. (1969a). Tetrodotoxin resistant electrical activity in presynaptic terminals. *J. Physiol.*, 203:459–488.

Katz, B., and Miledi, R. (1969b). Spontaneous and evoked activity of motor nerve endings in calcium Ringer. *J. Physiol.*, 203:689–706.

Katz, B., and Miledi, R. (1970): Further study of the role of calcium in synaptic transmission. *J. Physiol.*, 207:789–801.

Kusano, K., Livengood, C. R., and Werman, R. (1967): Correlation of transmitter release with membrane properties of the presynaptic fibre of the squid giant synapse. *J. Gen. Physiol.*, 50:2579–2601.

Landau, E. M. (1969): The interaction of presynaptic polarization with calcium and magnesium in modifying spontaneous transmitter release from mammalian motor nerve terminals. *J. Physiol.*, 203:281–299.

Liley, A. W. (1956): The effects of presynaptic polarization on the spontaneous activity at the mammalian neuromuscular junction. *J. Physiol.*, 134:427–443.

Maeno, T., and Edwards, C. (1969): Neuromuscular facilitation with low-frequency stimulation and effects of some drugs. *J. Neurophysiol.*, 32:785–792.

Miledi, R., and Slater, C. R. (1966): The action of calcium on neuronal synapses in the squid. *J. Physiol.*, 184:473–498.

Miledi, R., and Thies, R. (1971): Tetanic and post-tetanic rise in frequency of miniature end-plate potentials in low-calcium solutions. *J. Physiol.*, 212:245–257.

Quastel, D. M. J., Hackett, J. R., and Cooke, J. D. (1971). Calcium: Is it required for transmitter secretion? *Science*, 172:1034–1036.

Quastel, D. M. J., Hackett, J. T., and Okamoto, K. (1972): Presynaptic action of central depressant drugs: Inhibition of depolarization-secretion coupling. *Can. J. Physiol. Pharmacol.*, 50:279–284.

Rubin, R. P. (1970): The role of calcium in the release of neurotransmitter substances and hormones. *Pharmac. Rev.*, 22:389–428.

Weinreich, D. (1970): Post-tetanic potentiation at the neuromuscular junction of the frog in the presence of tetrodotoxin. *Brain Res.*, 17:527–529.

Synaptic Transmission and Neuronal Interaction
Raven Press, New York 1974

Kinetics of Postsynaptic Membrane Response at the Neuromuscular Junction

Charles F. Stevens

Department of Physiology and Biophysics, University of Washington School of Medicine, Seattle, Washington 98195

INTRODUCTION

The frog neuromuscular junction offers several advantages as a preparation in which to study the molecular mechanisms underlying membrane permeability changes. First, a very high density of receptors — as estimated by snake toxin binding sites — is present in a circumscribed area (Fambrough, Hartzell, Powell, Rash, and Joseph, *This Volume*). Because this density is so great, about three orders of magnitude higher than that estimated for sodium channels in axon membrane (Keynes, Ritchie, and Rojas, 1971), it should be possible to examine permeability mechanisms with other than standard electrophysiological techniques (e.g., with optical methods). Second, isolation and characterization of the acetylcholine receptor is being actively pursued in a number of laboratories and a good start on these problems has already been made (Klett, Fulpius, Cooper, and Reich, *This Volume;* Lindstrom and Patrick, *This Volume*). Thus, in the not too distant future, physiological and biochemical approaches to conductance changes may be correlated. Finally, end-plate channels may prove, as will be discussed below, a favorable system in which to study the influence of membrane electric fields on the behavior of gating macromolecules that control permeability.

Because of these and other advantages, my laboratory has been concentrating on electrophysiological investigations of permeability changes at the end plate in an effort to elucidate the molecular mechanisms involved in the gating of ionic channels. The work of Magleby, Anderson, Beam, and myself, together with that from other laboratories, has yielded the following tentative physical explanation for the end-plate conductance change: upon depolarization of the presynaptic terminal, acetylcholine (ACh) is released and diffuses to the postsynaptic membrane where it binds rapidly to its receptor. This binding reduces the energy barrier for a conformational change either in the receptor or in an associated gating macromolecule and, when the conformational change occurs, the end-plate channel conductance is increased from effectively zero to 2 to 3×10^{-11} mho. The cleft ACh concentration decreases rapidly because of diffusional losses and the hydrolytic action of acetylcholinesterase. As the time constant for closing of already opened channels is relatively long, on the order of 1 msec, the entire population of end-plate channels closes comparatively slowly after the cleft transmitter concentration has dropped essentially to zero; this relaxation of the gating molecules to their closed conformation is the rate-limiting step in end-plate conductance changes and is reflected in the decaying phase of end-plate currents measured under voltage clamp conditions.

As the gating molecule changes its conformation between its open and closed states, the dipole moment of the molecule is also somewhat altered. Since these dipole moment alterations occur in an electric field produced by the membrane potential, the energy of the gating molecule in a particular conformation is somewhat dependent upon membrane potential. Thus, the opening and closing rates are influenced by membrane potentials and these influences are detected by alterations in the decay time for end-plate conductance changes. The magnitude of the gating kinetics sensitivity to voltage suggests a dipole moment change between the open and closed conformations of about 50 Debye or more.

The purpose of this discussion is to summarize some of the experimental findings which have led to the physical picture just described. The first section of the results will deal with an analysis, carried out by Magleby and myself, of the end-plate permeability changes produced by nerve stimulation, and will be especially concerned with the effects of membrane potential on the time course of these permeability changes. The model, described above, was originally formulated to explain the results of investigations of this type. In more recent experiments, however, Anderson and I have further tested this model by examining the spontaneous fluctuations in end-plate permeability which are seen in end plates subjected to constant concentrations of ACh; some results of our experiments will be described in the second section. Finally, alternative interpretations of the data will be discussed briefly.

METHODS

The experiments described here were carried out on frog sartorius muscles which had been pretreated with hypertonic glycerol or ethylene glycol Ringer's solution to disrupt excitation-contraction coupling (see Eisenberg, Howell, and Vaughan, 1971; Sevcik and Narahashi, 1972). The muscles were placed in a glass-bottom chamber, transilluminated, and impaled with pairs of relatively low-resistance (2 to 5 MΩ) microelectrodes. These microelectrodes were positioned to be near end-plate regions as judged by the rapid rise and large amplitude of end-plate potentials and miniature end-plate potentials.

The postjunctional membranes were activated with ACh released from presynaptic terminals by nerve stimulation or from an ACh-filled microelectrode by iontophoresis. The iontophoresis microelectrode was placed approximately 40μ from the end-plate region to minimize the effect of any possible rapid fluctuations in ACh ejection by a relatively long diffusion distance. Voltage was held constant at levels between -140 and $+60$ mV by the feedback voltage clamp amplifier, and the resulting currents, or, strictly speaking, differences between resting and ACh-activated currents, were recorded. In early experiments analysis was carried out from photographic records, but in more recent studies a digital computer (PDP 11) was used.

Methods have been described in greater detail in Magleby and Stevens (1972*a*).

RESULTS

Analysis of the End-Plate Conductance Change

Before considering the mechanisms responsible for end-plate conductance changes, it will be necessary to characterize the properties of these conductances. The results to be presented show that, following nerve stimulation, end-plate conductance rises rapidly and then decays exponentially with a rate constant α, which itself depends exponentially on membrane potential; end-plate conductance decay is about two times slower for each 100 mV of hyperpolarization.

Examples of the end-plate conductance changes obtained from a voltage clamp experiment carried out and analyzed by Beam are shown in Fig. 1A and B; for A the membrane potential was -59 mV, and for B it was -123 mV. The data in Fig. 1 demonstrate the features of end-plate conductance changes seen at all membrane potentials: the end-plate conductance increases and decays more slowly as the membrane potential is made more negative. Furthermore, the peak conductance is somewhat smaller at the more negative membrane potentials than near zero.

Semilogarithmic plots of end-plate conductance reveal that it decays exponentially over the entire range for which reliable measurements can be made; the decay constant which characterizes the declining phase of end-plate conductance is denoted by α. End-plate conductances have been studied at a variety of membrane potentials between -140 and $+60$ mV, and throughout this entire voltage range the decaying phase is exponential, but α varies systematically with membrane potential. Semilogarithmic graphs of α as a function of membrane potential are linear as shown by Beam's data in Fig. 2, so α's dependence on membrane potential may be written as

$$\alpha(V) = Be^{AV} \tag{1}$$

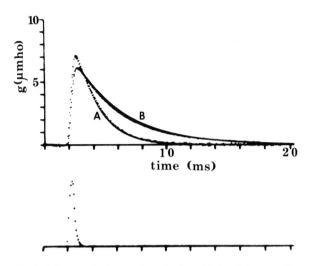

FIG. 1. Top: End-plate conductance transients, obtained from voltage-clamped frog sartorius nerve-muscle preparation, at membrane potentials of (A) −59 mV and (B) −123 mV. Temperature = 20°C. Theoretical curves, which have been superimposed on experimental data in both A and B, were calculated from equations (3) and (5) with the constants for (5) specified by least-squares lines in Fig. 2 and the concentration function $NC^n(t)/K$ shown in the lower part of this figure. The fit of theory to observation is sufficiently close that it is difficult to distinguish between theoretical and experimental curves. Bottom: The function $NC^n(t)/K$ for the same end plate from equation (3) plotted with arbitrary units on the ordinate as a function of time. This function was obtained from experimental data through equation (3), using the values of α in that equation as shown in Fig. 2, and represents the average of calculations from about 30 end-plate conductance transients obtained at different membrane potentials. Note that the values on the ordinate are known only to an undetermined multiplicative constant because β and $C^n(t)$ always appear as a product in equation (3) and cannot be determined independently. These data were obtained and analyzed by Dr. Kurt Beam.

In this equation V is membrane potential, and A and B are constants with average values (Magleby and Stevens, 1972a), $A = .008$ mV^{-1} and $B = 1.7$ msec^{-1}; for the data in Fig. 2 (obtained at a somewhat lower temperature), $A = .011$ mV^{-1} and $B = .88$ msec^{-1}.

Further interpretation of the end-plate conductance change depends upon identifying the mechanisms responsible for the decaying phase. The fact that conductance decreases according to a simple exponential suggests, but does not prove, that end-plate conductance decay predominantly reflects a single mechanism rather than a combination of mechanisms. Two general classes of mechanisms may be considered. The first possibility is that postjunctional processes (binding of ACh to its receptor and opening and closing of channels) are rapid and that the rate-limiting step is the decay of concentration in the cleft. The second alternative is that the cleft concentration decays rapidly and the rate-limiting steps are in postjunctional membrane processes. If the rates of both postjunctional processes and the decline of cleft ACh concentrations were comparable, one would not expect

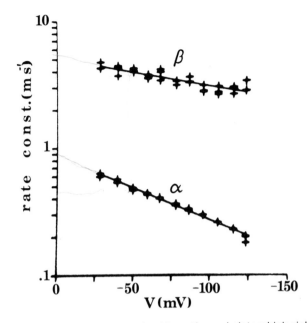

FIG. 2. Semilog plots of α and β, determined from the end plate which yielded the data in Fig. 1, as a function of membrane potential. Note that β is specified only to an undetermined multiplicative constant. The data have been fit with least-squares regression lines.

the observed single exponential decay of end-plate conductance over all voltages and over the rather wide temperature range (8 to 31°C) used in our experiments. These two classes of mechanisms will be considered in turn.

If the decaying phase of end-plate conductance reflects cleft ACh concentration, one must suppose either that the voltage dependence of α is an artifact of voltage clamping or that membrane potential in some way influences the decline of transmitter concentration. A number of arguments suggest that the voltage dependence of α is not a voltage clamp artifact: α has the same voltage dependence for both miniature end-plate currents and evoked end-plate currents so that area of activation is not important. Furthermore, any procedure which is known to decrease the accuracy of voltage clamping (e.g., decreasing feedback amplifier gain or moving electrodes away from the end-plate region) decreases rather than increases the voltage sensitivity of α as would be expected if voltage sensitivity were a clamp artifact. Finally, the voltage dependence of α persists at lowered temperatures where the clamp is certainly able to follow accurately the conductance changes. It appears, then, that the voltage sensitivity of α is related to the properties of the mechanisms responsible for the closing of end-plate channels, and does not arise from some artifact in the voltage clamping procedure.

If the decline in cleft ACh concentration is the rate-limiting step, the post-junctional membrane potential must thus influence the course of cleft ACh concentration. This could occur in at least two ways. First, because the magnitude and direction of end-plate currents depend on membrane potential, these currents might, depending on their direction, accelerate or retard the diffusional losses of ACh by iontophoresis. Under this hypothesis, the outward currents seen in depolarized muscles would sweep the positively charged ACh molecules away from their receptors and shorten the end-plate current duration whereas the large inward currents which occur with hyperpolarization would retard diffusional loss and prolong end-plate currents. Second, it might be that the membrane field influences the catalytic rate of acetylcholinesterase so that, as the membrane becomes more hyperpolarized, the enzyme hydrolizes ACh less rapidly, thereby prolonging the duration of transmitter action. We have examined both of these possibilities.

If the iontophoretic hypothesis is correct, the decay constant α should depend on membrane potential only through the magnitude and direction of end-plate currents. Since end-plate current amplitude is readily varied without changing membrane potential, this possibility is not difficult to investigate. If end-plate current magnitudes are decreased by application of curare or by the depression of transmitter release, or if they are increased by facilitation or raised extracellular calcium concentrations, the decay of end-plate currents at any voltage is unaffected. Thus, because an approximately fourfold change in end-plate current magnitude failed to produce a significant change in the voltage sensitivity of end-plate current decay, the iontophoretic hypothesis can be rejected.

According to a possible alternative version of the iontophoretic hypothesis, the effect of membrane potential might be mediated through holding currents, that is, through the steady current required to hold the membrane potential at the specified level. Holding currents could act either directly by causing iontophoretic movement of acetylcholine, or indirectly by altering local ionic concentrations which might be supposed to exert effects on, for example, the binding of acetylcholine to its receptor. This hypothesis also can be rejected, however, because holding current magnitude was unrelated to value of the decay constant α. For example, the holding current required for a particular potential would in some instances change markedly during the experiment (from zero to several hundred nanoamps) as the resting potential decreased because of damage to the membrane, but the decay constant α at that potential would be unaffected.

The second possibility is that membrane potential affects the catalytic rate of acetylcholinesterase, and that this rate in turn determines the time course of cleft ACh concentration and hence conductance. According to this hypothesis, the voltage sensitivity of end-plate current decay depends on acetylcholinesterase activity; if the cholinesterase is poisoned with an anticholinesterase, the linkage between membrane potential and voltage sensitivity of α should be removed and thus voltage sensitivity should disappear. Anticholinesterases can indeed have a dramatic effect on the time course of end-plate currents in that these agents produce results that are rather like cooling the end plate: the rising phase of end-plate current is slowed and usually, but not always (see Kordas, 1972), the decaying phase is prolonged. However, both reversible (prostigmine methylsulfate) and irreversible (sarin) inhibitors of acetylcholinesterase activity in concentrations up to about .2 mM, a concentration about three orders of magnitude above that required to cause 50% inhibition of the esterase *in vitro* (Goodman and Gillman, 1970), have very little if any effect on the voltage sensitivity of α. That is, B in equation (1) is affected by these anticholinesterases, but A in that equation is nearly unchanged. Thus, although anticholinesterases do alter the kinetics of end-plate processes, their action seems not to be consistent with the hypothesis that the voltage sensitivity of α is mediated through effects of membrane field on the catalytic rate of acetylcholinesterase.

It appears, then, that end-plate currents are not simply a reflection of cleft ACh concentration. We now turn to investigation of the possibility that properties exhibited by end-plate currents can be explained in terms of postjunctional mechanisms.

Acetylcholine acts by binding to its receptor and causing, presumably through a conformational change of the receptor or some related molecule, an increase in end-plate conductance. This process seems analogous to the first steps in enzyme-substrate interactions, and, in the absence of direct evidence about receptor properties, it is most natural to be guided by the results of rapid kinetic analysis of enzymes (see Hammes, 1968; Gutfreund, 1971). The early steps in the catalytic sequence of many enzymes are rapid binding followed by a conformational change; by analogy then

$$nT + R \xrightarrow{\text{K}} T_nR \underset{\alpha}{\overset{\beta}{\rightleftharpoons}} T_nR^* \qquad (2)$$

where T represents the ACh molecule, R the receptor, $T \cdot R$ the transmitter receptor complex in its closed state, $T \cdot R^*$ the transmitter receptor complex in an open conformation, and n ACh's are required to produce the conformational change. Because binding is assumed to be rapid and the conformational change to be rate limiting, the binding step may be characterized by an equilibrium constant K and the conformational change by forward and backward rate constants β and α.

If we make the simplifying approximation that only a small percentage of the receptors are occupied at any time, so that the number of receptors available for binding is never very different from the total number of receptors N, then standard kinetic arguments yield the differential equation which describes the number H of transmitter-receptor complexes in their open conformation:

$$\frac{dH(t)}{dt} + \alpha(V)H(t) = \frac{\beta(V)N}{K} C^n(t)$$

$C(t)$ in this equation is the cleft ACh concentration. On the assumption that each channel has a closed conductance of zero and an open conductance of γ, an equation for end-plate conductance $g(t)$ may be obtained from the preceding equation by multiplying both sides of that equation by γ:

$$\frac{dg(t)}{dt} + \alpha(V)g(t) = \frac{\beta(V)N}{K} C^n(t) \tag{3}$$

It should be noted that we have supposed that channels are identical and do not interact with one another.

Equation (3), which provides a description of end-plate response to applied ACh, was obtained by exploiting the analogy between postjunctional processes and enzyme-substrate interaction. How the voltage dependence of α and β in these reactions can occur is seen from considering more carefully the postulated rate-limiting steps in equation (2). When a macromolecule changes its conformation, its dipole moment is also generally altered by either or both of two mechanisms. First, because a spatial redistribution of bond dipoles and more importantly of ionic charges occurs with isomerization, the resultant total molecular dipole moment may be changed. Second, ionization constants of functional groups may vary with conformational state, so the number (as opposed to the spatial distribution) of charges and thus the molecular dipole moment may be affected by a conformational change. Since the receptor is apparently an integral part of the postjunctional membrane, it presumably is subjected to an electric field associated with membrane potential, so that dipole moment changes arising from altered conformations will give rise to different energies. Thus, for example, a particular conformation might be more favored at some membrane potentials than at others because of a tendency of the molecule to take on the conformational state which aligned its dipole with the field and thus lowered the energy.

Our model for voltage dependence of end-plate current decay basically depends on understanding how α and β in equation (3) vary with membrane potential. According to rate theory these rate constants should be given by the equation (see Magleby and Stevens, 1972b)

$$\alpha(V) = \nu e^{-F(V)/kT}$$

where ν is an effective vibration frequency, k is Boltzmann's constant, T is the temperature ($^\circ$Kelvin), and $F(V)$ is the free energy difference between the molecule's present conformation and the transition state through which it passes to a new conformation. The free energy of a dipole in an electric field is proportional to the product of the field strength and the dipole moment magnitude, so that the free energy term in the equation above is simply

$$F(V) = F_0 - \frac{V}{M} \mu(V)$$

with F_0 the free energy barrier at zero membrane potential, $\mu(V)$ the membrane normal component of the difference in the gate molecule's dipole moment between the present conformation and the transition state, and M the effective membrane thickness; V/M is the effective (average) field strength.

In general, the dipole moment $\mu(V)$ in this last equation would itself depend on membrane potential because dipoles tend to align with the applied field by any movements consistent with their present conformation. For a large, relatively rigidly fixed receptor molecule, however, one might anticipate that such alignment would be minimal so that we can expect μ to be approximately constant over a relatively large range of membrane potentials. Finally, as exactly similar arguments to those above apply also for β in scheme (2), the rate constants α and β should be governed by the equations

$$\alpha(V) = \nu e^{-F_0/kT} \, e^{(\mu/MkT)V} \tag{4a}$$

$$\beta(V) = \nu' e^{-F_0'/kT} \, e^{(\mu'/MkT)V} \tag{4b}$$

Primed symbols here have the same physical significance as their unprimed counterparts, but may have different numerical values. With the obvious definition of the constants A, B, A', and B', these equations become

$$\alpha(V) = Be^{AV} \tag{5a}$$

$$\beta(V) = B'e^{A'V} \tag{5b}$$

Altogether then, equations (3) and (4) provide us with a description of the postjunctional membrane response to ACh. We now wish to investigate the extent to which this description is able to account for end-plate response properties.

According to the model just presented, the rise and fall of cleft ACh concentration is rapid and the closing of opened channels is somewhat slower; the decaying phase of end-plate currents therefore reflects the gating molecule conformational change. In order to describe the decay of end-plate currents, then, equation (3) is to be solved with $C(t) = 0$, and, according to this solution, the decay will be exponential, a prediction in accord with the observations presented earlier. Further, the decay constant α should itself depend exponentially on voltage as described by equation (5a). As was pointed out in the preceding discussion, this exponential dependence is precisely the relationship observed (see Fig. 2). Thus, our model is able to account for at least the decaying phase of end-plate currents.

Because we have given a physical interpretation to the constants in equations (3) and (4), a preliminary check on the plausibility of our model can be made by examining the extent to which the physical parameters in these equations are reasonable. The conformational change of our hypothetical gating molecule takes place with a rate constant of approximately 1 msec. Although the conformational changes exhibited by enzymes occur with a rather large variety of rates, many enzymes do seem to show a value close to the 1 msec we have observed (see Hammes, 1968; Gutfreund, 1971). If the dipole moment change associated with the hypothesized conformational change is calculated from equation (4a) and data such as those in Fig. 3, an average value of approximately 40 Debyes results. Since macromolecules typically have dipole moments an order of magnitude greater than this (McClellan, 1963), our calculated value therefore seems plausible.

Equations (3) and (5) should, if our analysis is correct, account for the entire time course of the end-plate conductance change. Because the cleft ACh concentration cannot be determined independently, this function must be estimated from end-plate currents by using equation (3); the average (from about 30 end-plate currents) cleft concentration function, up to an undetermined multiplicative constant, is shown in the lower part of Fig. 1. The values of β, again up to a multiplicative constant, have been determined for the same end plate and are plotted in Fig. 2. Finally, to demonstrate that equations (3) and (5) do account adequately for the entire end-plate

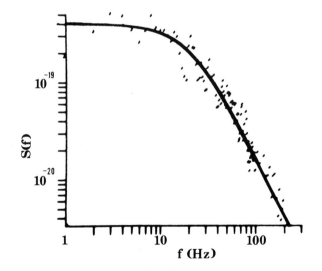

FIG. 3. Spectral density $S(f)$ of ACh-produced conductance fluctuations. Ordinate units are ohm^2 sec. The theoretical curve is drawn according to equation (6) with the parameters specified in the text. These data were obtained and analyzed by Dr. Charles Anderson.

conductance change, equations (3) and (5) have been solved with the cleft concentration $C(t)$ shown in the lower part of Fig. 1 and with the rate constants α and β given by the least-squares lines in Fig. 2. These solutions have been superimposed on the plots of measured end-plate conductance in Fig. 1A and B.

Our analysis to this point may be summarized as follows: models which assume that the rate-limiting step in production of end-plate currents is the relaxation of cleft ACh concentration seem not to be able to account for the observed data. On the other hand, a plausible model, derived by analogy from postjunctional processes to enzyme-substrate interactions, is able to account quantitatively for all of the observed properties of the end-plate conductance change. Our next task is to devise some further test of the model presented above.

Analysis of End-Plate Conductance Fluctuations

The most direct test of the mechanisms proposed here would be to observe the postulated conformational change in some independent way, for example, by light scattering or with fluorescent probes. Although this approach is certainly desirable and seems possible, it is not without its own difficulties. We decided therefore that the first step should be to test some other predictions made by the model. Katz and Miledi (1970, 1971, 1972) have discovered that relatively large fluctuations in current around the steady mean end-plate current occur in end plates subjected to a constant concentration of ACh. Because the physical picture we have presented should account for the character of these current fluctuations, we have examined ACh-produced conductance fluctuations in voltage-clamped end plates and have compared their properties to those predicted by the model described in the preceding section.

Although a detailed analysis is rather more complex, the basic mechanisms responsible for conductance fluctuations are apparent on consideration of the model, see scheme (2). With a constant cleft concentration of ACh, a certain fraction of the receptors will be in the completed form. The receptors with bound ACh are continually opening and closing in a probabilistic manner because the conformational change is an essentially probabilistic process. The mean number of open "gating" molecules is fixed, but the actual number open at any instant fluctuates somewhat around this mean value. The nature of these fluctuations should reflect the underlying molecular processes.

Fluctuations of the type we are discussing, conductance fluctuations in the present example, may be characterized by their *spectral densities*. The spectral density basically reflects the amplitude of each component frequency in the fluctuating conductance. More specifically, the spectral density is calculated by decomposing a specific record of conductance as a function of time into constituent sine and cosine components by Fourier analysis; the sum of the squared amplitudes of the sine and cosine waves of any frequency which result then gives the spectral density for that frequency. If the fluctuations are very rapid, large spectral densities will be present in the high-frequency range. On the other hand, if the fluctuations are very slow, only relatively large spectral densities will occur for low frequencies.

Analysis of the model presented earlier reveals that, for relatively small ACh concentrations, the spectral density should follow the equation (see Stevens, 1972):

$$S(f) = \frac{2\gamma\mu_g/\alpha}{1 + \left(\dfrac{2\pi f}{\alpha}\right)^2} \qquad (6)$$

Here $S(f)$ is the spectral density at frequency f, μ_g is the mean conductance, and γ is the conductance of one open channel, and α is the voltage-dependent, decay constant that appeared earlier, equation (5). The model we are discussing was developed for a situation in which the postsynaptic membrane was subjected to a rapid transient of cleft ACh concentration, whereas the predictions embodied in equation (6) apply to the case where ACh concentration is constant. In our experiments we have measured the spectral density of ACh-produced fluctuations in end-plate conductance and have examined the accuracy of equation (6) in accounting for them.

Figure 3 presents the spectral densities of conductance fluctuations for a voltage-clamped end plate at about 10°C (Anderson and Stevens, *unpublished observations*). The mean end-plate conductance in this instance was approximately 1.2 μmho, the membrane potential -100 mV. The smooth curve in the figure is the prediction of equation (6) with the parameters $\alpha = .12$ msec^{-1}, and $\gamma = 2 \times 10^{-11}$ mho^2. It is apparent that the shape of the spectrum is adequately specified by equation (6).

If our analysis is correct, the values of α estimated from spectra such as that in Fig. 3 should depend exponentially on voltage, and should agree with the values of α obtained from end-plate currents. In recent experiments Anderson and I have estimated α from spectral densities, from end-plate currents, and from miniature end-plate currents in the same preparation, and have found that all three estimates are in excellent agreement. The value for γ, the single channel conductance, is estimated to be 2 to 3 $\times 10^{-11}$ mho in these same experiments.

DISCUSSION

Equations (3), (5), and (6), derived from scheme (2), clearly provide an accurate description both of the end-plate conductance change produced by nerve stimulation and the conductance fluctuations which occur with constant ACh concentration. Insofar as the physical picture from which these equations were derived can be accepted, a molecular mechanism for post-junctional conductance changes has been provided, the voltage dependence of gating behavior in one system is accounted for, the conductance increase produced by the opening of a single channel has been measured, and estimates of the dipole moment change—or more correctly, its membrane normal component—associated with the opening and closing of the gating molecule have been made. At least, we have provided a formal description of postjunctional mechanisms, and, at most, we have provided a physical explanation of end-plate channel gating behavior.

Nevertheless, it must be emphasized that this physical picture, however plausible, has not yet been established because other mechanisms could lead to the same formal description. For example, we have assumed that ACh-receptor binding is rapid and that the rate-limiting step is a subsequent conformational change. The same equation can result, however, from the opposite assumption, namely that the conformational change is rapid and that binding is rate limiting and voltage dependent. Doubtless many other models could also be proposed which would yield, to satisfactory approximation, precisely the same equations we have developed. Our description, then, must remain hypothetical until some further and more direct test of the underlying assumptions, with optical measurements, for example, can be made. Our theory is specific and, in principle, testable, and we hope that properties of the frog neuromuscular junction will ultimately make the scheme presented here testable in practice.

REFERENCES

Eisenberg, R. S., Howell, J. N., and Vaughan, P. C. (1971): The maintenance of resting potentials in glycerol-treated muscle fibres. *J. Physiol.*, 215:95–102.

Goodman, L. S., and Gilman, A. (1970): *The Pharmacological Basis of Therapeutics*. Macmillan Company, New York.

Gutfreund, H. (1971): Transients and relaxation kinetics of enzyme reactions. *Ann. Rev. Biochem.*, 40:315–344.

Hammes, G. G. (1968): Relaxation spectrometry of biological systems. *Adv. Protein Chem.*, 23:1–58.

Katz, B., and Miledi, R. (1970): Membrane noise produced by acetylcholine. *Nature*, 226:962–963.

Katz, B., and Miledi, R. (1971): Further observations on acetylcholine noise. *Nature New Biol.*, 232:124–126.

Katz, B., and Miledi, R. (1972): The statistical nature of the acetylcholine potential and its molecular components. *J. Physiol.*, 224:665–700.

Keynes, R. D., Ritchie, J. M., and Rojas, E. (1971): The binding of tetrodotoxin to nerve membranes. *J. Physiol.*, 213:235–254.

Kordas, M. (1972): An attempt at an analysis of the factors determining the time course of the end-plate current. II. Temperature. *J. Physiol.*, 224:333–348.

Magleby, K. L., and Stevens, C. F. (1972a): The effect of voltage on the time course of end-plate currents. *J. Physiol.*, 223:151–171.

Magleby, K. L., and Stevens, C. F. (1972b): A quantitative description of end-plate currents. *J. Physiol.*, 223:173–197.

McClellan, A. L. (1963): *Tables of Experimental Dipole Moments*. W. H. Freeman, San Francisco.

Sevcik, C., and Narahashi, T. (1972): Electrical properties and excitation contraction coupling in skeletal muscle treated with ethylene glycol. *J. Gen. Physiol.*, 60:221–236.

Stevens, C. F. (1972): Inferences about membrane properties from electrical noise measurements. *Biophys. J.*, 12:1028–1047.

Synaptic Transmission and Neuronal Interaction
Raven Press, New York 1974

Morphology of Synaptic Vesicle Discharge and Reformation at the Frog Neuromuscular Junction

J. E. Heuser* and T. S. Reese

Laboratory of Neuropathology and Neuroanatomical Sciences, National Institute of Neurological Diseases and Stroke, National Institutes of Health, Bethesda, Maryland 20014

A study of the morphological changes in the frog neuromuscular junction that accompany repetitive nerve stimulation led us to propose that during quantal release of transmitter, synaptic vesicles are discharged and reformed in the manner illustrated in Fig. 1 (Heuser and Reese, 1973). The major steps in this sequence are:

1. Synaptic vesicle contents are discharged by exocytosis.
2. The membrane of discharged vesicles remains fused with the plasma membrane and moves to recovery sites located at a distance from discharge sites.
3. At recovery sites, surface membrane is returned to the inside of the terminal by endocytosis of coated vesicles.
4. Under conditions of rapid sustained stimulation, coated vesicles lose their coats and coalesce to form elongated compartments called cisternae.
5. New synaptic vesicles are subsequently re-formed by division of cisternae.

The evidence which suggested this particular sequence of synaptic vesicle discharge and reformation was purely morphological. It consisted of a quantitative evaluation of changes seen with the electron microscope in chemically fixed nerve terminals that had been stimulated for various periods at 10 Hz. Stimulation was performed *in vitro* at 10°C on isolated frog sartorius muscles attached to their sciatic nerves, which had been sectioned at their exit from the spinal column.

As stimulation progressed, a regular sequence of morphological changes occurred in the finger-like terminal branches of each motor axon (Figs. 2 and 3). After the first minute of stimulation, the terminals already appeared

---

* Current address: Department of Biophysics. University College, London, England.

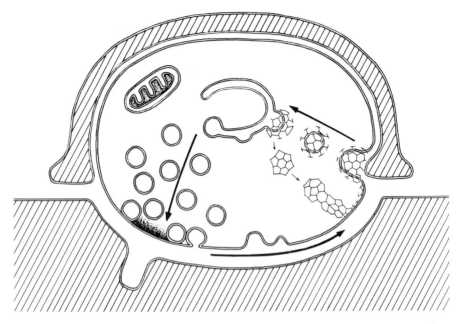

FIG. 1. Diagrammatic summary of a hypothesis for synaptic vesicle membrane recycling at the frog neuromuscular junction. (1) Synaptic vesicles discharge their content of transmitter as they coalesce with the plasma membrane at specific regions adjacent to the muscle. (2) Equal amounts of membrane are then retrieved when coated vesicles pinch off from regions of the plasma membrane adjacent to the Schwann sheath. (3) Finally, the coated vesicles lose their coats and coalesce to form cisternae which accumulate in regions of vesicle depletion and slowly divide to form new synaptic vesicles. (Figs. 1–14 are reprinted from The Journal of Cell Biology with permission of the Rockefeller University Press.)

to be slightly enlarged and depleted of synaptic vesicles. Planimetric measurements of representative micrographs revealed that brief stimulation had produced a 30% depletion of synaptic vesicles and that the loss of vesicle membrane had been nearly compensated by an increase in area of the plasma membrane (Fig. 8), suggesting that during stimulation some vesicle membrane had promptly coalesced with the plasma membrane. After 15 min of stimulation, the terminals appeared even more depleted of vesicles and more irregular in profile (Fig. 3). Measurements revealed that the additional stimulation had produced a further 30% depletion of vesicles, but no more increase in plasma membrane area than after brief stimulation. Nevertheless, the total amount of membrane composing the nerve terminal

$\longrightarrow$

FIG. 2. Longitudinal section of an unstimulated terminal. The terminal contains a large number of synaptic vesicles on the side facing the muscle (right); and neurofilaments, dense mitochondria, and axonal endoplasmic reticulum on the side facing the Schwann sheath (left). Presynaptic densities (arrow) occur opposite folds (f) in the muscle surface, and Schwann processes (s) periodically insinuate between the nerve and muscle. Osmium fixation. × 34,000.

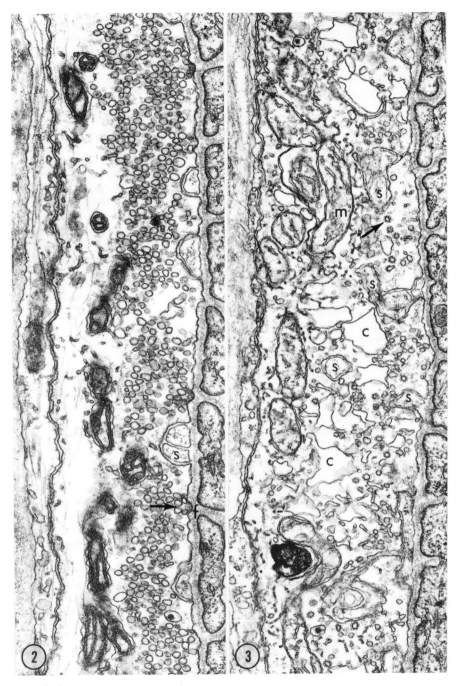

FIG. 3. Longitudinal section of a terminal stimulated for 15 min at 10°C. The terminal contains many cisternae (c) and coated vesicles (arrow) in place of the missing synaptic vesicles, appears less organized, and at several points is invaginated by Schwann processes (s). Coated vesicles and filamentous material occasionally forming discrete baskets are particularly prominent around the invaginating Schwann processes. Mitochondria (m) are swollen and pale. Osmium fixation. × 25,500.

remained constant because the further loss of vesicle membrane had been compensated by a large increase in the size and number of intracellular cisternae (Figs. 3 and 4), suggesting that during prolonged stimulation some vesicle membrane ultimately formed cisternae. Such vesicle membrane relocations did not represent irreversible damage to the terminals because, after 2 hr of rest, stimulated terminals returned to their original dimensions and vesicle content (Figs. 4–7).

Similar experiments were performed in the presence of the cytological tracer horseradish peroxidase (HRP), an enzyme with a molecular weight of 40,000 that was added to the muscle bath in a concentration of 0.25 mM. After different schedules of stimulation and rest, HRP could be localized by histochemical methods in the extracellular spaces around the nerve terminals and trapped in certain organelles within the terminals (Figs. 9–14). Since HRP is not known to cross membranes (Graham and Karnovsky, 1966) and did not appear to do so in any of these experiments, its appearance in a particular intracellular organelle indicated that, at some point during the experiment, this compartment had been open to the extracellular space or to some other HRP-containing or "labeled" compartment.

HRP permeated muscles rapidly to reach the nerve terminals, but little appeared in internal compartments until the terminals were stimulated. Upon stimulation, HRP first appeared in cisternae and coated vesicles (Figs. 9 and 10). HRP also appeared in a few ordinary synaptic vesicles, but it did not label a large percentage of them until stimulation was stopped and the terminals were allowed to reform their resting complement of vesicles (Figs. 11–13). Thereafter, labeled synaptic vesicles remained in the terminals for several hours, even after HRP was washed out of the extracellular space; they did not appear to become sequestered or digested. Only when washed terminals were stimulated a second time did labeled vesicles finally disappear. Since there was no indication that all these labeled vesicles moved up the axon or fused with the new, unlabeled cisternae which formed as a result of the second stimulation (Fig. 14), it seemed probable that they

---

$\longrightarrow$

FIG. 4. Cross section of a terminal stimulated for 15 min and fixed immediately. Cisternae, either vesicular (c) or flattened (arrow), replace a large proportion of the synaptic vesicles. Osmium fixation. × 26,250.

FIG. 5. Cross section of a terminal stimulated for 15 min and then rested for 30 min at 10°C. The rest has resulted in partial recovery of synaptic vesicle numbers and disappearance of cisternae. Some cisternae appear to be dividing into vesicles (arrow). Mitochondria remain swollen. Osmium fixation. × 26,250.

FIG. 6. Cross section of a terminal stimulated for 15 min and then rested for 60 min at 10°C. Synaptic vesicle numbers have nearly recovered and cisternae (arrow) have been reduced to short lengths. Mitochondria have returned to nearly normal size and density. Lateral invaginations of the plasma membrane containing Schwann fingers (s) are prominent during this period of recovery. Osmium fixation. × 26,250.

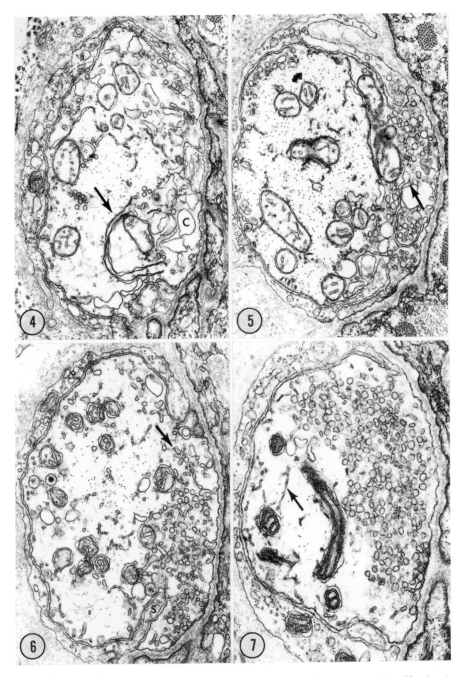

FIG. 7. Cross section of a terminal stimulated for 15 min and then rested for 60 min at room temperature to demonstrate the reversibility of the changes occurring during stimulation. Synaptic vesicles have been recovered, most of the cisternae have disappeared, and mitochondria have returned to normal size and density. Arrow indicates an element of the tubular endoplasmic reticulum, which can be distinguished from microtubules or cisternae. Osrnium fixation. × 30,625.

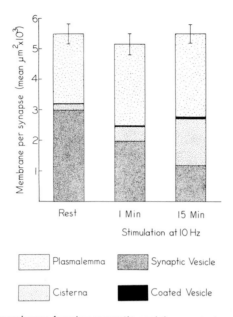

FIG. 8. Amounts of membrane forming synaptic vesicles, coated vesicles, cisternae, and plasmalemma in an average frog neuromuscular junction at rest, 1 min of stimulation, and 15 min of stimulation. The total amount of membrane forming an average end plate did not change appreciably during stimulation even though the relative amounts of membrane forming different components of the end plate changed dramatically. As discussed in the text, this suggests that synaptic vesicle membrane remained visible and simply became redistributed during stimulation. The values for average whole end plates were derived from planimetric measurements on individual sections and by multiplying these measurements by 9,090, the number of 55-nm sections in a 500-mm-long end plate. Ranges on tops of bars are standard errors of the total membrane area which was computed separately for each section of a terminal. Osmium fixation.

FIG. 9. Cross section of a terminal soaked in HRP for 30 min and stimulated for 1 min. The dense histochemical reaction product that indicates HRP location is present in the newly formed cisternae and the one coated vesicle lying along the lateral edge (arrow), but is not present in synaptic vesicles lying near the synaptic cleft. Inset is from terminal stimulated for 1 min and illustrates the coalescence of a coated vesicle with a cisterna in a terminal soaked in HRP. We presume that very little of the space inside these labeled compartments was actually occupied by HRP. With 0.25 mM HRP present outside, a coated vesicle would acquire only about 10 molecules of HRP as it formed; the dense histochemical reaction product, however, appears to fill the vesicle. × 38,250. Inset (c), 85,000.

FIG. 10. Cross section of a terminal soaked in HRP and stimulated for 2 min. Cisternae have become more numerous and all contain HRP. However, no synaptic vesicles near the cleft (right) contain HRP which is evidence that they do not carry it to cisternae. × 34,000.

FIG. 11. Cross section of a terminal soaked in HRP, stimulated in HRP for 15 min, and

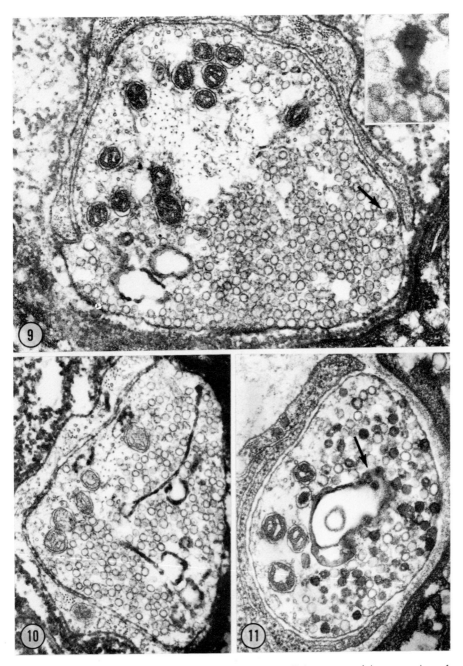

rested for 1 hr while HRP was washed from the extracellular spaces. A large number of synaptic vesicles containing HRP have appeared, presumably by division of labeled cisternae (arrow). Since this cisterna still contains HRP, it must not have been connected to the plasmalemma while the HRP was washed from the extracellular space. × 42,500.

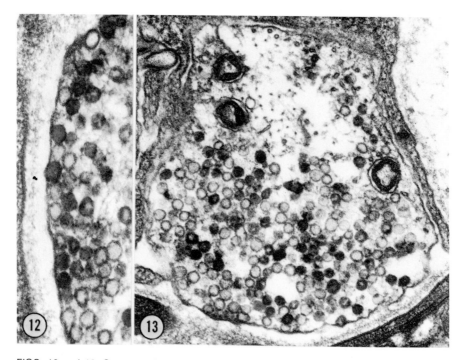

FIGS. 12 and 13. Cross sections through normal regions of terminals stimulated in HRP and then rested to produce labeled synaptic vesicles. Nearly 50% of the vesicles contain HRP, which corresponds to the number which should have been depleted by the stimulation and reformed from labeled cisternae. Figure 13 illustrates that the labeled vesicles appear to be distributed randomly within the nerve terminal, including the area near the presynaptic surface, which is shown in more detail in Fig. 12 to illustrate that labeled vesicles in contact with the plasma membrane do not discharge HRP, even though the tracer has been washed out of the synaptic cleft. Fig. 12, × 72,250. Fig. 13, × 28,050.

had discharged their HRP by exocytosis, but this was not actually visualized.

These, briefly, were the morphological data from the frog neuromuscular junction which suggested that synaptic vesicles were discharged and reformed in a particular manner that could be called "recycling" (Heuser, 1971). The vesicle-recycling hypothesis holds that reversible morphological changes during stimulation represented accumulations of membrane at slow points along a continuous path of synaptic vesicle membrane movement, and that HRP uptake during stimulation represented the sequential formation of particular intracellular membranous compartments along this path. The critical feature of this recycling hypothesis is that vesicle discharge and recovery are spatially separate, one-way interactions with the presynaptic plasma membrane.

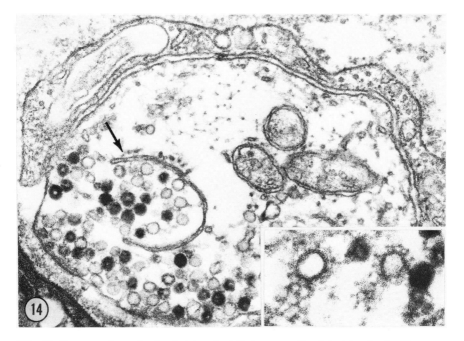

FIG. 14. Cross section of a loaded terminal that was restimulated for 1 min. The new cisterna (arrow) and coated vesicles (inset) formed as a result of the second stimulation do not contain HRP, indicating that they have formed from the surface and have accumulated tracer-free extracellular fluid, and have not formed by coalescence of labeled synaptic vesicles. × 59,500. Inset, × 127,500.

Step 1: Exocytosis

The plasma membrane expansion which occurred as synaptic vesicles became depleted suggests that during stimulation synaptic vesicles coalesced with the plasma membrane to such an extent that they lost their identity as synaptic vesicles. Presumably, synaptic vesicles break open onto the surface to discharge transmitter, or undergo exocytosis, and then completely flatten out. There was no indication that discharged vesicles remained as open flasks connected to the plasma membrane or pulled back directly from the surface, because HRP did not selectively label vesicles near the surface as it would if discharged vesicles were recovered by an immediate reversal of exocytosis. This experimental result did not rule out the possibility that after exocytosis the vesicles usually pull back directly from the surface without acquiring HRP and only occasionally flatten into the surface membrane to such an extent that they must be reformed by a separate process which traps HRP. However, if this were so, then the total number of exocytoses, estimated from the number of quanta discharged by stimulation, would be much larger than the number of vesicles that transiently disappear into the surface membrane and take up HRP as they reform. As well as we could determine, these numbers were not very different (Heuser and Reese, 1973). This correlation, although it rested on the assumption that each exocytosis produced one physiological quantum and would be invalid if, in fact, several vesicles undergo synchronous exocytoses to produce one quantum (M. Kreibel, *personal communication*), suggested that exocytosis of synaptic vesicles is an irreversible process that is accompanied by a physically separate process of vesicle reformation that can trap extracellular tracers.

Since surface membrane expanded promptly during the first minute of stimulation and did not increase further during longer stimulation, it appeared that the rate of exocytotic addition of vesicle membrane to the surface membrane exceeds the rate of vesicle recovery from the surface only during the first moments of stimulation. In part, these differences in rate could result from a brief delay between the time of arrival of vesicle membrane at the surface and its eventual recovery elsewhere. Unfortunately, since the surface membrane did not expand beyond 20% with longer stimulation, it probably would be difficult to detect such addition of vesicle membrane to the plasma membrane by biochemical analysis of fractionated synaptosomes (Hosei, 1965). Furthermore, since the surface membrane expansion was not accompanied by much swelling of the nerve terminals (at least was not accompanied by a significant change in the volume of 100 terminals fixed after 15 min of stimulation), it probably would be difficult to detect this morphological change in living nerve terminals viewed with the light microscope during stimulation.

Since the volume of stimulated terminals did not increase as their surface membrane expanded, it was natural to find that they became more convoluted or varicose (Fig. 3). Most stimulated terminals billowed out laterally between the muscle and the overlying Schwann cell until their plasma membrane reached the outer edge of the synaptic gutter (Fig. 5). Apposition between nerve and muscle was thus increased; but there is no reason to suspect that this increase altered synaptic "effectiveness;" probably the plasma membrane simply expanded along the plane of least resistance. Other stimulated terminals developed deep evaginations or invaginations which, in all cases, remained closely enveloped or filled by Schwann cell processes (Figs. 3, 5, 6). It remains to be determined whether Schwann cells passively expand and flatten to retain close contact with terminals as they change shape, or whether they actively sculpt the shape changes.

In contrast to such shape changes in terminals fixed immediately *after* stimulation, terminals fixed in hypertonic aldehydes *during* stimulation developed a different form of surface expansion which produced a severe distortion. This expansion consisted of repeated, large inward bulges of the surface membrane away from the underlying muscle or Schwann cell (Fig. 15). Similar bulges have only previously been reported after prolonged

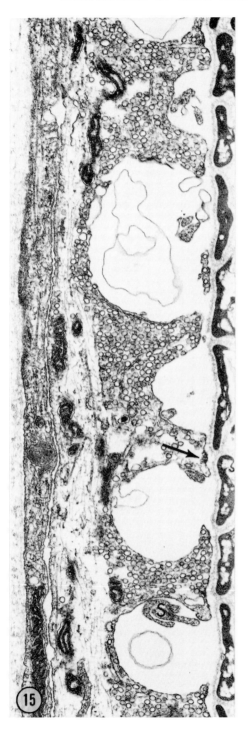

FIG. 15. Longitudinal section of a terminal placed in aldehyde fixative and then stimulated. Its plasma membrane facing the muscle (right) is expanded and bulges away from the adjacent muscle and Schwann processes (s) except at the presynaptic densities (arrow) located opposite the muscle folds. × 267,000.

stimulation with black widow spider venom (Clark et al., 1972), but in the present experiments they appeared whenever massive transmitter release was ongoing at the moment of hypertonic fixation. Inward bulges could usually be produced by placing muscles in fixative and then stimulating their nerve, in which case evoked transmitter release could be recorded with an intracellular microelectrode for nearly a minute. Inward bulges were also produced by soaking muscles in lanthanum or potassium ions, or black widow spider venom[1] for just a few minutes before fixation. Such bulges may simply represent an altered distribution of the usual surface membrane expansion that accompanies transmitter release, produced by osmotic shrinkage of the terminals at the moment of fixation. However, further planimetric measurements may reveal that the bulges are particularly localized, which could indicate that addition of vesicles to the surface continued while the plasma membrane became less fluid during fixation, or are particularly extensive, which could indicate that addition of vesicles to the plasma membrane continued after vesicle recovery was blocked by fixation.

In addition to these large shifts of synaptic vesicle membrane into the plasma membrane, stimulation appeared to reduce the number of vesicles that contact the plasma membrane adjacent to the presynaptic densities. This change was not apparent in previous studies of lanthanum-stimulated muscles fixed in osmium (Heuser and Miledi, 1971), where even the control terminals had few vesicles contacting a plasma membrane that was typically wrinkled (Fig. 18). However, these control terminals may not have been resting; they may have been agonally stimulated by the fixative itself. We have since noticed that osmium fixatives cause a transient muscle fasiculation which is blocked by curare and exacerbated by prostigmine, so osmium may directly stimulate transmitter release from these nerve terminals. In contrast, isotonic aldehyde fixatives do not cause fasiculation and, presumably, do not stimulate as much transmitter release, so they should be more suitable for determining the resting morphology of these terminals. In aldehyde-fixed resting terminals, the plasma membrane appeared quite smooth and many vesicles contacted the plasma membrane, including whole rows of vesicles on either side of the presynaptic dense bands (Fig. 16).

Such vesicle contacts occurred less frequently in OsO_4-fixed terminals (Fig. 17), unless they were first soaked long enough in isotonic magnesium to block transmitter release completely (Heuser et al., 1971). At the point of vesicle contact, the cytoplasmic leaflets of adjacent membranes were joined to form a single dense line that became even more dense when 20 mM calcium was added to the fixative, perhaps because this interface has an affinity for calcium.

There is no reason to suspect that such contact between a vesicle and the plasma membrane increases their combined permeability sufficiently to

---

[1] Spiders furnished by Dr. H. L. Stahnke, Arizona State University.

allow discharge of transmitter without actual coalescence or exocytosis. Neither HRP nor microperoxidase (mol. wt. 1800) entered vesicles that contacted the plasma membrane when muscles were soaked in these tracers, and HRP inside vesicles did not exit when they contacted the plasma membrane (Fig. 12). However, the contact could respresent a preliminary adherence of vesicle to surface membrane before actual coalescence; indeed, contacting vesicles in stimulated terminals fixed with aldehydes were less frequent and were largely replaced by wrinkles and depressions in the plasma membrane (Fig. 19) such as those found in most OsO_4-fixed terminals (Fig. 18). Where vesicles contact or adhere to the plasma membrane at rest seems in general to be where distortions and enlargements of the plasma membrane first appear during stimulation (Couteaux and Pecot-Dechavassine, 1970).

Vesicles contacting or adhering to the plasma membrane form a particular sub-population of synaptic vesicles, about 1% of the total number, that are in a particularly favorable position to be affected by changes in the plasma membrane. Thus, they could be the morphological counterpart of the hypothetical "immediately available" pool of transmitter, which physiological experiments suggest is the immediate source of transmitter released in response to plasma membrane changes (Elmqvist and Quastel, 1965). Fatigue or depression of transmitter release is generally interpreted to result from depletion of this immediately available pool of transmitter (del Castillo and Katz, 1954; Hubbard et al., 1969), and could be reflected in the rapid and severe reduction in number of vesicles that contact the plasma membrane which typically results from stimulation or from OsO_4 fixation. Recovery from depression is an exponential process with a Q_{10} of 1.7 (Takeuchi, 1958) which has been interpreted as repletion of the immediately available pool of transmitter by slow diffusion (Hubbard et al., 1969). This could be reflected in slow movement of vesicles up to contact the plasma membrane at vacated spots (Shea and Karnovsky, 1966). If so, variations in the size of the available pool might be expected to fall in a Poisson distribution since the few vesicles that adhere to the appropriate spots on the plasma membrane could be independently drawn from a large population of vesicles milling about in the terminals, and this might explain why evoked transmitter release at some synapses still appears to be a Poisson process even when a large fraction of the pool is released with each nerve impulse (Vere-Jones, 1966; Auerbach and Bennett, 1969).

Nevertheless, unless vesicles adhering to the plasma membrane can be demonstrated by means other than chemical fixation, such as freeze fracture (Pfenninger et al., 1971), and unless the number of adhering vesicles can be shown to vary in parallel with variations in the size of the evoked synaptic potential (Hubbard and Kwanbunbumpen, 1968), it would be premature to conclude that vesicles adhering to the plasma membrane represent a distinct, immediately available pool of transmitter.

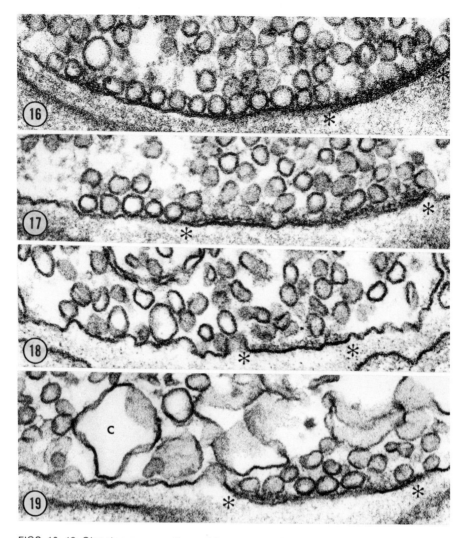

FIGS. 16–19. Glancing cross sections of the presynaptic dense bands (between asterisks), to show the association of synaptic vesicles with the plasma membrane in this region. Under all conditions the plasma membrane at the presynaptic density appears smooth. Figure 16 is an unstimulated terminal fixed in aldehydes; here a row of vesicles contacts the plasma membrane adjacent to the density, which may represent the resting condition. Figure 17 is an unstimulated terminal fixed in osmium; here, too, a short row of vesicles contacts the plasma membrane adjacent to the density. However, Fig. 18 is also an unstimulated terminal fixed in osmium, in which contacting vesicles are replaced by wrinkles in the plasma membrane, which may result from stimulation of transmitter release by the osmium fixative. Figure 19 is a terminal stimulated for 15 min and fixed in aldehydes, in which the vesicles contacting the plasma membrane are also replaced by pits or by overlying cisternae (c), except immediately over the presynaptic density where some vesicles typically remain. × 86,000.

Step 2: Endocytosis

Expansion of the plasma membrane during stimulation indicated that vesicle recovery from the surface initially lagged behind addition of vesicle membrane to the surface by exocytosis, but it did not indicate exactly how vesicle recovery eventually came about. Morphological signs of this process could be found in terminals fixed after brief intense stimulation, when vesicle recovery was presumably operating at a maximum rate. Such terminals contained more coated vesicles and cisternae than usual (Fig. 8). These new intracellular compartments apparently formed from the surface membrane because they trapped HRP when it was present outside the terminal (Figs. 9 and 10).

Synaptic vesicles near the surface of these terminals did not become selectively labeled with HRP (Fig. 10), so there was no indication that discharged vesicles could be recovered directly from the surface to form the new cisternae. Instead, coated vesicles appeared to provide the actual means of membrane recovery from the plasma membrane, since they were often found connected to it. Cisternae, in turn, appeared to form indirectly by coalescence of coated vesicles, since they were often connected to coated vesicles but never directly connected to the plasma membrane (Figs. 9, 10, 21). Some of the plasma membrane convolutions that persist after stimulation have been described as deep invaginations of the surface (Clark et al., 1972; Ceccarelli et al., 1973), which raises the possibility that they could pinch off to form cisternae directly, but these structures, in fact, represent deep folds of the surface membrane and invariably contain Schwann cell processes which would prevent them from pinching off.

The nature of the cytoplasmic material that forms the coat and the role it plays in endocytosis of vesicle membrane remain to be elucidated. It might transduce energy or transmit force needed to deform the plasma membrane and pinch off vesicles from it (Roth and Porter, 1964; Kanaseki and Kadota, 1969). Alternatively, it might maintain whatever chemical differences exist between the plasma membrane and vesicle membrane (Eichberg et al., 1964; Hosei, 1965), by selectively gathering components of the vesicle membrane and excluding components of the plasma membrane as it pinched off vesicles. Also, it might confer special protein-uptake capabilities upon endocytotic vesicles and allow the terminal to recover any soluble protein it might have lost during exocytosis (Bowers, 1964; Musick and Hubbard, 1972).

It also remains to be determined whether the coat is a discrete basket of fine cytoplasmic filaments which attaches to the plasma membrane, pinches off a vesicle, and then recycles itself to repeat that process (Heuser and Reese, 1973) or whether it is a local contraction in a more diffuse cytoplasmic network which attaches to certain regions of the plasma membrane (Gray, 1973) (Fig. 20). In any case, in the frog motor nerve terminals, some

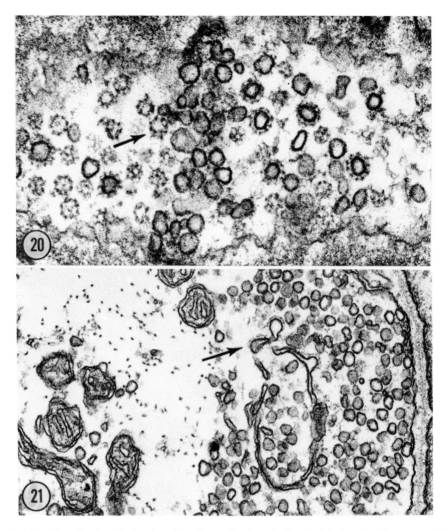

FIG. 20. Glancing longitudinal section through a terminal stimulated for 1 min. Adjacent to the presynaptic dense band and its overlying cluster of synaptic vesicles are several coated vesicles and many empty coats or baskets (arrow). If coats were this frequent along most of the surface, then each end plate would contain more than 10,000 free coats at rest, and they could retrieve membrane as fast as it was added to the surface during stimulation so long as each coat took no more than a minute to attach to the plasma membrane, pinch off a vesicle, and detach from the vesicle as it coalesced with a cisterna. Our count of nearly 10,000 coated vesicles in terminals stimulated for 15 min fits well with the estimated number of free coats, and may indicate that when membrane retrieval is active, coated vesicles can form faster than they can find cisternae to coalesce with. Osmium fixation. × 80,000.

FIG. 21. Terminal stimulated for 1 min. Synaptic vesicles are not obviously depleted, mitochondria are slightly expanded, and only one cisterna has formed. However, even at this early stage the cisterna lies far away from the plasma membrane and appears to have formed indirectly by the coalescence of coated vesicles (arrow). Osmium fixation. × 55,000. Inset, × 100,000.

sort of filamentous cytoplasmic structure seems to be needed to recover vesicle membrane from the surface, since synaptic vesicles do not appear to be recovered directly.

Usually, coated pits or coated invaginations of the plasma membrane were found around the periphery of the synaptic contacts, where Schwann cell processes girdled the terminal, whereas signs of vesicle exocytosis were found more centrally near the presynaptic density. Such spatial separation of the endocytotic from the exocytotic processes would require that synaptic vesicle membrane can slide or diffuse through the plasma membrane from the point where it joins the surface to where it is recovered. Such mobility seems feasible (Singer and Nicolson, 1972).

Step 3: Vesicle Reformation

In intensely stimulated nerve terminals, cisternae appeared to represent an intermediate step in the reformation of synaptic vesicles. They accumulated during rapid, prolonged stimulation and appeared to divide into synaptic vesicles during periods of rest (Fig. 4–7). Thus, they appeared to represent a temporary repository for vesicle membrane, like the Golgi apparatus in other secretory cells, which accumulated when the rate of endocytotic recovery of vesicle membrane from the surface exceeded the rate of reformation of new synaptic vesicles.

What limits the rate of vesicle reformation from cisternae is not known but it could be slowed and cisternae made to persist for several hours by extremely prolonged stimulation or by cooling to 4°C (Heuser and Miledi, 1971). One factor which could limit the rate of vesicle reformation from cisternae might be the acetylcholine content of the cisternae. If cisternae had to accumulate acetylcholine before they could divide, then stimulating cholinergic nerve terminals in hemicholinum-3 (HC3), which deprives them of choline for new transmitter synthesis, would produce unusually severe vesicle depletion and accumulation of cisternae. HC3 did not have this effect on frog motor nerve terminals (Heuser and Reese, 1973), although it is not yet certain that it completely arrested new transmitter synthesis at this synapse (Bevan and Heuser, *unpublished*). HC3 has been reported to exacerbate vesicle depletion at mammalian synapses where it is known to arrest transmitter synthesis (Jones and Kwanbunbumpen, 1970; Csillik and Bense, 1971), but other reports disagree and none has shown that cisternae accumulate in the presence of HC3 (Green, 1966; Pysh and Wiley, 1972).

Recognizable cisternae are not a necessary step in vesicle reformation, since they apparently do not form in frog motor nerve terminals stimulated at slow rates (Ceccarelli et al., 1973). However, it remains to be determined whether, under more physiological conditions, coated vesicles directly form mature synaptic vesicles, or whether they still briefly coalesce with each other or with small, fixed internal membrane compartments that represent persistent intermediates in vesicle reformation, like small Golgi apparatuses. In any case, the fact that cisternae appeared under conditions of intense stimulation illustrated that final vesicle reformation from the original endocytotic compartments is a potential slow step in vesicle recycling.

Contribution of the cell body to local recycling

The recycling hypothesis illustrates how local reformation of synaptic vesicles could help maintain a supply of vesicles in the nerve terminal at various rates of transmitter release, but it sheds no light on how synaptic vesicles are originally formed and supplied to the terminal. In particular, it remains to be determined how large a contribution synthesis or degradation of synaptic vesicles in the cell body makes to the total synaptic vesicle economy in the terminal. On the one hand, synapses which recover from depression sluggishly may recycle only a small proportion of their vesicles locally, and may depend upon a supply of new membrane from the axon. On the other hand, frog motor terminals which have been severed from their cell bodies promptly recover from depression, and in a few hours can release several times more quanta than the number of vesicles they contained to begin with (Heuser and Miledi, 1971; Ceccarelli et al., 1973). They appear to be able to reform each vesicle many times before replacing it with a new one. No information is available on how or where new membrane might be injected into the local cycle, but the fine tubular endoplasmic reticulum found in these terminals is an obvious source. Movement of membrane from the endoplasmic reticulum to some step in the local cycle would probably be unidirectional, because HRP never appears in this endoplasmic reticulum during vesicle recycling and tracer uptake (Heuser and Reese, 1973).

It is also likely that some of the coated vesicles and cisternae produced by stimulation may not reform synaptic vesicles but may instead form multivesicular bodies or other autoplagic organelles which move up the axon. The retrograde transport of HRP to the cell bodies of motor neurons could be a manifestation of such a process (Kristensson et al., 1971; La Vail and La Vail, 1972). The relative rates of anterograde transport of axonal endoplasmic reticulum or other membranes needed by the terminal to form new vesicles and retrograde transport of old vesicle membrane could control the total stock of synaptic vesicles in the nerve terminal.

REFERENCES

Auerbach, A. A., and Bennett, M. V. L. (1969): Chemically mediated transmission at a giant fiber synapse in the central nervous system of a vertebrate. *J. Gen. Physiol.*, 53:183–210.
Bowers, B. (1964): Coated vesicles in the pericardial cells of the aphid. *Protoplasma*, 59:351–367.

Ceccarelli, B., Hurlbut, W. P., and Mauro, A. (1973): Turnover of transmitter and synaptic vesicles at the frog neuromuscular junction. *J. Cell Biol.*, 57:499–524.

Clark, A. W., Hurlbut, W. P., and Mauro, A. (1972): Changes in the fine structure of the neuromuscular junction of the frog caused by black widow spider venom. *J. Cell Biol.*, 52:1–14.

Couteaux, R., and Pecot-Dechavassine, M. (1970): Vesicules synaptiques et poches au niveau des "zones actives" de la jonction neuromusculaire. *Comptes Rendus Acad. Sci. (Paris)* D, 271:2346–2349.

Csillik, B., and Bense, S. (1971): Function-dependent alterations in the distribution of synaptic vesicles. *Acta. Biol. Acad. Sci. Hung.*, 22:131–139.

del Castillo, J., and Katz, B. (1954): Statistical factors involved in neuromuscular facilitation and depression. *J. Physiol.*, 124:574–585.

Eichberg, J., Whittaker, V. P., and Dawson, R. M. C. (1964): Distribution of lipids in subcellular particles of guinea pig brain. *Biochem. J.*, 92:91–100.

Elmqvist, D., and Quastel, D. M. J. (1965): A quantitative study of end-plate potentials in isolated human muscle. *J. Physiol.*, 178:505–529.

Graham, R. C., and Karnovsky, M. J. (1966): The early stages of absorption of injected horseradish peroxidase in the proximal tubule of the mouse kidney; ultrastructural cytochemistry by a new technique. *J. Histochem. Cytochem.*, 14:291–302.

Gray, E. G. (1973): Are the coats of coated vesicles artifacts? *J. Neurocytol.*, 1:363–382.

Green, K. (1966): Electron microscopic observations on the relationship between synthesis of synaptic vesicles and acetylcholine. *Anat. Rec.*, 154:351.

Heuser, J. E. (1971): Evidence for recycling of membrane accompanying transmitter release at the frog neuromuscular junction. First Annual Meeting, Society for Neuroscience, p. 112.

Heuser, J. E., Katz, B., and Miledi, R. (1971): Structural and functional changes of frog neuromuscular junctions in high calcium solutions. *Proc. Roy. Soc. London B*, 178:407–415.

Heuser, J. E., and Miledi, R. (1971): Effect of lanthanum ions on function and structure of frog neuromuscular junctions. *Proc. Roy. Soc. London B*, 179:247–260.

Heuser, J. E., and Reese, T. S. (1973): Evidence for recycling of synaptic vesicles membrane during transmitter release at the frog neuromuscular junction. *J. Cell Biol.*, 57:315–344.

Hosei, R. J. A. (1965): The localization of adenosine triphosphatases in morphologically characterized subcellular fractions of guinea-pig brain. *Biochem. J.*, 96:404–412.

Hubbard, J. I., and Kwanbunbumpen, S. (1968): Evidence for the vesicle hypothesis. *J. Physiol.*, 194:407–420.

Hubbard, J. I., Llinas, R., and Quastel, D. M. J. (1969): *Electrophysiological Analysis of Synaptic Transmission*. Edward Arnold, London.

Jones, S. F., and Kwanbunbumpen, S. (1970): The effects of nerve stimulation and hemicholinium on synaptic vesicles at the mammalian neuromuscular junction. *J. Physiol.*, 207:31–50.

Kanaseki, T., and Kadota, K. (1969): The "vesicle in a basket." *J. Cell Biol.*, 42:202–220.

Kristensson, K., Olsson, Y., and Sjostrand, J. (1971): Axonal uptake and retrograde transport of exogenous proteins in the hypoglossal nerve. *Brain Res.*, 32:399–406.

La Vail, J. H., and La Vail, M. M. (1972): Retrograde axonal transport in the central nervous system. *Science*, 176:1416–1417.

Musick, J., and Hubbard, J. I. (1972): Release of protein from mouse motor nerve terminals. *Nature*, 237:279–281.

Pfenninger, M., Albert, K., Moor, H., and Sandri, C. (1971): Freeze-fracturing of presynaptic membranes in the central nervous system. *Phil. Trans. Roy. Soc. Lond. B*, 261:387–389.

Pysh, J. J., and Wiley, R. G. (1972): Morphologic alterations of synapses in electrically stimulated superior cervical ganglia of the cat. *Science*, 176:191–193.

Roth, T. F., and Porter, K. R. (1964): Yolk protein uptake in the oocyte of the mosquito *Aedes aegypti* L. *J. Cell Biol.*, 20:313–332.

Shea, S. M., and Karnovsky, M. J. (1966): Brownian motion; a theoretical explanation for the movement of vesicles across the endothelium. *Nature*, 212:353–355.

Singer, S. T., and Nicolson, G. L. (1972): The fluid mosaic model of the structure of cell membranes. *Science*, 175:720–725.

Takeuchi, A. (1958): The long lasting depression in neuromuscular transmission of frog. *Jap. J. Physiol.*, 8:103–113.

Vere-Jones, D. (1966): Simple stochastic models for the release of quanta of transmitter from a nerve terminal. *Aust. J. Statist.*, 8:53–63.

Synaptic Transmission and Neuronal Interaction
Raven Press, New York 1974

Factors in Efficacy of Central Synapses

Motoy Kuno

*Department of Physiology, University of North Carolina School of Medicine, Chapel Hill,
North Carolina 27514*

This chapter is concerned with analysis of the factors which may be responsible for determination of synaptic efficacy in the mammalian central nervous system. One of the major obstacles to the analysis of central synaptic action is the complexity of neuronal interconnections. Each mammalian central neuron may receive about 10,000 synaptic contacts, and these synapses are formed by presynaptic fibers arising from different sources. Under these conditions, it is practically impossible to study central synaptic action at the level of individual synapses unless the neuron network is untangled. For this purpose, our experiments were designed mainly for spinal motoneurons of the cat, which are large enough to permit intracellular recording and receive direct synaptic connections from primary sensory fibers arising in the muscle. The advantage of this preparation is that the sensory input to motoneurons can be dissected into single fibers for stimulation, so that the synaptic mechanism can be analyzed in a single motoneuron in response to an impulse in a single sensory fiber. The situation is then almost analogous to the neuromuscular junction in which the end plate on each muscle fiber is formed by a single motor nerve fiber.

I. DEFINITION OF SYNAPTIC EFFICACY

Group Ia afferent fibers arising from a muscle make monosynaptic connections to the motoneurons which innervate the muscle or its synergists (Lloyd, 1943). Therefore, when intracellular potentials are recorded from a motoneuron, stimulation of appropriate muscle nerves produces excitatory postsynaptic potentials (EPSP's) with a monosynaptic latency (Brock, Coombs, and Eccles, 1952). The amplitude of EPSP's so produced increases as the intensity of sensory stimulation is increased, and when the EPSP amplitude reaches the threshold for excitation, the motoneuron initiates an action potential. It is obvious that the efficacy of synaptic excitation is determined by the EPSP amplitude and the threshold level of the postsynaptic neuron. The EPSP amplitude depends entirely on the intensity of the input as well as on the postsynaptic responsiveness to the input, and this is the definition of synaptic efficacy to be described in this chapter. It should be noted that synaptic efficacy thus defined is not identical with the efficacy of impulse transmission across the synapse. The former reflects the efficiency of the processes involved only in synaptic action, whereas the latter includes an additional factor which depends on excitability of the post-synaptic neuron. Therefore, it is possible that the efficacy of synaptic excitation may increase even with the reduced synaptic efficacy under certain conditions. For example, chronic axotomy results in a significant decrease of the amplitude of monosynaptic EPSP's in the motoneuron (Eccles, Libet, and Young, 1958; McIntyre, Bradley, and Brock, 1959; Shapovalov and Grantyn, 1968; Kuno and Llinás, 1970b). However, the axotomized motoneurons show an increase in the efficacy of the synaptic excitation (Downman, Eccles, and McIntyre, 1953; McIntyre et al., 1959) presumably because of the generation of "dendritic spikes" at the lowered threshold level (Kuno and Llinás, 1970a).

II. PARAMETERS FOR THE EPSP AMPLITUDE

As mentioned above, the amplitude of monosynaptic EPSP's is proportional to the number of Group Ia afferent fibers stimulated. Therefore, at first approximation, the EPSP amplitude (E) may be described by

$$E = F \cdot \overline{E}_1 \tag{1}$$

where $\overline{E}_1$ is the mean amplitude of EPSP's evoked by impulses in a single afferent fiber, and F is the number of Group Ia fibers activated by a given stimulus intensity. It is known that each Group Ia fiber arising from a muscle makes monosynaptic connections with almost all (100%) of the motoneurons that innervate the muscle (Mendell and Henneman, 1971). On the other hand, the ratio of synaptic connections from one Group Ia fiber is approximately 50% for the motoneurons which innervate the synergists (Mendell and Henneman, 1971; also, Kuno and Miyahara, 1969b; Jack, Miller, Porter, and Redman, 1970). Therefore, the actual input to a given motoneuron depends on the convergence ratio of the sensory nerve under test as well as on the number of sensory fibers stimulated. Thus, the relationship (1) may be corrected by

$$E = a \cdot F \cdot \overline{E}_1 \tag{2}$$

where a is convergence ratio which may be given by the number of Group Ia fibers converging on to the motoneuron under study relative to the total number of Group Ia fibers in the muscle nerve stimulated. It has been shown (Eccles, Eccles, and Lundberg, 1957) that an afferent volley from a muscle produces larger monosynaptic EPSP's in the motoneuron which innervates the muscle (homonymous) than in motoneurons subserving the synergists (heteronymous). The difference in synaptic efficacy between homonymous and heteronymous pathways may be accounted for by the difference in the convergence ratio (Kuno and Miyahara, 1969*b*).

Monosynaptic EPSP's evoked in motoneurons by stimulation of a single afferent fiber show a random fluctuation in amplitude with occasional failures of synaptic response (Katz and Miledi, 1963; Kuno, 1964*a;* Burke, 1967*a*). This behavior is essentially identical with that observed at the neuromuscular junction depressed by high Mg and/or low Ca (del Castillo and Katz, 1954). Information has recently accumulated which indicates that transmitter release at central synapses occurs in quantal steps (Kuno, 1971) as is the case at the neuromuscular junction (del Castillo and Katz, 1954). It may be assumed that the transmitter is stored in the presynaptic terminals in the form of a great number of quanta and that each quantum is released with a small probability in response to a presynaptic impulse. Therefore, the amount of transmitter released by a presynaptic impulse can be quantified in terms of the mean number of quanta liberated by the impulse *(m)*. The release of each quantum generates a unit EPSP *(v₁)* of a certain amplitude. Thus, the mean amplitude of EPSP's evoked by impulses in a single afferent fiber $(\overline{E}_1)$ may be described by the product of m and v_1. The relationship (2) is then given by

$$E = a \cdot F \cdot m \cdot v_1 \qquad (3)$$

The two parameters (m and v_1) included in this relationship are the factors which determine the efficacy at individual synapses.

III. UNIT EPSP's (v_1)

The mean amplitude of unit EPSP's measured in motoneurons varies from about 0.1 mV (Kuno, 1964*a*) to 0.7 mV (Burke, 1967*a*). If the size of individual quanta of transmitter is identical, the release of each quantum should be associated with a constant change of leakage conductance in the postsynaptic membrane. The resultant synaptic current (I_1) then flows across the input resistance (R) of the postsynaptic membrane at the recording site to generate the unit EPSP (v_1). In agreement with the results obtained from the neuromuscular junction (Katz and Thesleff, 1957), the average amplitude of unit EPSP's has been found to be linearly related to the input resistance of motoneurons (Kuno and Miyahara, 1969*b*). This implies that the synaptic current produced by the release of each quantum of transmitter is approximately constant. Therefore, there is no need to postulate that the size of individual quanta is different from one synapse to another on motoneurons. The parameter, v_1, in relationship (3) is then described in terms of I_1 and $R;$ thus

$$E = a \cdot F \cdot m \cdot I_1 \cdot R \qquad (4)$$

The implication of this relationship is that synaptic efficacy depends in part on the input resistance of central neurons. The input resistance of motoneurons is inversely related to the axonal conduction velocity (Kernell, 1966; Burke, 1967*b*). The higher synaptic efficacy in slowly conducting motoneurons than in fast conducting motoneurons (Denny-Brown, 1929; Granit, Henatsch, and Steg, 1956; Kuno, 1959; Henneman, Somjen, and Carpenter, 1965) may be attributed to the large amplitude of unit EPSP's as a result of the high input resistance.

It has recently been noted that the unit EPSP amplitude is significantly smaller in axotomized motoneurons than in normal motoneurons (Kuno and Llinás, 1970*b*). This change was not associated with any appreciable alteration in the input resistance (Eccles et al., 1958; Kuno and Llinás, 1970*a*). In axotomized motoneurons the presynaptic terminals located on the cell body are displaced from the postsynaptic membrane by glial invasion into the synaptic cleft (Blinzinger and Kreutzberg, 1968; Hamberger, Hansson, and Sjostrand, 1970). A decrease in the unit EPSP amplitude of axotomized motoneurons was therefore suggested to be due to the restriction of synaptic location to remote dendrites (Kuno and Llinás, 1970*b*). Under these conditions, the EPSP evoked at the synaptic site would be subjected to electrotonic attenuation during the passive spread to the recording site (Rall, 1960). Theoretically, there is little doubt that the degree of electrotonic attenuation increases with an increase in the distance between the synaptic site and the cell body where the recording electrode is presumably located (Rall, 1960, 1962, 1967). However, the input resistance of motoneuron dendrites would increase with distance from the cell body as the dendrites taper. Therefore, the unit EPSP's at the dendritic synaptic sites may be considerably greater than those evoked at the cell body (Kuno and Miyahara, 1969*a*). At present, it seems difficult to quantify the degree of attenuation of the unit EPSP amplitude in relation to the synaptic site (Kuno, 1971).

IV. MEAN QUANTUM CONTENT *(m)*

The mean number of quanta of transmitter released by a single Group Ia impulse *(m)* at different motoneuron synapses varies from less than one to approximately 15 with the average between two and three (Kuno and Miyahara, 1969*a*). The mean quantum content *(m)* seems to be the only factor which is responsible for alterations of synaptic efficacy produced by various conditioning stimuli. It has been shown that facilitation and depression of monosynaptic EPSP's during repetitive stimulation of the presynaptic fiber are associated with an increase and a decrease in the mean quantum content (Kuno, 1964*b*). Similarly, potentiation of EPSP's following tetanic stimulation of a presynaptic fiber (posttetanic potentiation) is accompanied by an increase in *m* (Kuno, 1964*b*), and the conditioning volleys which lead to presynaptic inhibition decrease the mean quantum content (Kuno, 1964*b*). In addition, it has also been reported that the decrease of EPSP amplitude observed after the application of barbiturates is due to a reduction in the mean quantum content (Weakly, 1969). The quantal nature of transmitter release has recently been demonstrated for the synapses on motoneurons formed by excitatory (Kuno and Weakly, 1972*a*) and inhibitory (Kuno and Weakly, 1972*b*) interneurons. Facilitation of excitatory and inhibitory synaptic potentials evoked by internuncial impulses has also been attributed to an increase in the mean quantum content (Kuno and Weakly, 1972*a,b*). The mean quantum content is entirely determined by the presynaptic properties (Katz, 1962). Therefore, any alteration in the mean quantum content indicates that the alteration results from the changes confined to the presynaptic level.

At the neuromuscular junction, the mean quantum content has been shown to be positively correlated with the size of motor nerve terminals (Kuno, Turkanis, and Weakly, 1971). A question that may be posed is whether a similar relationship exists at central synapses. Suggestive evidence for this notion may be provided by the high-quantum content of monosynaptic EPSP's observed in Clarke's column neurons (Kuno and Miyahara, 1968; Eide, Fedina, Jansen, Lundberg, and Vyklický, 1969), which coincides with the presence of "giant" synaptic terminals on these neurons (Szentágothai and Albert, 1955). However, a sensory fiber often terminates on each Clarke's column neuron with multiple synaptic contacts in the form of *boutons de passage* (Szentágothai and Albert, 1955; Réthelyi, 1970). A question may then arise as to whether the high *m* value observed in Clarke's column neurons is due to the large number of multiple synaptic contacts arising from a single presynaptic fiber rather than the large size of individual terminals (Réthelyi, 1970). The giant terminals on Clarke's column neurons are located on or very close to the cell body (Szentágothai and Albert, 1955; Kuno, Muñoz-Martinez, and Randić, 1973). If the giant synapses are responsible for the generation of large EPSP's, one may expect that the EPSP amplitude is sensitive to polarizing currents applied through the cell body and that the large EPSP's are shorter in time-to-peak and decay time than small EPSP's. In contrast, the large EPSP showed no detectable increase in amplitude during postsynaptic hyperpolarization, and the large and small EPSP's were comparable in time-to-peak (Kuno et al., 1973). Thus, there has been no evidence that the generation of large EPSP's in Clarke's column neurons is directly related to the presence of "giant" terminals observed on the cell body. In addition, the large EPSP's showed a longer time-to-peak than small EPSP's. It may be suggested that the large EPSP's are associated with a longer duration of transmitter action and that the prolonged transmitter action results from conduction time of an afferent impulse along the terminal axon which makes multiple contacts on a Clarke's column neuron (Kuno et al., 1973). It is likely that the high-quantum content observed in Clarke's column neurons is largely due to the large number of multiple synaptic contacts formed by a single sensory fiber. However, it should be noted that a large number of small terminals arising from one fiber is essentially the same in effect as a single large terminal. Therefore, the conclusion deduced from the observations on Clarke's column does not conflict with that obtained from the neuromuscular junction.

ACKNOWLEDGMENT

Assistance in preparation of this report was provided by research grant NS 10319 from the U.S. Public Health Service.

REFERENCES

Blinzinger, K., and Kreutzberg, G. (1968): Displacement of synaptic terminals from regenerating motoneurons by microglial cells. *Z. Zellforsch. Mikroskop. Anat.*, 85:145–157.

Brock, L. G., Coombs, J. S., and Eccles, J. C. (1952): The recording of potentials from motoneurones with an intracellular electrode. *J. Physiol.*, 117:431–460.

Burke, R. E. (1967a): Composite nature of the monosynaptic excitatory postsynaptic potential. *J. Neurophysiol.*, 30:1114–1137.

Burke, R. E. (1967b): Motor unit types of cat triceps surae muscle. *J. Physiol.*, 193:141–160.

del Castillo, J., and Katz, B. (1954): Quantal components of the end-plate potential. *J. Physiol.*, 124:560–573.

Denny-Brown, D. (1929): On the nature of postural reflexes. *Proc. Roy. Soc. B*, 104:252–301.

Downman, C. B. B., Eccles, J. C., and McIntyre, A. K. (1953): Functional changes in chromatolysed motoneurones. *J. Comp. Neurol.*, 98:9–36.

Eccles, J. C., Eccles, R. M., and Lundberg, A. (1957): The convergence of monosynaptic excitatory afference on to many different species of alpha motoneurones. *J. Physiol.*, 137:22–50.

Eccles, J. C., Libet, B., and Young, R. R. (1958): The behaviour of chromatolysed motoneurones studied by intracellular recording. *J. Physiol.*, 143:11–40.

Eide, E., Fedina, L., Jansen, J., Lundberg, A., and Vyklický, L. (1969): Unitary components in the activation of Clarke's column neurons. *Acta Physiol. Scand.*, 77:145–158.

Granit, R., Henatsch, H.-D., and Steg, G. (1956): Tonic and phasic ventral horn cells differentiated by post-tetanic potentiation in cat extensors. *Acta Physiol. Scand.*, 37:114–126.

Hamberger, A., Hansson, H., and Sjostrand, J. (1970): Surface structure of isolated neurons. Detachment of nerve terminals during axon regeneration. *J. Cell Biol.*, 47:319–331.

Henneman, E., Somjen, G., and Carpenter, D. O. (1965): Functional significance of cell size in spinal motoneurons. *J. Neurophysiol.*, 28:560–580.

Jack, J. J. B., Miller, S., Porter, R., and Redman, S. J. (1970): The distribution of group Ia synapses on lumbosacral spinal motoneurones in the cat. In: *Excitatory Synaptic Mechanisms*, edited by P. Andersen and J. K. S. Jansen, pp. 199–205. Universitetsforlaget, Oslo.

Katz, B. (1962): The transmission of impulses from nerve to muscle and the subcellular unit synaptic action. *Proc. Roy. Soc. B*, 155:455–477.

Katz, B., and Miledi, R. (1963): A study of spontaneous miniature potentials in spinal motoneurones. *J. Physiol.*, 168:389–422.

Katz, B., and Thesleff, S. (1957): On the factors which determine the amplitude of the "miniature end-plate potential." *J. Physiol.*, 137:267–278.

Kernell, D. (1966). Input resistance, electrical excitability and size of ventral horn cells in cat spinal cord. *Science*, 152:1637–1639.

Kuno, M. (1959): Excitability following antidromic activation in spinal motoneurones supplying red muscles. *J. Physiol.*, 149:374–393.

Kuno, M. (1964a): Quantal components of excitatory synaptic potentials in spinal motoneurones. *J. Physiol.*, 175:81–99.

Kuno, M. (1964b): Mechanism of facilitation and depression of the excitatory synaptic potential in spinal motoneurones. *J. Physiol.,* 175:100–112.

Kuno, M. (1971): Quantum aspects of central and ganglionic synaptic transmission in vertebrates. *Physiol. Rev.,* 51:647–678.

Kuno, M., and Llinás, R. (1970a): Enhancement of synaptic transmission by dendritic potentials in chromatolysed motoneurones of the cat. *J. Physiol.,* 210:807–821.

Kuno, M., and Llinás, R. (1970b): Alterations of synaptic action in chromatolysed motoneurones of the cat. *J. Physiol.,* 210:823–838.

Kuno, M., and Miyahara, J. T. (1968): Factors responsible for multiple discharge of neurons in Clarke's column. *J. Neurophysiol.,* 31:624–638.

Kuno, M., and Miyahara, J. T. (1969a): Non-linear summation of unit synaptic potentials in spinal motoneurones of the cat. *J. Physiol.,* 201:465–477.

Kuno, M., and Miyahara, J. T. (1969b): Analysis of synaptic efficacy in spinal motoneurones from "quantum" aspects. *J. Physiol.,* 201:479–493.

Kuno, M., Muñoz-Martinez, E. J., and Randić, M. (1973): Synaptic action on Clarke's column neurones in relation to afferent terminal size. *J. Physiol.,* 228:343–360.

Kuno, M., Turkanis, S. A., and Weakly, J. N. (1971): Correlation between nerve terminal size and transmitter release at the neuromuscular junction of the frog. *J. Physiol.,* 213:545–556.

Kuno, M., and Weakly, J. M. (1972a): Facilitation of monosynaptic excitatory synaptic potentials in spinal motoneurones evoked by internuncial impulses. *J. Physiol.,* 224:271–286.

Kuno, M., and Weakly, J. N. (1972b): Quantal components of the inhibitory synaptic potential in spinal motoneurones of the cat. *J. Physiol.,* 224:287–303.

Lloyd, D. P. C. (1943): Neuron patterns controlling transmission of ipsilateral hindlimb reflexes in cats. *J. Neurophysiol.,* 6:293–314.

McIntyre, A. K., Bradley, K., and Brock, L. G. (1959): Responses of motoneurons undergoing chromatolysis. *J. Gen. Physiol.,* 42:931–958.

Mendell, L. M., and Henneman, E. (1971): Terminals of single Ia fibers; location, density, and distribution within a pool of 300 homonymous motoneurons. *J. Neurophysiol.,* 34:171–187.

Rall, W. (1960). Membrane potential transients and membrane time constant of motoneurons. *Exptl. Neurol.,* 2:503–532.

Rall, W. (1962). Electrophysiology of a dendritic neuron model. *Biophys. J.,* 2:146–167.

Rall, W. (1967): Distinguishing theoretical synaptic potentials computed for different soma-dendritic distributions of synaptic input. *J. Neurophysiol.,* 30:1138–1168.

Réthelyi, M. (1970): Ultrastructural synaptology of Clarke's column. *Exptl. Brain Res.,* 11:159–174.

Shapovalov, A. I., and Grantyn, A. A. (1968): Suprasegmental synaptic influences on chromatolyzed motoneurons. *Biofisika,* 13:260–269.

Szentágothai, J., and Albert, A. (1955): The synaptology of Clarke's column. *Acta Morphol. Sci. Hung.,* 5:43–51.

Weakly, J. N. (1969): Effect of barbiturates on "quantal" synaptic transmission in spinal motoneurones. *J. Physiol.,* 204:63–77.

Synaptic Transmission and Neuronal Interaction
Raven Press, New York 1974

Synaptic Arrangements in the Vertebrate Retina: The Photoreceptor Synapse

John E. Dowling

The Biological Laboratories, Harvard University, Cambridge, Massachusetts 02138

The vertebrate retina is an accessible part of the central nervous system that is particularly advantageous for the study of neuronal interactions. It is made up of just five types of neurons whose cell perikarya are arranged in three nuclear layers. Virtually all the synapses in the retina are confined to two synaptic (plexiform) zones, and in each plexiform layer the processes of three cell types interact.

Recent studies, employing mainly electron microscopy and intracellular recording, have focused on identifying synaptic contacts, tracing neural pathways, and describing electrical activity of the various retinal cells (Missotten, 1965; Dowling and Boycott, 1966; Dowling, 1968; Werblin and Dowling, 1969; Kaneko, 1970). From such studies it is now possible to postulate a simplified scheme for the synaptic organization of the vertebrate retina (Fig. 1) (Dowling, 1970; Dowling and Werblin, 1971). A detailed description of this scheme is given in the legend to Fig. 1. It is important to note, however, that several rather unconventional features have been brought out by these studies on retinal structure and function (only some of which are illustrated in the figure). For example, distal retina neurons (receptor, bipolar, and horizontal cells) respond to light with sustained, graded, mostly hyperpolarizing potentials (Werblin and Dowling, 1969; Kaneko, 1970). Not until the level of amacrine and ganglion cells are depolarizing potentials and nerve impulses observed. A second unconventional feature of retinal organization is that both receptors and bipolar cells make synapses that are characterized by electron-dense ribbons presynaptically and multiple elements postsynaptically (DeRobertis and Franchi, 1956; Sjostrand, 1958; Missotten, 1965; Dowling and Boycott, 1966). Also, serial and reciprocal synaptic arrangements have been observed in all retinas so far studied, and anatomical evidence further suggests that the processes of amacrine and horizontal cells may be both pre- and postsynaptic along their length (Kidd, 1962; Dowling, 1968).

These unusual anatomical and physiological features raise interesting

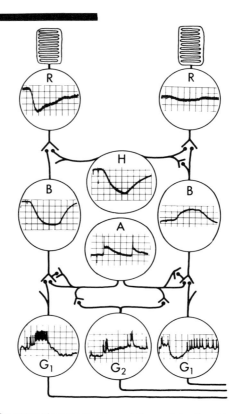

FIG. 1. A scheme of the synaptic organization of the vertebrate retina. The drawing correlates a wiring diagram of the synaptic pathways in the vertebrate retina with responses
obtained from the mudpuppy retina. The figure indicates the responses expected in each
neuron following a 0.5- 1-sec flash of light presented to the receptor on the left. The
left-hand receptor *(R)* responds to the light with a sharp hyperpolarization. The receptor
on the right shows no significant potential change after the flash, indicating that the
receptors in mudpuppy probably do not interact to any considerable extent. The horizontal cells *(H)* also hyperpolarize in response to light. These cells summate inputs from
a wide retinal area, and show response latencies similar to those of most bipolar cells *(B)*,
indicating that both cell types are driven by the receptors. The bipolar cell illustrated on
the left strongly hyperpolarizes in response to the light, reflecting the direct receptor-
bipolar synaptic interaction; the bipolar cell on the right shows a small depolarizing
potential, reflecting the antagonistic receptor-horizontal-bipolar synaptic pathway.
(There are also bipolar cells that depolarize in response to direct receptor-bipolar stimulation; these depolarizing potentials are likewise antagonized by horizontal-bipolar
interactions.) Amacrine cells *(A)* are driven by bipolar cells at reciprocal synaptic junctions, and they respond to light with transient, depolarizing potentials at both the onset
and cessation of illumination. One or two spikes are observed typically superimposed on
the large transient slow potentials of the amacrine cells. Two major classes of ganglion
cells are recognized in the mudpuppy retina. One class (G_1), thought to receive its input
mainly from the bipolar cells, responds mainly tonically to illumination. Its light response
shows numerous spikes superimposed on a small sustained depolarization or a small
sustained hyperpolarization with inhibition of spike firing for the duration of the light. In
the example, the cell on the left shows activity for the duration of the flash through a
direct receptor-bipolar-ganglion cell synaptic pathway. The cell on the right shows

questions concerning the mechanisms of synaptic action in the retina. At present, little is known about the mechanism of any retinal synapse. In this chapter I will focus on the photoreceptor synapse and discuss aspects of its anatomy and physiology. This is the first synapse along the visual pathway. Understanding of this junction appears prerequisite for any analysis of synaptic mechanisms in the vertebrate retina.

I. ANATOMY OF THE PHOTORECEPTOR SYNAPSE

The striking feature of the photoreceptor terminal when observed by electron microscopy is the densely stained synaptic ribbon or bar, which is usually situated in a ridge above a deep invagination into the receptor terminal (Figs. 2, 4, and 5). Numerous synaptic vesicles are scattered rather evenly throughout the receptor terminal, but a precisely arranged array of synaptic vesicles is invariably found around the synaptic ribbons [see Gray and Pease (1971) for a discussion on the origin and fate of photoreceptor synaptic vesicles]. Some increase of membrane density on both pre- and postsynaptic membranes may often be observed in the region adjacent to the synaptic ribbons, and a widened extracellular gap is typically seen between pre- and postsynaptic elements.

Three or more processes penetrate into each invagination of the receptor terminal, and in most species there is a rather precise arrangement of the processes in the invaginations (Sjostrand, 1958; Missotten, 1965; Dowling, 1970). Two deeply inserted processes are positioned on either side of the ridge containing the synaptic ribbon, although one or two processes lie more centrally in the invagination, directly under the ribbon. It has now been established in a variety of species that the lateral elements in the invagination are horizontal cell processes whereas the central elements are bipolar cell dendrites (Stell, 1965; Missotten, 1965; Kolb, 1970). It is generally assumed that both horizontal and bipolar cell processes receive input from the receptors within the invagination.

---

inhibition for the duration of illumination through a receptor-*horizontal*-bipolar-ganglion cell pathway. (Ganglion cells that show tonic inhibition in response to direct receptor-bipolar-ganglion cell interaction are also found; activation of these cells via the receptor-*horizontal*-bipolar pathway results in spike firing for the duration of the light.) The second class of ganglion cells (G_2) responds transiently to static retinal illumination, much as amacrine cells do. It is believed that this type of ganglion cell receives its input mainly from amacrine cells. Many of these transient ganglion cells respond very well to motion, and many show directionally selective responses (Werblin, 1970). In summary, the outer plexiform layer of the retina appears concerned with the static and spatial aspects of retinal illumination; the inner plexiform layer with the dynamic and temporal aspects of illumination. The two (physiological) types of ganglion cells found in vertebrate retina appear closely related to either bipolar or amacrine cell activity, and they transmit information to higher visual centers concerning the transformations occurring in the two synaptic layers (from Dowling, 1970; Dowling and Werblin, 1971).

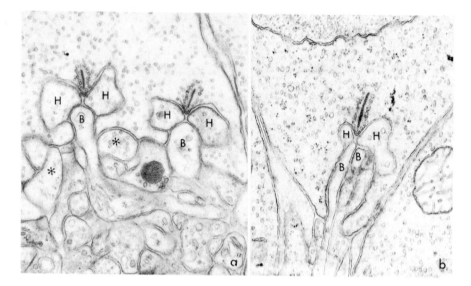

FIG. 2. Electron micrographs of ribbon synaptic complexes in the receptor terminals. In cone terminals (a), three processes penetrate into each invagination along the receptor terminal base; in rod terminals (b), four (or more) processes are observed in the single invagination. The elements that lie laterally and deeper in the invaginations are horizontal cell processes (H); the central elements are bipolar cell dendrites (B). Processes apparently making superficial contacts onto the base of the cone terminal are marked by asterisks. (a) Monkey cone terminal (× 27,300); (b) cat rod (× 29,400) (from Dowling, 1970).

Most vertebrate retinas contain two types of photoreceptors, rods and cones. Cone receptor terminals (called pedicles) tend to be larger and have numerous invaginations and synaptic ribbons (Missotten, 1965; Dowling and Boycott, 1966). Rod terminals (spherules) are smaller and usually have only a single invagination (Fig. 2). An additional important difference between rod and cone receptor terminals in many species is the occurrence of a second type of junction between the cone terminals and certain bipolar cell processes (Missotten, 1965; Dowling, 1968; Lasansky, 1969; Kolb, 1970). These junctions are observed usually along the base of the receptor pedicle (between the invaginations), and they have been called superficial, flat, or basal contacts (Figs. 2 and 3). Not much specialization is ordinarily seen at these junctions, which are usually distinguished by (1) a slight denting of the pedicle base at the site of the junction; (2) some membrane densification on both sides of the contact (often more prominent on the presynaptic side), and (3) occasional filamentous material within and extending across the extracellular cleft (Fig. 3). No aggregation of vesicles is observed in association with the presynaptic membrane, and only in the mudpuppy retina have synaptic ribbons been seen at such junctions (Dowling and Werblin, 1969). However, since certain bipolar cells (the flat bipolars) make *only* this type of contact with the receptors (Missotten, 1965;

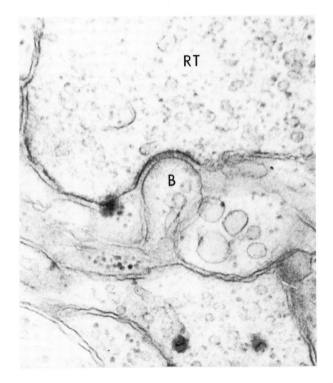

FIG. 3. A basal contact of a flat bipolar *(B)* onto a receptor terminal *(RT)* in the frog retina. These are relatively unspecialized junctions. No synaptic ribbon or aggregation or synaptic vesicles are observed on the presumed presynaptic side of these junctions which are characterized principally by some membrane densification on both sides of the contact, and by filamentous material within and extending across the synaptic cleft. Frog (× 67,000).

Kolb, 1970), it is generally assumed that these junctions also are synaptic in nature.

Most of the above observations were made originally in mammalian retinas. Studies of receptor terminals in cold-blooded vertebrates have suggested that some of their synaptic junctions may be somewhat different, and perhaps more complex (Kalberer and Pedler, 1963; Lasansky, 1971). However, serial section analysis is now revealing the presence of ribbon and superficial junctions in the terminals of nonmammalian vertebrates which are very similar to those observed in the mammalian retina. An illustration of this point is provided by an examination of the photoreceptor terminals found in the skate (*Raja erinacea* or *R. oscellata*) (Dowling and Ripps, *in preparation*). The skate retina appears to have only rod receptor cells; its receptor terminals are typically small, and they have but a single invagination (Fig. 4). However, in a single section three synaptic ribbons are typically observed in association with the single invagination, and numerous processes (15 to 25) are observed within the invagination (Fig. 4).

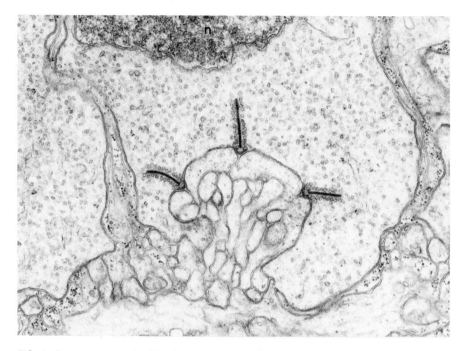

FIG. 4. A receptor terminal in the skate retina. Three synaptic ribbons are observed in association with the single invagination. Numerous profiles (15 to 25) are observed within the invagination. *n*, nucleus (× 17,700).

Analysis of these terminals shows that a triad of postsynaptic processes can always be associated with every synaptic ribbon provided serial sections are examined (Fig. 5*a*). The lateral elements have been traced to horizontal cells; the central elements have cytoplasmic characteristics typical of bipolar cell dendrites. Commonly, one lateral element is shared by two synaptic ribbons. Serial sections also reveal that a number of the processes observed in the invagination are derived from the receptor terminal itself (Fig. 5*a,b*). These extensions of receptor terminal found in the invaginations usually contain no synaptic vesicles; if continuity between process and terminal is not observed in a section, the origin of such processes is not apparent. Some suggestion that these receptor processes surround and partially isolate the multiple synaptic sites in the invagination is provided by serial section reconstruction.

Serial section analysis also reveals that a superficial type of junction is made by these receptor terminals along the presynaptic membrane *within* the invagination (Fig. 5*b*). Certain processes (probably bipolar cell dendrites) penetrate into the invagination but avoid the synaptic ribbon complexes. Instead, they approach the presynaptic membrane between the ribbon complexes and form a junction of the superficial type. A particularly

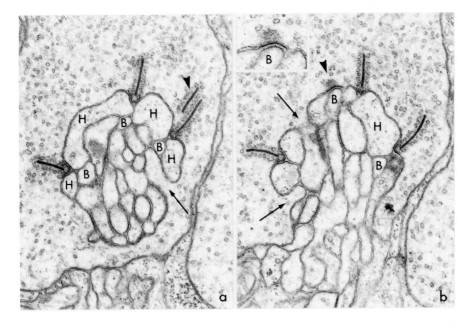

FIG. 5. Example micrographs from a serial-section analysis of a skate receptor terminal. In *(a)* (section number 10), three postsynaptic processes are observed in association with each of the three synaptic ribbons positioned around the invagination. A small fourth synaptic ribbon is observed in this section *(arrowhead)*. This ribbon did not approach closer to the receptor terminal membrane in any section, and did not appear involved with the synaptic junctions. The thin arrow marks a process from the receptor terminal extending into the invagination. Such processes appear (as here) to surround and partially isolate the synaptic complexes. In *(b)* (section number 4), a superficial type of junction is observed within the invagination, between the ribbon complexes *(arrowhead)*. Such contacts in the skate are marked by some membrane densification on both sides of the junction and an accumulation of granular material on the presynaptic side *(insert)*. The thin arrows mark two processes from the terminal extending into the invagination and surrounding a ribbon synaptic complex. Note that, in this single section, it appears that only two processes are postsynaptic to the ribbon. *H*, horizontal cell processes; *B*, bipolar cell dendrites (× 21,600; insert, × 42,350).

interesting feature of these superficial junctions in the skate terminal is the finding of an aggregation of fine granular material in the presynaptic cytoplasm adjacent to the junction (Fig. 5*b, insert*). This granular material is found only adjacent to these junctions and provides a clear marker for them.

A schematic diagram of the organization of the skate receptor terminal is presented in Fig. 6 and shows the basic similarity of the photoreceptor synaptic organization in the skate with that observed in the mammal. It is interesting to note that even though skates appear to have only rod receptors, they have both types of receptor terminal junctions. This indicates that there are in this retina, as in retinas containing both rods and cones, different types of bipolar cells that make junctions of either one type or the other with the receptor terminals.

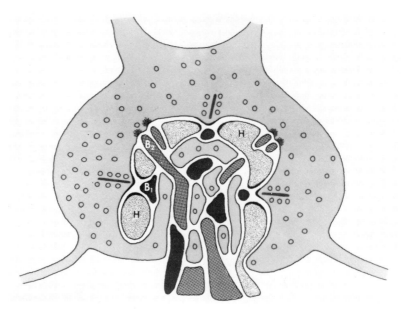

FIG. 6. A summary diagram of the receptor terminals in the skate based on serial section reconstruction. Three ribbons are positioned around the single invagination. Three processes are observed postsynaptic to each ribbon synapse. The elements laterally positioned with regard to the synaptic ribbons *(H)* have been traced back to horizontal cells; the centrally placed elements appear to be bipolar dendrites *(B₁)*. In addition, a superficial type of junction is observed within the invagination, between the synaptic ribbon complexes. These junctions usually occur in pairs and are marked by an aggregation of granular material on the presynaptic side of the contact. The postsynaptic elements at these contacts appear to be dendrites from a second class of bipolar cell *(B₂)*. A number of the profiles observed within the invagination are derived from the receptor terminal itself. These processes appear to surround and isolate the synaptic complexes. Fine processes from the receptor terminal also extend out laterally to contact nearby receptor terminals. These junctions between receptor terminals are currently under study; preliminary observations suggest that they may be gap junctions.

II. PHYSIOLOGY OF THE PHOTORECEPTOR SYNAPSE

The anatomy of the photoreceptor synapse, which shows numerous synaptic vesicles in the presynaptic terminal and a prominent gap between junctional elements, suggests that synaptic transmission between vertebrate photoreceptors and the second-order neurons (horizontal and bipolar cells) is chemically mediated. Intracellular recordings from receptors, bipolar and horizontal cells show significant latency differences between pre- and postsynaptic responses (Werblin and Dowling, 1969), a finding also consistent with chemical transmission.

Horizontal cells in many vertebrate species are extraordinarily large, which permits intracellular recordings to be made from these postsynaptic units rather routinely (Fig. 7). The electrical properties of horizontal cells in both light and dark have been extensively examined and a number of these studies have led to the interesting suggestion that photoreceptors release a depolarizing transmitter in the dark and that light decreases the flow of this transmitter (Trifonov and Byzov, 1965; Trifonov, 1968; Tomita, 1970). Thus, it is proposed that horizontal cells are maintained in a partially depolarized condition in the dark, and that light causes repolarization of the cell. Evidence in support of this suggestion includes the following: (1) horizontal cells in a healthy retina exhibit low resting potentials (−25 to −40 mV) (Svaetichin and MacNichol, 1958; Dowling and Ripps, 1970). In anoxic or metabolically poisoned retinas, on the other hand, the membrane potentials of horizontal cells are considerably greater (−60 to −80 mV) (Fatehchand, Svaetichin, Negishi, and Drujan 1966; Negishi and

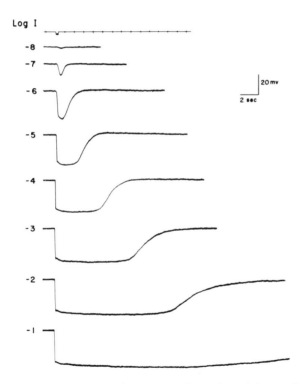

FIG. 7. Horizontal cell potentials recorded from the dark-adapted skate retina in response to 0.2-sec test flashes. The resting potential of the unit was approximately −30 mV. Light flashes of increasing intensity caused the cell to hyperpolarize in a graded fashion to a maximum membrane potential level of approximately −65 mV. More intense light flashes prolonged the duration of the response, but did not increase the response magnitude (from Dowling and Ripps, 1971b).

Svaetichin, 1966). (2) Most horizontal cells only hyperpolarize in response to light stimulation,* to a level of −60 to −80 mV (Svaetichin and Mac-Nichol, 1958). Intense light flashes prolong the duration of the response hyperpolarization (Fig. 7), but do not increase its magnitude (Dowling and Ripps, 1970). (3) An increase of input resistance of the horizontal cell usually accompanies the hyperpolarization induced by light (Toyoda, Nosaki, and Tomita, 1969; Nelson, 1972). Although, the resistance increase is small and somewhat variable in onset (Tomita, 1965), never has a resistance *decrease* been shown to accompany the light-evoked hyperpolarization. (4) Current passed throught the retina in a direction appropriate to depolarize the receptor terminals induces a depolarizing response in the horizontal cells (Trifonov and Byzov, 1965; Trifonov, 1968).

The view that transmitter may be released continuously in darkness at these receptor synapses is supported also by recent studies on the electrical properties of the photoreceptors. In the dark there is a steady inward flow of sodium across the plasma membrane of the outer segment of the rod receptors; light decreases the sodium conductance of the outer segment, causing the receptor to hyperpolarize (Penn and Hagins, 1969; Hagins, Penn, and Yoshikami, 1970; Tomita, 1970). Thus, the photoreceptors also appear to be partially depolarized in the dark, a condition consistent with the notion of transmitter release from receptor synapses in darkness.

Ripps and I have recently further examined this hypothesis by determining the influence of magnesium on the electrical properties of skate horizontal cells (Dowling and Ripps, 1973). We assumed that, as in other chemically mediated synapses, high levels of extracellular magnesium block neurotransmitter release from the presynaptic (i.e., receptor) terminal (Del Castillo and Engbaek, 1954; Takeuchi and Takeuchi, 1962; Katz and Miledi, 1967). Intracellular recordings from horizontal cells were obtained from the eyecup preparation, and, after a cell was satisfactorily impaled, a drop of elasmobranch Ringer, in which 100 mm MgCl was substituted for an equivalent amount of NaCl, was gently pressure-injected onto the surface of the retina. In this way recordings before, during, and after exposure to the high-magnesium Ringer's solution were obtained.

Figure 8 shows the effects of the test solution on two horizontal cells. Resting potentials of 25 and 30 mV were recorded initially in the two cells, and light flashes of constant duration and intensity gave hyperpolarizing

---

* Horizontal cells that show both hyperpolarizing and depolarizing potential shifts (the polarity of response depending on the wavelength of the stimulating light) have been observed in several species (Svaetichin and MacNichol, 1958). It has been found, however, that the depolarizing potentials of these cells have longer response latencies than the primary hyperpolarizing responses (Spekreijse and Norton, 1970), suggesting that the depolarizing potentials do not result from direct receptor input. Metabolic inhibitors cause these horizontal cells also to hyperpolarize to a level of −60 to −80 mV; and while this occurs, both hyperpolarizing and depolarizing components are abolished (Santamaria, Drujan, Svaetichin, and Negishi, 1971).

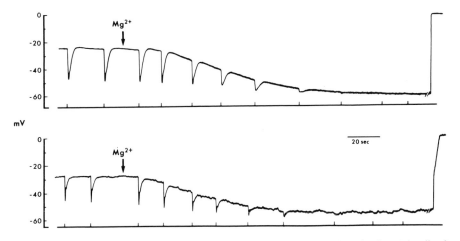

FIG. 8. Two experiments showing the effects of magnesium on skate horizontal cells. A drop of magnesium Ringer's was applied to the eyecup *(arrows)*, and within 15 to 25 sec, the cells began to hyperpolarize. Over the next 3 min, the cells hyperpolarized to a level of approximately -60 mV and light-evoked activity was lost. A break in the trace indicates the time at which the pipettes were withdrawn from the cells. The rapid, positive shifts of potential of 55 to 60 mV confirmed the increase in membrane potential of the horizontal cells in the presence of high levels of magnesium. Flash intensity (filter density of 5.5) and duration (0.2 sec) were kept constant throughout both experiments. The markers along the lower trace of each record indicate flash presentations (from Dowling and Ripps, 1973).

responses of 15 to 20 mV. These test stimuli were approximately 1.5 log units above threshold; flashes of saturating intensity evoked responses of 25 to 30 mV in these cells.

About 15 to 25 sec after a drop of magnesium Ringer's was applied to the eyecups *(arrows,* Fig. 8), the membrane potentials of the horizontal cells began to hyperpolarize and there was a corresponding decrease in the amplitudes of the light-evoked responses. Within 3 min, the membrane potentials had fallen to approximately -60 mV and the response to light was abolished. In these two experiments, the micropipettes were withdrawn from the cells after the resting potentials had stabilized. Positive shifts of potentials of 55 to 60 mV signaled the exit of the pipettes from the cells and confirmed the intracellular measurements of large membrane potentials in the presence of high magnesium.

These results strongly support the notion that skate horizontal cells are maintained in a partially depolarized state in the dark. We suggest that high magnesium, like light, decreases the release of neurotransmitter from the receptors, causing the horizontal cell to hyperpolarize. It is interesting to note that as the horizontal cells hyperpolarize in response to a high magnesium environment, there is a distinct increase in baseline fluctuations. This is particularly clear in the lower record of Fig. 8. It is possible that these fluctuations indicate the presence of spontaneous miniature postsynaptic potentials in the horizontal cells, which are uncovered under conditions of high extracellular magnesium. In muscle it has been shown that miniature end-plate potentials persist in the presence of high magnesium (del Castillo and Katz, 1954; Hubbard, 1967).

The effects of a drop of magnesium Ringer's on the skate eyecup preparation are transient. Figure 9 illustrates an experiment in which a horizontal cell was monitored for more than 30 min after the test solution was added to the eyecup. In this experiment the horizontal cell did not fully hyperpolarize and light-evoked responses were not entirely abolished. Thirty sec after application of the magnesium Ringer's, the membrane potential of the cell became more negative and responses to light decreased in amplitude. After 3 to 5 min, the resting potential stabilized, and only small light-evoked potentials could be recorded. For the next 5 to 10 min, no significant changes were noted. Between 15 and 30 min, however, the horizontal cell membrane depolarized to its former level ($\sim$ -30 mV) and light-evoked activity regained its original amplitude.

The evidence at hand points toward the release of a depolarizing transmitter from receptors in darkness. This evidence, however, has been obtained primarily from studies on horizontal cells. Is it consistent with what we know of bipolar cell activity? Two types of bipolar cell responses have been described in vertebrate retinas (Werblin and Dowling, 1969;

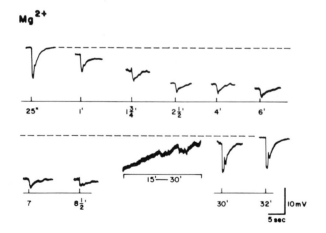

FIG. 9. Long-term recordings illustrating the transient nature of the effects of magnesium on skate horizontal cells. The times after the application of the test solution at which light stimuli were presented are indicated along the lower line. The level of each trace relative to the dashed line shows the extent to which the cell was hyperpolarized. Since the cell was not completely hyperpolarized by the drop of test solution, a small response could be elicited even after 8½ min. Between 15 and 30 min (shown on the contracted time base), the membrane potential of the cell depolarized and the responses at the end of this time had returned to normal amplitudes (from Dowling and Ripps, 1973).

Kaneko, 1970). Like horizontal cell responses, these are both sustained, graded potentials; one is hyperpolarizing in polarity, the other depolarizing. The receptive fields of both types of bipolar cells are organized in such a way that surround or annular illumination antagonizes central stimulation (Fig. 1). It has been postulated that the response to central stimulation is mediated by direct receptor-bipolar cell junctions, whereas the surround antagonism is mediated by horizontal-bipolar cell interactions (Werblin and Dowling, 1969; Naka, 1972).

The hyperpolarizing bipolar cells exhibit an increase in membrane resistance during light stimulation of the center of their receptive fields (Tomita, 1970; Nelson, 1972); thus generation of these responses could be similar to that of horizontal cell potentials. The responses of depolarizing bipolar cells, on the other hand, provide a more difficult problem. Nelson (1972) has recently found that the center response of these cells in the mudpuppy is accompanied by a decrease in membrane resistance. If these bipolar cells also receive their central input directly from receptors, this finding implies that the effect of the receptor neurotransmitter is to *decrease* conductance of the cell. Thus, in the light when transmitter release is decreased, a conductance increase would be observed in the bipolar cell. Although unconventional action for a neurotransmitter, recent experiments suggest that this does occur in neurons in the frog sympathetic ganglion (Weight, 1973). Alternatively, it is possible that depolarizing cells do not receive any direct synaptic input from receptors but instead are activated entirely through horizontal cells. In support of this notion, there is some suggestion that depolarizing bipolar cells have longer response latencies than do hyperpolarizing bipolar cells (Tomita, 1970; Nelson, 1972).

What can be said, finally, about possible photoreceptor transmitters? It has been shown recently that certain acidic amino acids powerfully depolarize horizontal cells in the skate (Dowling and Ripps, 1971a; Cervetto and MacNichol, 1971). L-Na aspartate is particularly potent in this regard and would appear to be a likely candidate for the photoreceptor transmitter. Figure 10 shows the effects of L-Na aspartate on a skate horizontal cell. This experiment was similar in design to those described in detail earlier. A drop of elasmobranch Ringer's, in which 100 mm L-Na aspartate was substituted for an equivalent amount of NaCl, was applied to the eyecup preparation *(arrow)*, and some 15 to 25 sec later the impaled cell began to depolarize. During the initial phase of the depolarization, the light-evoked responses were significantly larger than the control responses. However, as the cell depolarized further, light-evoked responses diminished in amplitude and eventually disappeared. The unit was depolarized by the aspartate to a level of -5 to -7 mV. This low level of membrane potential was confirmed by withdrawal of the pipette from the cell (shown at the end of the record).

Much work is needed to establish rigorously the identification of the photoreceptor transmitter. However, it is of interest to note that evidence

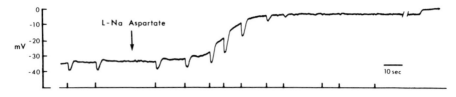

FIG. 10. The depolarizing effect of L-Na aspartate on a skate horizontal cell. Approximately 15 to 25 sec after a drop of aspartate-substituted Ringer's was applied to the surface of the retina, the cell began to depolarize. The light-evoked responses were first larger than control potentials, but then they diminished in amplitude and gradually disappeared. The cell was depolarized by the aspartate to a membrane potential level of −5 to −7 mV. This low level of membrane potential was confirmed by the withdrawal of the pipette from the cell shown at the end of the record (from Dowling and Ripps, 1972).

has been presented in this volume suggesting that L-glutamate is the transmitter at the electroreceptor synapses in the skate (Steinbach, 1973). These receptor synapses are also characterized by a synaptic ribbon in the presynaptic terminal, and they too appear to release transmitter when they are partially depolarized.

III. CONCLUSIONS AND COMMENTS

Although the anatomy of the photoreceptor terminals shows many unconventional features, including invaginated junctions, presynaptic ribbons, multiple postsynaptic elements at single junction sites, unspecialized superficial contacts, the physiology so far suggests that rather conventional synaptic mechanisms may operate at these junctions. The photoreceptors appear to release transmitter when they are partially depolarized, and this transmitter release is magnesium sensitive. Certain acidic amino acids, especially aspartate, powerfully depolarize postsynaptic elements (horizontal cells) and could well serve as the photoreceptor transmitter.

More work is clearly indicated before these conclusions can be fully accepted. For example, study of bipolar cell activity in the presence of high magnesium is a critical experiment that should be undertaken in the near future. Study of the effects of aspartate and other possible transmitter substances on bipolar cell activity is a second important experiment to attempt. Other questions of considerable interest concerning the photoreceptor synaptic junctions appear more difficult to approach at present. These include (1) the function of the synaptic ribbon in the receptor terminal; (2) the physiological differences (if any) between the ribbon and superficial junctions; (3) the reasons why vesicles (or synaptic ribbons) are not observed in association with the superficial contacts; (4) the significance of the invaginated contacts; and (5) the reasons for the precise arrangement of horizontal and bipolar cell processes within the invaginations. These latter queries may relate to a whole new group of questions concerning the mechanisms of horizontal and bipolar cell synaptic interaction in the outer plexiform layer of the retina, about which we know virtually nothing at the moment (Werblin and Dowling, 1969).

A final comment concerns the curious finding that the distal retinal elements appear to be maintained "on" in the dark, and that light turns them "off." It is obvious that most vertebrates spend a considerable amount of time in the dark, and under these conditions it appears that there is a considerable metabolic drain on the visual system, especially on the photoreceptors. Hagins et al. (1970) have calculated, for example, that in the dark, the rate of ion exchange across the photoreceptor membranes is so high that the cell will fail in less than a minute if it is metabolically poisoned. Thus, darkness acts as a powerful stimulus for the vertebrate photoreceptor and, presumably, the postsynaptic cells. One might have expected that visual systems would have evolved in such a way as to avoid long periods of continual activation. In the invertebrate visual system, receptors depolarize in response to light and appear to release transmitter only when in the light (Hartline, Wagner, and MacNichol, 1952; MacNichol, 1956; Chappell and Dowling, 1972). Many invertebrates are highly visually dependent and extremely sensitive to light (Reichardt, 1965). Thus, it is difficult at the moment to assign an advantage to the vertebrate system of being highly active in the dark.

ACKNOWLEDGMENTS

The research reported in this chapter was supported by grants from the National Eye Institute (EY-00811 and EY-00824). Patricia A. Sheppard provided excellent technical assistance and prepared the figures.

REFERENCES

Cervetto, L., and MacNichol, E. F., Jr. (1971): Pharmacology of horizontal cells in the isolated perfused skate retina. *Biol. Bull.*, 141:381.

Chappell, R. L., and Dowling, J. E. (1972): Organization of the medial ocellus of the dragonfly: I. Intracellular electrical activity. *J. Gen. Physiol.*, 60:121–165.

del Castillo, J., and Engbaek, L. (1954): The nature of the neuromuscular block produced by magnesium. *J. Physiol.*, 124:370–384.

del Castillo, J., and Katz, B. (1954): The effects of magnesium on the activity of motor nerve endings. *J. Physiol.*, 124:553–559.

DeRobertis, E., and Franchi, C. M. (1956): Electron microscopic observations on synaptic vesicles in synapses of the retinal rods and cones. *J. Biophys. Biochem. Cytol.*, 2:307–318.

Dowling, J. E. (1968): Synaptic organization of the frog retina: An electron microscopic analysis comparing the retinas of frogs and primates. *Proc. Roy. Soc. B*, 170:205–227.

Dowling, J. E. (1970): Organization of vertebrate retinas. *Invest. Ophthal.* 9:655–680.

Dowling, J. E., and Boycott, B. B. (1966): Organization of the primate retina: Electron microscopy. *Proc. Roy. Soc. B*, 166:80–111.

Dowling, J. E., and Ripps, H. (1970): Visual adaptation in the retina of the skate. *J. Gen. Physiol.*, 56:491–520.

Dowling, J. E., and Ripps, H. (1971a): Aspartate isolation of receptor potentials in the skate retina. *Biol. Bull.*, 141:384.

Dowling, J. E., and Ripps, H. (1971b): S-Potentials in the skate retina: Intracellular recordings during light and dark adaptation. *J. Gen. Physiol.*, 58:163-189.

Dowling, J. E., and Ripps, H. (1972): Adaptation in skate photoreceptors. *J. Gen. Physiol.*, 60:698-719.

Dowling, J. E., and Ripps, H. (1973): Effect of magnesium on horizontal cell activity in the skate retina. *Nature*, 242:101-103.

Dowling, J. E., and Werblin, F. S. (1969): Organization of retina of the mudpuppy, *Necturus maculosus*. I. Synaptic structure. *J. Neurophysiol.*, 32:315-338.

Dowling, J. E., and Werblin, F. S. (1971): Synaptic organization of the vertebrate retina. *Vis. Res. Suppl.*, 3:1-15.

Fatehchand, R., Svaetichin, G., Negishi, K., and Drujan, B. (1966): Effects of anoxia and metabolic inhibitors on the S-potential in isolated fish retinas. *Vision Res.*, 6:271-283.

Gray, E. G., and Pease, H. L. (1971): On understanding the organization of the retinal receptor synapses. *Brain Res.*, 35:1-15.

Hagins, W. A., Penn, R. D., and Yoshikami, S. (1970): Dark current and photocurrent in retinal rods. *Biophys. J.*, 10:380-412.

Hartline, H. K., Wagner, H. G., and MacNichol, E. F. (1952): The peripheral origin of nervous activity in the visual system. *Cold Spring Harb. Symp. Quant. Biol.*, 17:125-141.

Hubbard, J. I. (1961): The effect of calcium and magnesium on the spontaneous release of transmitter from mammalian motor nerve endings. *J. Physiol.*, 159:507-517.

Kalberer, M., and Pedler, C. (1963): The visual cells of the alligator: An electron microscopic study. *Vis. Res.*, 3:323-329.

Kaneko, A. (1970): Physiological and morphological identification of horizontal, bipolar, and amacrine cells in the goldfish retina. *J. Physiol.*, 207:623-633.

Katz, B., and Miledi, R. (1967): A study of synaptic transmission in the absence of nerve impulses. *J. Physiol.*, 192:407-436.

Kidd, M. (1962): Electron microscopy of the inner plexiform layer of the retina in the cat and the pigeon. *J. Anat.*, 96:179-188.

Kolb, H. (1970): Organization of the outer plexiform layer of the primate retina: Electron microscopy of Golgi-impregnated cells. *Phil. Trans.*, 258:261-283.

Lasansky, A. (1969): Basal junctions at synaptic endings of turtle visual cells. *J. Cell. Biol.*, 40:577-581.

Lasansky, A. (1971): Synaptic organization of cone cells in the turtle retina. *Phil. Trans.*, 262:365-381.

MacNichol, E. F., Jr. (1956): Visual receptors as biological transducers. In: *Molecular Structure and Functional Activity of Nerve Cells*, edited by R. G. Grenell and L. J. Mullins. Am. Inst. Biol. Sci., Washington, D.C.

Missotten, L. (1965): *The Ultrastructure of the Retina*. Arscia Uitgaven N.V., Brussels.

Naka, K. I. (1972): The horizontal cells. *Vis. Res.*, 12:573-588.

Negishi, K., and Svaetichin, G. (1966): Effects of anoxia, CO_2 and NH_3 on S-potential producing cells and on neurons. *Pflügers Arch.* 292:177-205.

Nelson, R. (1972): Ph.D. Thesis, Johns Hopkins University.

Penn, R. D., and Hagins, W. A. (1969): Signal transmission along retinal rods and the origin of the electroretinographic a-wave. *Nature*, 223:201-205.

Reichardt, W. E. (1965): Quantum sensitivity of light receptors in the compound eye of the fly, *Musca. Cold Spring Harb. Symp. Quant. Biol.*, 30:501-515.

Santamaria, L., Drujan, B. D., Svaetichin, G., and Negishi, K. (1971): Respiration, glycolysis, and S-potentials in teleost retina: A comparative study. *Vis. Res.*, 11:877-887.

Sjostrand, F. S. (1958): Ultrastructure of retinal rod synapses of the guinea pig eye as revealed by three-dimensional reconstructions from serial sections. *J. Ultrastruct. Res.*, 2:122-170.

Spekreijse, H., and Norton, A. L. (1970): The dynamic characteristics of color-coded S-potentials. *J. Gen. Physiol.*, 56:1-15.

Steinbach, A. B. (1974): This Volume.

Stell, W. K. (1965): Correlation of retinal cytoarchitecture and ultrastructure in Golgi preparations. *Ana. Rec.*, 153:389-397.

Svaetichin, G., and MacNichol, E. F., Jr. (1958): Retinal mechanisms for chromatic and achromatic vision. *Ann. N.Y. Acad. Sci.*, 74:385-404.

Takeuchi, A., and Takeuchi, N. (1962): Electrical changes in pre- and post-synaptic axons of the giant synapse of *Loligo. J. Gen. Physiol.*, 45:1181-1193.

Tomita, T. (1965): Electrophysiological study of the mechanisms subserving color coding in the fish retina. *Cold Spring Harb. Symp. Quant. Biol.*, 30:559–566.

Tomita, T. (1970): Electrical activity of vertebrate photoreceptors. *Quart. Rev. of Biophys.*, 3:179–222.

Toyoda, J., Nosaki, H., and Tomita, T. (1969): Light-induced resistance changes in single photoreceptors of *Necturus* and *Gekko*. *Vis. Res.*, 9:453–463.

Trifonov, Y. A. (1968): Study of synaptic transmission between the photoreceptor and the horizontal cell using electrical stimulation of the retina. *Biofizika*, 13, 5:809–817.

Trifonov, Y. A., and Byzov, A. L. (1965): The response of the cells generating S-potential on the current passed through the eyecup of the turtle. *Biophysica, Moscow*, 10:673–680.

Weight, F. F. (1974): *This Volume*.

Werblin, F. S. (1970): Response of retinal cells to moving spots: Intracellular recording in *Necturus maculosus*. *J. Neurophysiol.*, 33:342–351.

Werblin, F. S., and Dowling, J. E. (1969): Organization of the retina of the mudpuppy *Necturus maculosus*. II. Intracellular recording. *J. Neurophysiol.*, 32:339–355.

Synaptic Transmission and Neuronal Interaction
Raven Press, New York 1974

Transmission from Receptor Cells to Afferent Nerve Fibers

Alan B. Steinbach

Marine Biological Laboratory, Woods Hole, Massachusetts 02543

INTRODUCTION

In three of the five main vertebrate sense systems (visual, acoustico-lateralis, and taste), specialized non-neuronal cells receive and transduce sensory information. These receptor cells are in close contact with nerve processes whose bodies lie nearer to or within the CNS. The term "sensory synapse" or "receptor-nerve synapse" is used here to mean the contacts that relay information from receptor cell to afferent nerve process. The mechanisms involved in such synapses are the subject of this chapter. The visual system is dealt with by Dowling *(This Volume)*.

What we know about synaptic physiology stems from study of nerve-nerve and nerve-muscle synapses, primarily in the motor output system. A regenerative, depolarizing, sodium-dependent action potential in the pre-synaptic nerve terminal triggers calcium entry which facilitates a brief increase in release of quantal packets of transmitter chemical, and, as a result of the interaction of transmitter with receptor molecules located on the postsynaptic membrane, there is a local increase in postsynaptic membrane conductance and a resulting postsynaptic potential (psp) (Katz, 1969). Similar events occur in CNS synapses, although cell geometry and the large number of inputs to each cell often make it hard to figure out what is going on (see Kuno, *This Volume*). Our knowledge of synaptic structure is similarly based on study of motor and CNS synapses, although a number of studies of sensory synapses have been made. Clusters of presynaptic vesicles, a narrow synaptic cleft, and membrane specialization at contact points are all characteristic of chemically transmitting synapses.

Motor synapses relay well-coded monotypic nerve commands from CNS to effector cells. Sensory synapses link non-neuronal cells (which are responding to and coding external stimuli) to afferent nerves that must provide abundant, reliable, and specific inputs (coded as spikes) to the CNS. The first part of this chapter provides a brief view of how various sensory systems work. In the second part, I want to present new information gained from study of electroreceptors. Finally, I will attempt to consider the major question: to what extent does transmission at a sensory synapse involve mechanisms common to motor synapses?

I. VERTEBRATE SENSORY SYSTEMS INVOLVING SENSORY SYNAPSES

Introduction

Sensory receptors are complex in structure (Fig. 1). A number of cell types are involved, and all are important in function (see Bennett, 1971a). For the limited purpose of this chapter, I will consider the structure and function of receptor cells, the cells believed to transduce sensory information. In the systems that I will consider, the culmination of transduction is probably always a depolarization or a hyperpolarization of the receptor cell. At chemically transmitting receptor synapses depolarization elicits transmitter release and hyperpolarization may reduce any ongoing release. I will minimize discussion of transduction. As a general paradigm, the systems to be considered reduce to a group of receptor cells, usually with microvilli or cilia on their outer (distal, or apical) faces, and with synapses usually at their inner (proximal or basal) faces.

Electroreceptors

Electroreceptors occur in a number of fish, including most electric fish (see reviews by Bennett, 1967, 1971a,b). There are two general types of electroreceptors (Fig. 1). In the tuberous (phasic) type, receptor cells are clustered in a cavity, surrounded by supporting cells, and covered by a layer of loosely packed epithelial cells. In the ampullary (tonic) type, receptor cells also lie in a cavity, but the cavity is at the end of a tube or canal which is open to the surface. The canal is generally short in freshwater forms, and long in marine forms. In both types the nonreceptor cells lining the cavity and supporting the electroreceptor cells form a high-resistance layer that channels current through the receptor cells.

Ampullary receptors are tonic in function. *In vivo*, a tonic spike frequency is recorded from an afferent nerve. Electrical stimuli increase or decrease spike frequency depending on whether they lead to depolarization or hyperpolarization of the inner face of the receptor cells. There are initial and terminal transient effects of stimulation but adaptation is slow and generally incomplete for ordinary stimulus durations. In teleosts, one or more nerve fibers innervate a number of receptor cells in each electroreceptor. In elasmobranchs five to eight nerve fibers innervate several hundred to a thousand receptor cells in a single ampulla of Lorenzini. Only one type of synapse is found between receptor cells and nerves, and only afferent nerves enter the receptors (Barets and Szabo, 1962; Wachtel and Szamier, 1966,

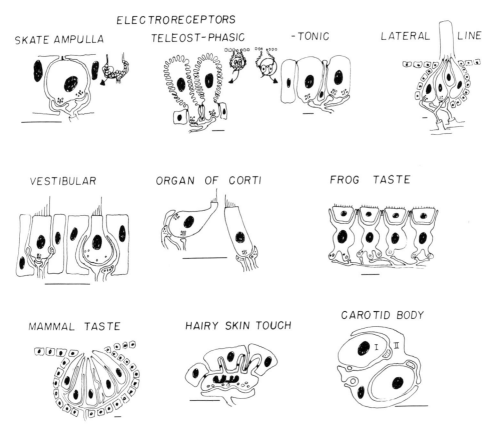

ELECTRORECEPTORS

SKATE AMPULLA   TELEOST-PHASIC   -TONIC   LATERAL LINE

VESTIBULAR   ORGAN OF CORTI   FROG TASTE

MAMMAL TASTE   HAIRY SKIN TOUCH   CAROTID BODY

FIG. 1. Semischematic drawings of receptor cell-nerve relationships in vertebrate sensory systems (excluding visual systems). The size of receptor cells is in accord with the 10-micron scale shown next to each drawing. Skate ampulla: Electroreceptor cell from skate (after Murray, 1965a,b) with inset to right showing the proximal end of an ampulla of Lorenzini where these cells occur. Teleost-phasic: Two electroreceptor cells from a typical tuberous (phasic) receptor (inset) found in many teleost electric fish (after Fig. 20, Bennett, 1971a). Tonic: Two electroreceptor cells from a typical ampullary (tonic) receptor (inset) in teleost fishes including nonelectric fish (from Fig. 11, Bennett, 1971a). Lateral line: Neuromast typical of lateral line organs in fish and amphibians; cells are this large only in *Necturus*. Note both afferent (presynaptic body in receptor) and efferent (vesicles in nerve terminal) synapse (modified from Fig. 1, Harris et al., 1970). Vestibular: The two types (cylindrical on left, bottle-shaped on right) of receptor cells found in vertebrate vestibular system. Note chalice form afferent synapse surrounding bottle-shaped cell, and cilia, as in lateral line (from Wersäll et al., 1965). Organ of Corti: Inner (left) and outer (right) receptor (hair) cells from vertebrate acoustical organ (Wersäll et al., 1965). Frog taste: Portion of the cells in the taste plate of frog fungiform papillae. Associate cells form superficial layer with receptor cell processes (linked by gap junctions) between them; synapses have dense cored vesicles and no presynaptic dense bodies (after DeHan and Graziadei, 1971). Mammal taste: Section through mammalian taste bud, showing taste cells with apical microvilli, nerve branches, and ill-defined synapses (based on figures in Graziadei, 1969). Hairy skin touch: Tactile receptor studied by Iggo and Muir (1969) showing overlying epithelial cells, desmosomes between receptor cell (with invaginations) and epithelial cells, lobed nucleus, dense cored vesicles, and nerve plate (after Iggo and Muir, 1969). Carotid body: Portion of carotid body showing the type I cells, surrounded by type II cells, with vesicle containing nerve endings on type I cells and nerve terminals nearby (after Biscoe, 1971).

1969; Szamier and Wachtel, 1969, 1970). There are presynaptic bars, ribbons, or rods located in the receptor cell, and vesicles line up near these bodies. The vesicles are clear. A single nerve terminal is involved in each synapse, although receptor cells may synapse with more than one terminal, and vice versa.

Intracellular recordings have been made from one tonic electroreceptor cell in *Kryptopterus* (see Bennett, 1971*b*). Small depolarizing receptor potentials without regenerative components were seen. In marine elasmobranch ampullae of Lorenzini, receptor cells produce a regenerative response (Waltman, 1968; Obara and Bennett, 1972).

Tuberous electroreceptors are phasic in function. There is generally no tonic spike discharge in afferent nerves. Long-lasting stimuli excite only at the beginning and/or end. This high pass filter effect results from the outer face of the receptor cell acting as a series blocking capacity (Bennett, 1971*a*). The number of receptor cells and afferent nerves per receptor is variable from species to species. Synapses between receptor cells and nerves are similar to those in tonic receptors. In Mormyrid "medium" receptors there are two cavities and two types of receptor cell (Szabo and Wersäll, 1970).

Evidence that transmission is chemically mediated in both tuberous and ampullary electroreceptors has been reviewed by Bennett (1971*a*). Briefly, (a) there is a synaptic delay of 0.6 msec or longer, (b) afferent spike frequency increases greatly outlast effective brief stimuli and cannot be blocked by strong inhibitory stimuli, (c) divalent ions greatly alter synaptic function, (d) antidromic spikes do not invade receptor cells, (e) synaptic structure suggests chemical transmission. Transmission in Mormyrid "large" electroreceptors may be electrically mediated (Bennett, 1967; Steinbach and Bennett, 1971).

Lateral Line Receptors

Lateral line receptors or neuromasts occur in both teleost and elasmobranch fishes, and in some amphibians. In fish the neuromasts are often placed singly in the walls of lateral line tubes or canals which direct water movements to the receptors; in amphibians and fish they can be exposed directly to the exterior, and in amphibians neuromasts occur in rows known as stitches. A neuromast consists of a cluster of receptor cells, each with a compact array of cilia on the outer face. The cilia project upward into a gelatinous dome or cupola which covers the entire neuromast (Fig. 1). In fish each neuromast contains 10 to 50 cells and may be innervated by several afferent and efferent nerve fibers (Flöck and Wersäll, 1962*a*; Hama, 1965). In amphibians each neuromast contains about eight cells, and there are two to six neuromasts per stitch, all innervated by one or two afferent and one or more (Fig. 3) efferent nerves (Jande, 1966; Harris, Frishhopf, and Flöck,

1970). In both fishes and amphibians, two types of synapse can be seen (Hama, 1965; Wersäll, Flöck, and Lundquist, 1965; Jande, 1966). At the presumed afferent synapse, vesicles cluster in the receptor cell side, associated with a dense presynaptic body. The vesicles are clear, and are not seen in the postsynaptic nerve terminal. At the efferent synapse, many vesicles without a dense body are found in the nerve terminal. Few vesicles are found in the adjacent receptor cell, but there is generally a flattened cistern or sac, apparently not connected to the external membrane, lying adjacent to the synapse.

Mechanical displacement of the cupola over the neuromast produces spikes in the afferent nerve; in amphibians, there may be a tonic spike frequency without stimulation (Russell, 1968; Harris and Milne, 1966). The direction of stimulation in relation to the orientation of the receptor cell cilia is critical (Flöck and Wersäll, 1963; Wersäll et al., 1965). Single receptor cells respond to unidirectional movement, and single afferent nerves may innervate only one receptor cell type. After the onset of a step movement, adaptation in spike frequency takes place (Harris and Milne, 1966). Efferent stimulation decreases the spike frequency (Russell, 1968) apparently without qualitatively changing receptor response characteristics.

Very small (30 to 800 μvolt), nonadapting, potential changes in response to stimulation have been recorded in the relatively large receptor cells of *Necturus* lateral line (Harris et al., 1970). Cell damage is likely, and the amplitude of the recordings may not be an accurate measure of the receptor potential in intact cells.

Some lateral line organs in fish have been shown to respond to chemical stimuli, and may serve that function physiologically (Katsuki, Hashimoto, and Kendall, 1971).

Vestibular System

The receptor cells of the vertebrate vestibular labyrinth are used to monitor the animal's orientation; in fish some cells are sensitive to sound. Ciliated receptor cells (hair cells) line the surface of selected areas of the labyrinth, and movements affect the position of an otolith (stone) and the flow of fluid in the labyrinth and thereby cause a deflection of the receptor cell cilia. In birds and mammals two kinds of cell are seen; one cylindrical and the other bottle shaped (Fig. 1; Wersäll et al., 1965). The afferent nerve associated with the bottle-shaped cell type forms a large chalice enclosing the basal portion of each cell. Transmission here may be in part electrically mediated (see Bennett, 1971a). Efferent endings in this cell type are said to be on the chalice rather than on the receptor cell. In the cylindrical type of cell, both afferent and efferent endings are on the receptor cell, and there are presynaptic dense bodies equivalent to those seen in electroreceptor cells (Wersäll et al., 1965). In fish and amphibians, only the cylindrical type occurs. The most comprehensive physiological studies have been made on fish.

Some receptor cells in the anterior portion of the fish saccular macula are innervated by large (15 micron diameter) nerves, called Sl nerves by Furukawa and Ishii (1967). There are no tonic spikes in Sl nerves, but sound stimuli evoke psp's with a 0.6-msec latency in response to compression or rarefaction or both (the cilia on receptor cells synapsing with a single Sl nerve can be oppositely oriented (Fig. 2) (Furukawa and Ishii, 1967; Hama, 1969). Each psp appears to be composed of "quantal" units (Ishii, Matsuura, and Furukawa, 1971a). Large enough psp's elicit a single spike. The input-output relationship between stimuli and psp amplitude has been well studied, and is fairly linear over a range near threshold (Ishii, Matsuura, and Furukawa, 1971b; Fig. 3).

In studies of the saccular macula receptors, microphonic potentials were recorded as monitors of receptor cell response (Furukawa and Ishii, 1967). Microphonic potentials are also associated with the function of neuromasts of the lateral line (Flöck and Wersäll, 1962b, 1963) and with receptor cells in the mammalian vestibular and auditory system. Although microphonics do not give detailed information about the electrical polarity or magnitude of receptor cell activity, the tight coupling of microphonics to stimuli suggests that regenerative mechanisms, with associated temperature dependence and refractory periods, are not involved.

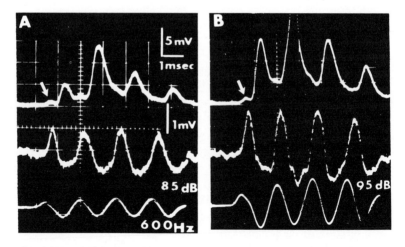

FIG. 2. Recordings from micropipette placed in an S1 nerve fiber (top trace) which is postsynaptic to receptor cells that generate microphonics (middle trace). The sound stimulus is shown in the bottom trace. The arrows indicate the low-amplitude coupling potential coinciding with the microphonic potential. Weaker (A) and stronger (B) stimuli. Note variability and brief duration of the psp's (top trace). Taken from Figure 1 in Ishii et al., 1971b.

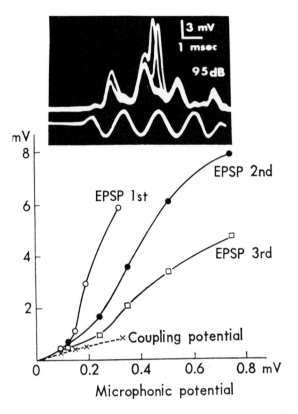

FIG. 3. Input-output relationships in the vestibular system of goldfish. The inset shows microphonics (lower trace) and psp's with several traces superimposed. The plot is mean amplitude of postsynaptic response (ordinate) versus amplitude of microphonic potential (abscissa). The relationship varies for the first, second, and third psp (EPSP) in a series (Fig. 3B in Ishii et al., 1971*b*).

The Organ of Corti

In lower vertebrates the vestibular apparatus has portions specialized for sound reception; in higher vertebrates this function is carried out by the receptor cells in the organ of Corti in the cochlea. In this system the receptor cells are of two distinct types, called outer and inner hair cells because of their location (Fig. 1). Although the total number of cells, approximately 30,000 (Spoendlin, 1972; Harris and Milne, 1966) may be about the same as the total number of cells in amphibian lateral line organs, they are placed in a tonotopic lamina richly supplied with both afferent and efferent nerves. There are said to be about 20 afferent fibers per single inner hair cell, and about 10 outer hair cells per single afferent fiber (Spoendlin, 1972). Thus the inner hair cell system, at least, is not convergent. Efferent terminals are said to be larger and more numerous on the outer hair cell (Wersäll et al., 1965). In most general respects, both afferent and efferent synapses resemble those in other systems mentioned (Smith and Sjöstrand, 1961). Because of the small size of the receptor cells (Fig. 1) and the gross structure and location of the organ of Corti, electrophysiological studies have not provided much information about sensory synapses in this system. There is a considerable amount of histological and pharmacological evidence concerning transmitter chemicals, but most of this pertains to the efferent innervation (see below).

Mammalian Tactile (Hairy Skin) Receptor

Iggo and co-workers (Fjälbrant and Iggo, 1961; Iggo and Muir, 1969) have studied the structure and function of a receptor in the hairy skin of cats that appears to have a synapse between receptor cell and afferent nerve. There is a capsule of supporting cells, and an overlying group of epithelial cells (Fig. 1). Receptor cells lie beneath the epithelial cells, and small tubular processes of receptor cells invaginate the epithelial cells. A single nerve entering the receptor branches and forms a single end plate with each receptor cell. Dense cored vesicles are found in the receptor cell, but are said not to be affected by reserpine treatment (Iggo and Muir, 1969). No presynaptic dense bodies are seen. Mechanical deformation of the receptor from the outside direction produces an irregular discharge of spikes in the afferent nerve. Initial spike frequencies adapt, probably in two phases lasting several seconds, to a tonic level that is said to persist for up to 30 min with continued stimulation. The system is thus tonic, with adaptation, but the structure of the receptor-nerve synapse is different from that of any other system considered here.

Taste

In the taste system of vertebrates, non-neuronal cells are definitely involved in reception, but the rather straightforward picture of receptor cells synapsing with nerve terminals is modified (Murray and Murray, 1960; Uga, 1966; Uga and Hama, 1967; Graziadei, 1969; Murray, 1969; Graziadei and DeHan, 1971; DeHan and Graziadei, 1971). Often several receptor cell types are seen; cells other than receptor cells synapse with nerves, and the synapses are often less distinct. Taste systems in frogs and in mammals have been studied most extensively.

A. Frogs

Taste receptors occur in fungiform papillae (Uga, 1966; Uga and Hama, 1967; Graziadei and DeHan, 1971; DeHan and Graziadei, 1971). These are flat-topped discs, about 100 microns in diameter. Each is bounded by a corona of ciliated cells. The superficial layer is primarily composed of a single type of cuboidal microvillous cell called supporting cells by Uga (1966) and associate cells by Graziadei and DeHan (1971). Beneath this layer is a layer of receptor cells that sends processes up between associate cells to the surface of the papillae, and down to mingle with nerve fiber terminals (Fig. 1). The processes reaching the surface are coupled morphologically by what are said to be gap junctions (Graziadei and DeHan, 1971). Synapses between these cells and nerve terminals are similar to synapses in the CNS; they lack a presynaptic dense body, and have dense cored vesicles. The vesicles are said to be depleted by reserpine and to appear as catecholamine-containing by histological methods (DeHan and Graziadei, 1971). Nonmyelinated nerve fibers also enter the taste papillae; their function is unknown. There are muscle fibers in the base of the papillae which may be able to alter taste function (Graziadei and DeHan, 1971). Frog taste cells have a finite lifetime, and undergo atrophy after nerve section (Robbins, 1967). They and the receptor cells of fish may be somewhat longer lived than vertebrate taste cells (Uga and Hama, 1967).

In fish, taste receptor cells are located more superficially, and form synapses with nerve terminals, but there is also a type of basal cell (Uga, 1966; Uga and Hama, 1967) that synapses with nerve terminals, although it does not send processes to the surface. Uga and Hama (1967) suggest that this cell may modify taste perception, perhaps in the way that the laterally running elements of the retina modify visual perception (see Dowling, *This Volume*).

B. Mammals

Taste reception occurs in taste buds, which are often but not always located in papillae of several sorts (Murray and Murray, 1960; Graziadei, 1969; Murray, 1969). Each bud is 20 to 100 microns in cross section, and composed of supporting cells plus elongated spindle-shaped receptor cells, whose distal (apical) ends have microvilli and contact a central pore (Fig. 1). In the rat, taste cells have a lifetime of about 11 days (Kimura and Beidler, 1961). This may be part of the reason that more than one cell type has been noted (see earlier references, also Fugimoto and Murray, 1970). Any given taste bud appears to contain several cell types; there is disagreement as to whether this primarily represents stages in one cell type, or differentiation of several cell types from one beginning type. Although some investigators have found more synapses than others (compare Murray, 1969, and Graziadei, 1969), it seems certain that there are not only fewer synapses between receptor and nerves than one might expect, but that the synaptic structure seems to be less differentiated. There are no presynaptic dense bodies; vesicles seem to be clear and show erratic clustering. Nerve fibers are often seen in grooves in the taste receptor cells, and often penetrate to very near the surface of the taste bud (Fig. 1).

Fishman (1957) recorded spikes in single afferent nerves connected to mammalian taste buds. There was not much tonic activity in the absence of stimulation, and a single nerve was found to respond to any of the basic four tastes: bitter (quinine), salt (NaCl), sour (HCl), and sweet (sucrose). Afferent nerves to taste buds not only branch to innervate several papillae, but also innervate a number of receptor cells within a given taste bud (Miller, 1971; Rapuzzi and Casella, 1965). This leads to interactions between taste buds (Miller, 1971). Single receptor cells also have been shown to respond to all four tastes in both mammals (Ozeki, 1971) and frogs (Sato, 1969, 1971). If frog taste cells are electrically coupled, single penetrations would *not* record from single cells. In the rat, Ozeki (1971) measured receptor cell membrane resistance as well as potential change. Salt, sour, and sweet stimulation produced a conductance increase, and bitter (quinine) produced a conductance decrease. All four taste stimuli generally produced a depolarizing response, although the reversal potential differed for each stimulus type. Ozeki (1971) suggested that there were, therefore, at least two taste receptive mechanisms; this seems a reasonable interpretation of the results. Resistance changes have not been recorded in other taste cells.

Spike frequency in taste nerves shows adaptation during stimulation (Fishman, 1957). In frogs Sato (1971) found that adaptation was more pronounced for spike frequency than for the receptor potential. In the rat Ozeki (1971) found that adaptation of the receptor potential was more pronounced than adaptation of the receptor conductance change. Thus it seems that adaptation in the taste systems involves several mechanisms.

Because taste stimuli take effect slowly, it is hard to test for a synaptic delay. Nomura and Sakada (1969) report slow potential changes associated with spikes in taste nerves and suggest that the slow potentials are psp's. TTX abolished spikes but did not affect the slow potentials. The results are a little puzzling since (a) the slow potentials did not clearly precede spikes in all cases, and (b) the slow potentials appear as unitary events lasting about 20 to 40 msec during continuous stimulation above threshold.

Beidler (1965) and others have established a semiquantitative relationship between taste stimuli and response. Because this relationship describes adapted responses, and because it holds for both nerve spikes and receptor cell potential changes, it is of little direct use in evaluating synaptic function. The relationship could be used to compare, for example, effects of divalent ions applied topically and intraarterially. This sort of experiment appears not to have been done.

Carotid Body Receptors

The carotid body is a chemoreceptor that monitors the blood supply. Because of its importance in regulation of cardiovascular function, it has been extensively studied; however, there is not yet a clear picture of how it works. At least three types of cell seem to be involved in receptor function (Fig. 1). The glomus or type I cells are complex in shape and are enveloped by the type II cells, which also envelop small nerve fibers. Type I cells contain dense core vesicles; reserpine treatment seems to deplete them. Type I and II cells have cilia, but they are not located at one pole or face of the cell as in accoustico-lateralis systems. Synapses between type I cells and nerve terminals are seen; recent evidence (Biscoe, 1971; Biscoe and Pallot, 1972) indicates that these nerve endings contain vesicles and are probably efferent (sympathetic nerves). A number of thin nerve fibers are seen near both type I and type II cells. Unlike other systems discussed, this receptor is not organized as a laminar epithelium, but as a complex body.

Eyzaguirre, Leitner, Nishi, and Fidone (1970) have studied an *in vitro* preparation of the carotid body and nerve, and have accumulated a large body of data on the effects of various chemicals on spike frequency in the carotid nerve and also slow potentials measured between carotid nerve and body. From these studies they have concluded that type I cells are receptor cells, that there are afferent synapses with nerve terminals, and that the afferent transmitter is ACh. It would not be possible to do justice to their work in a short space. Biscoe has written a critical review. His recent ultrastructural studies led him to conclude that the only synapses between nerves and type I cells are efferent (Biscoe and Pallot, 1972). He also points out some inconsistencies between any hypothesis of afferent transmission and the available physiological data (Biscoe, 1971). He suggests that type I cells may modify direct reception by nerve terminals. However, recordings from cells in the glomus have failed to reveal changes in potential during stimuli that excite afferent nerve spikes (Eyzaguirre et al., 1971) *or* during efferent stimulation (Goodman and McCloskey, 1972). Eyzaguirre et al. (1971) recorded slow potentials between carotid body and nerve by several methods, but the occurrence of such potentials does not necessitate an afferent synapse. It seems to me quite possible that the initial events in reception in this system may not result in a depolarization of either type I or II cells, but rather in some other change. For example, oxygen levels alter the function of the electron transport mechanism of one or more cell types (Mills and Jöbsis, 1972) and this might itself constitute a transduction process (see Biscoe, 1971). At present there is no physiological evidence that afferent synaptic transmission contributes to carotid body chemoreception.

Summary

Based on the preceding brief survey, I think that some generalizations are possible.

(1) In the acoustico-lateralis system and in electroreceptors, receptor

cells make well-formed synapses with nerve terminals in which there are clear presynaptic vesicles associated with dense rods, bars, or ribbons. Synaptic delays are consistent with chemically mediated transmission. Afferent spike frequency may show rapid adaptation, some of which is attributable to the synapse. In several cases, depolarizing psp's can be recorded directly. Many receptor cells contact each nerve (convergence of input).

(2) In hairy skin receptors there is a well-formed, polarized afferent synapse, but vesicles are dense cored, and there are no presynaptic dense bodies. Afferent spikes show a slow adaptation, but physiological evidence is not very revealing concerning the function of the synapse.

(3) In vertebrate taste the picture is even more complex. In frogs, associate cells are located distally to presumed receptor cells, and the receptor cells resemble neurons in that they have both proximal and distal processes. Afferent synapses show dense cored vesicles in the receptor cells, and no presynaptic dense bodies. In fish there are apparently non-receptor basal cells that also synapse with nerve terminals and that may modify reception. Single receptor cells respond to all four basic tastes; in mammals at least two receptor cell mechanisms seem to be involved. Many receptor cells may contact one nerve. Synapses between taste cells and nerves in mammals are indefinite, perhaps because the taste cells have a lifetime of about 11 days, and seem to undergo considerable change in structure during this short lifetime. More than one basic type of taste cell may occur. Physiologically, a synapse is indicated, at least in frogs, by a different rate of adaptation of nerve spike frequency and receptor potentials, and by what may be psp's.

(4) Morphological and physiological evidence concerning function of the carotid body does not allow one to make any firm statements at this time. If afferent synapses are involved, they may utilize mechanisms that are very different from those in the other systems considered.

At this point, I will turn to studies on electroreceptors that were intended to clarify the function of the afferent synapse.

II. STUDIES ON SYNAPTIC TRANSMISSION IN ELECTRORECEPTORS

Teleost Electroreceptors

Most studies of electroreceptors have utilized intact fish (see Bennett, 1967, 1971*a,b* for reviews). This favors survival of the receptor system, but makes it difficult to change the chemical composition of solutions. We made a semi-isolated preparation from Mormyrid fish, consisting of a piece of skin carrying many receptors, and then teased out nerves to single receptors (Fig. 4) (Steinbach and Bennett, 1971). Using extracellular

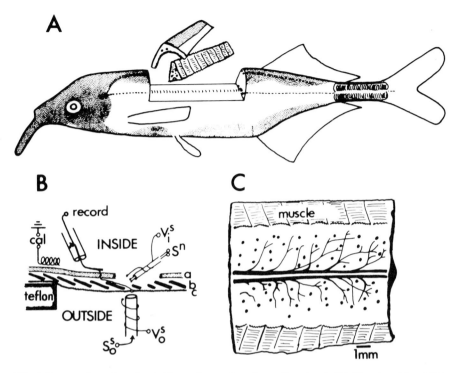

FIG. 4. Preparation of excised skin and receptors from *G. petersii.* (A) Chunk cut from the dorsal surface that includes an area of skin bearing electroreceptors (stippled areas) and both dorsal and medial pairs of lateral line nerves (dotted lines). The electric organ is in the caudal region as indicated. (B) Simplified side view of a portion of the preparation pinned over a window cut in the Teflon bottom of the experimental chamber. Three layers of skin shown are (a) fascia, (b) scales, and (c) epidermis. Fascia and scales are removed over a receptor. The nerve bundle containing the fiber(s) to the receptor studied is picked up to record impulses relative to the indifferent electrode in the bath. The transskin potential produced by stimuli applied between a second indifferent electrode (not shown) and the capillary on the external surface of the skin (S_o^s) is measured by Ag-AgCl electrodes ($V_s = V_o^s - V_i^s$). A bipolar electrode (S^n) is used to stimulate nerves directly. (C) Drawing of the inside of excised skin that was flattened following removal of attached muscle; d.l.l. nerves and branches to receptors (black dots) are shown (from Steinbach and Bennett, 1971).

electrodes, we recorded afferent spikes, but were unable to record psp's (Fig. 5). Our failure is not too surprising considering the relatively small area of postsynaptic membrane involved. We were able to directly stimulate nerve terminals with focal electrodes (Fig. 4) and thus could compare effects of solution changes on the nerve spikes produced by receptor stimulation (we called these synaptically evoked responses) and those produced by nerve stimulation (called directly evoked responses) (Fig. 5). We confirmed (see Bennett, 1967) a synaptic delay of about 0.7 msec in medium receptors, and a delay of about 0.25 msec in large receptors. Threshold for synaptically evoked responses in medium electroreceptors was greatly increased by

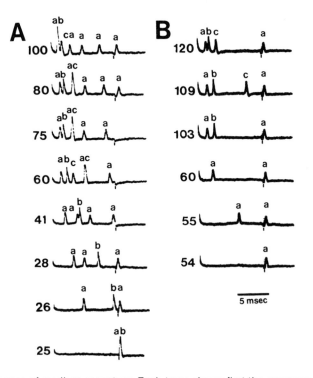

FIG. 5. Responses of medium receptors. Each trace shows first the response to a 2-msec rectangular pulse applied across the skin (amplitude in millivolts is shown by the number to the left of the trace). The records begin with termination of the stimulus. Also shown on each trace is the response to direct stimulation of the afferent nerve (artifact indicated under each trace). The synaptically evoked response involved impulses in three fibers, designated *a, b,* and *c,* as indicated by examination of records in both (A) and (B). The directly evoked response was adjusted to involve only fiber *a.* (A) Response in physiological saline (3.0 mM Ca^{+2} and 1.5 mM Mg^{+2}) after treatment with excess Mg^{+2} and washing. Fibers *a* and *b* were first excited at about the same stimulus strength; fiber *c* required stronger stimulation. All fibers responded at shorter latency as stimulus strength was increased; the response of fiber *a* also increased in number of impulses. The directly evoked response was blocked by closely preceding impulses in fiber *a* (traces 41, 60, 75), but not in fiber *b* (trace 26). (B) Records in saline with 15 mM Mg^{+2} and 3.0 mM Ca^{+2} taken before (A). Compared to records in (A), threshold was increased (from 26 to 55 mV, approximately) and number of impulses in fiber *a* was reduced to one without change in minimum impulse delay (from Steinbach and Bennett, 1971).

raising external Mg (Figs. 5 and 6). Lowering external Ca produced a decrease in apparent threshold (the opposite expected if transmission requires Ca), which could be attributed to increased nerve excitability. High levels of Mg and ostensibly zero Ca did not completely block synaptically evoked responses; we felt that either a part of transmission was not Mg sensitive or that Mg might partially substitute for Ca. We tested the effects of several chemicals, and found that L-glutamic acid, L-aspartic acid, and homocysteic

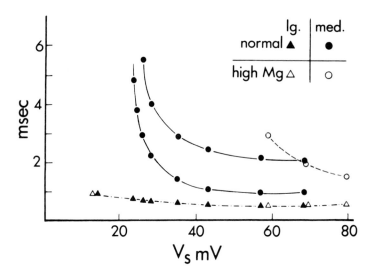

FIG. 6. Effects of high Mg^{+2} on synaptically evoked response. Abscissa, stimulus strength (V_s); ordinate, latency in milliseconds for impulses in a single fiber. Filled symbols: 3.0 mM Ca^{+2}, 1.5 mM Mg^{+2}, open symbols: 3.0 mM Ca^{+2}, 15 mM Mg^{+2}, 25 min after solution changes; round symbols: impulses from a medium receptor (in normal saline two impulses were evoked by stimuli just above threshold); triangular symbols: impulses from a large receptor. High Mg^{+2} had no effect on the responses of the large receptor but raised the threshold and reduced the number of impulses in responses of the medium receptor. A stimulus larger than 80 mV in high Mg^{+2} presumably would have reduced the latency of the medium receptor response (see Fig. 5) (from Steinbach and Bennett, 1971).

acid could reversibly alter synaptically evoked responses (Fig. 7). However, the concentrations we used were in the 10^{-3} M range. We also found that shortly after the beginning of a glutamate treatment, directly evoked responses became depressed for a few minutes. They then returned to normal threshold, while synaptically evoked responses remained blocked (Fig. 8). We interpreted this sequence of events as depression following the large initial depolarization of the spike generating region, and later repolarization and recovery of electrical excitability during desensitization. Synaptically evoked responses from large receptors were only slightly altered by any of the treatments mentioned (Fig. 6), which we took as a further indication of electrically mediated transmission.

From our studies of Mormyrid medium electroreceptors, we concluded that (1) receptor excitation (depolarization of the inner face) produces a release of chemical transmitter, (2) the release is decreased but perhaps not completely eliminated by Mg, and (3) the transmitter chemical is probably related to the L- form of a dicarboxylic amino acid, perhaps L-glutamic acid. We did not record psp's directly, and were not able to establish that transmission required calcium.

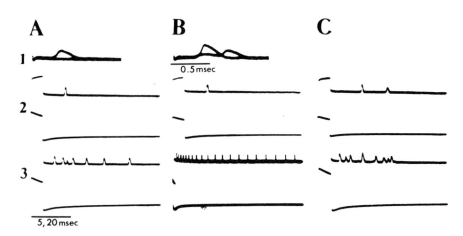

FIG. 7. Effect of 0.5 mM L-glutamate on responses of a medium receptor: (A) normal saline, (B) 30 sec after perfusing with 0.5 mM L-glutamate, (C) 7 min after perfusing with 0.5 mM L-glutamate. *1,* Directly evoked response (in B1 there are signs of separate components, perhaps due to nodes of Ranvier). *2* and *3,* Upper trace: synaptically evoked responses; lower trace: stimulating voltage. Stimulation was near threshold in *2* and suprathreshold in *3.* Time calibrations, 20 msec for B3, 5 msec for A2, A3, B2, C2, and C3, 0.5 msec for A1 and B1. This concentration of L-glutamate produced a transient hyperexcitability and reduced threshold. The directly evoked response after 7-min perfusion (C1) is not shown; it was normal but a suitable photograph was not taken during the experiment (from Steinbach and Bennett, 1971).

Skate Ampullae of Lorenzini

During the past two summers I have studied skate ampullae *in vitro.* Previous work had already revealed a good deal of information related to synaptic function.

(a) Current passing *outward* across the receptor cell layer (from basal to apical faces, see Fig. 1) stimulates receptor cells and synaptic transmission (Murray, 1965*a,b;* Obara and Bennett, 1972). Apparently there is a regenerative depolarizing response in the receptor cells involving the outer (apical) faces (Waltman, 1968; Obara and Bennett, 1972). This activity depolarizes the inner faces and leads to the release of transmitter. Very strong stimuli of the opposite polarity (inward current) can also cause a depolarizing psp which can be explained by assuming that the stimuli directly depolarize the inner faces and cause them to release transmitter.

(b) There are usually tonic spikes in afferent nerves studied *in vivo.* They are probably caused by tonic transmitter release, as a result of sporadic, or perhaps periodic, depolarizing activity of the outer faces of the receptor cells (Obara and Bennett, 1972). Because of the extreme convergence of input (several hundred to a thousand receptor cells synapse with branches of five to eight nerve fibers), the contributions of single synapses are not

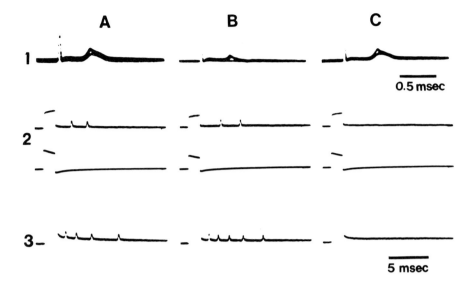

FIG. 8. Effect of 2 mM L-glutamate on responses of a medium receptor: (A) normal saline, (B) 30 sec after perfusing with L-glutamate, except for direct response (B1) taken after synaptically evoked responses had failed, about 3 min after beginning perfusion, (C) after 7-min perfusion. *1*, Directly evoked responses, note second small fiber excited by slight increase in stimulus in A and C; only the small fiber was excited in B. *2*, Upper trace: synaptically evoked responses; lower trace: stimulating voltage near threshold (7 mV for A2, lower for B2). *3*, Synaptically evoked response at about five times threshold. The second fiber in the direct response did not respond synaptically nor was it affected by glutamate, perhaps because its receptor was covered by connective tissue or was not functionally connected to its synaptic region. This concentration of L-glutamate first reduced the threshold for synaptic excitation, then blocked both synaptic and direct excitation. During continued perfusion the directly evoked response returned, but synaptically evoked responses did not recover (from Steinbach and Bennett, 1971).

resolved. Spike frequency in the afferent nerve is linearly related to stimulus strength over a considerable range (Murray, 1965*a,b*).

(c) Depolarizing and hyperpolarizing psp's can be recorded with intra-cellular micropipettes from nerve fibers in response to receptor stimulation (Obara and Bennett, 1972).

The preparation I studied consisted of a short length of ampullary canal, the alveoli containing the receptor cells, and a short length of nerve. The canal was electrically isolated with a suction pipette. Presynaptic recording and stimulation using a bridge circuit was thus possible. Postsynaptic responses were recorded with a second suction pipette. The waveform of the relatively low-amplitude, "extracellular" responses thus obtained closely resembled the intracellular recordings of Obara and Bennett (Fig. 9). Skate saline contained NaCl 245 mM, KCl 3 mM, urea 350 mM, dextrose 5 mM, and TRIS 5 mM adjusted to pH 7.2 to 7.6. Divalent ion concentration was varied in many experiments, usually in the range Ca 0 to 10 mM and

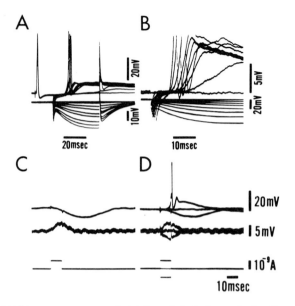

FIG. 9. Postsynaptic responses recorded intracellularly from single afferent fibers in the ampulla of Lorenzini of the skate. First trace: intracellular recording. Second trace: potential across the receptor cell layer (recorded lumen negativity down). Third trace (omitted in A and B): stimulating current (recorded outward down). (A) An antidromic spike precedes the responses to graded outward current pulses (superimposed sweeps). Increasing stimulus strength evokes psp's that shorten in latency and increase in amplitude until a spike is evoked. (B) As in A but at higher gain and faster sweep speed. (C) From a different preparation. An inward current pulse evokes a hyperpolarization of the nerve. (D) Superposition of equal amplitude inward and outward pulses. The outward pulse evokes a depolarizing psp and spike.

Mg 0 to 30 mM. The drugs used were obtained commercially, made up in concentrated form, and diluted shortly before use. Acidic amino acids were brought to neutral pH with NaOH. Solution changes took a few seconds because the bath had a volume of 0.5 ml, but equilibration at synapses seemed to take longer. Most experiments were made at 21°C; temperature was sometimes decreased with precooled solutions.

The general form of response is indicated in Fig. 10. An outward current across the receptor epithelium (from basal to apical faces of the cells) produced a depolarizing psp; inward current produced a hyperpolarizing psp. The receptor cells generated a response when stimulated with outward current (Obara and Bennett, 1972). In many experiments, spikes in the nerve were eliminated with TTX (10^{-5} to 10^{-7} w/v; Fig. 11). TTX did not alter psp's or the presynaptic response.

A. The Hyperpolarizing psp

Hyperpolarizing psp's presumably result from a decrease of transmitter release. DC current inward across the receptor cell layer reduces pre-

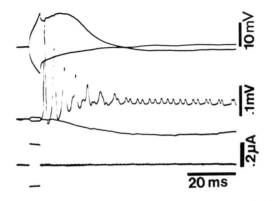

FIG. 10. Responses in the ampullae of Lorenzini recorded and evoked using extracellular electrodes (see text). Top trace: voltage recorded across the presynaptic cell layer (lumen positivity upward). Middle trace: response of the afferent nerve (terminal depolarization upward). Bottom trace: current applied across the receptor epithelium (outward, excitatory recorded downward). Two sweeps are superimposed. The postsynaptic response to outward current was the depolarizing psp and superimposed spikes, and to inward current the hyperpolarizing psp of slower time course. The receptor cells produced a regenerative response to outward current.

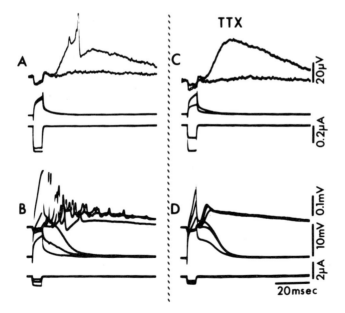

FIG. 11. TTX eliminates spikes but does not affect the psp in skate ampullae. Each set of records shows the psp (top trace), potential across the presynaptic cell layer (middle traces), and stimulating current (bottom traces, outward current downward). A, B: Responses to near threshold (A) and larger (B) stimuli in saline with Ca 3 mM, Mg 3 mM. B and C responses to similar stimuli after adding TTX 10^{-6}M. Note transient phase of psp produced by strong stimuli. Calibrations as shown, lower gains in B and D except for middle traces. Several superimposed sweeps in each record.

synaptic regenerative activity and eliminates the hyperpolarizing response. DC inward current also increases the apparent threshold of the depolarizing psp. In most experiments it was found that such a DC "holding" stimulus prolonged the viability of the preparation. Exhaustion (or, at least, a long-lasting depression of response) could be produced by outward DC current.

B. The Depolarizing psp

At least partly because electrical insulation of the ampullary canal was not perfect leading to reduction in recorded potentials, thresholds measured in the experiments reported here varied from less than 1 mV to greater than 10 mV. Moreover, the term "threshold" is a tricky one to use in this context. The membrane potentials of single receptor cells were clearly not under control, since the effective stimulus was an outward current that usually evoked oscillations and regenerative presynaptic activity. An obvious regenerative response was not required for the production of a psp, and in general there was no consistent relationship between amplitude of the presynaptic regenerative response and psp amplitude. In many cases the psp peak preceded the presynaptic response peak. Nevertheless, presynaptic regenerative responses presumably gave rise to the postsynaptic activity (Obara and Bennett, 1972). I shall use threshold to refer to the recorded presynaptic voltage deflection at which the first sign of a psp was seen. The threshold of a single receptor cell is not known at present.

Using brief pulses, the time between onset of an outward stimulus and the initial rise of a psp was 10 to 15 msec at threshold, decreasing to about 5 msec at two to three times threshold. The long latency reflects the time constant of the receptor cell layer and the delay in outer face activation, as well as the conventional synaptic delay (Obara and Bennett, 1972 and unpublished). Psp duration at threshold was governed by a 10 to 15 msec rise time and a comparable half-time of fall. There was considerable variation in both parameters from preparation to preparation. Solution changes did not generally alter the duration of threshold psp's. With stronger stimuli, psp amplitude increased, and, in general, two phases of the psp could be distinguished: an initial fast transient phase and a later prolonged phase which sometimes declined into a hyperpolarizing phase (see Figs. 11 and 12). In part this was an effect of the AC recording system used, but similar psp's were seen using a DC system. The cause of the later hyperpolarizing phase is not clear. The occurrence of two depolarizing phases of the psp might be the result of either pre- or postsynaptic processes, or both. In an effort to resolve this point, solution temperature was lowered to between 5° and 8°C. During temperature decrease, the initial transient amplitude remained stable or increased slightly, while the prolonged phase decreased steadily. At low temperature the threshold for eliciting a detectable psp was decreased (Fig. 12). At threshold, the psp's elicited consisted of brief

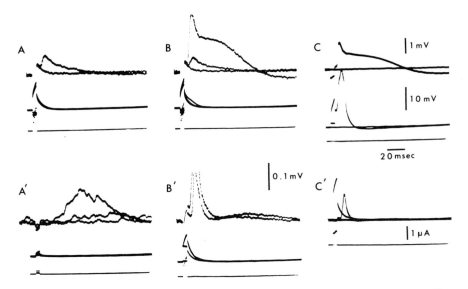

FIG. 12. Low temperature greatly alters the psp in skate ampullae. Records similar to Fig. 11, but outward current (bottom traces) is upward. TTX was present. A–C. Responses to increasingly large stimuli at 21°C. A'–C'. Similar stimuli at 5 to 7°C. A, A'. Responses to near threshold stimuli. B, B'. Responses to stronger stimuli. C, C'. Responses to very large stimuli. In C', pre- and postsynaptic response traces are brought to common baseline. Calibrations as shown; the postsynaptic gain is lower in C, C'.

and asynchronous "lumps." Spontaneous lumps were also seen (Fig. 12A'). With stronger stimuli, the asynchronous lumps built up into a brief synchronous transient whose amplitude was similar to the transient at room temperature. A prolonged phase, if present, was always very small (Figs. 12 and 18). Warming reversed these effects. The effects seem difficult to explain unless one postulates either a fairly dramatic change in release function with stimulus strength, or two release processes.

In response to a long stimulus pulse, synaptic delays could be as long as 40 to 60 msec at threshold. Threshold levels were always less for long pulses compared to short pulses. Because an AC amplifier (low-frequency time constant 1 sec) was routinely used, the duration of very long-lasting psp's was usually not determined accurately. When a DC system was used, instabilities interfered with long-term recording, but psp's showed little adaptation for long-lasting low-amplitude stimulation. With stronger stimuli (two to three times threshold) a transient similar to that seen with short pulses developed. In some cases several such transients could be evoked; they were usually seen to follow presynaptic oscillations.

C. The Depolarizing psp Results from a Conductance Increase

In several experiments an AC bridge (1 to 2 kHz stimulus frequency) and band pass filter system were used to test for a postsynaptic conductance change during the psp. In successful experiments a conductance increase was measured. This change appeared to have a duration similar to that of the psp (Fig. 13), although series resistance in the system made accurate determinations impossible due to low signals and instability. The conductance increase was eliminated by raised Mg solutions that eliminated the psp (see below). The presence of a conductance increase is also indicated by reduction in antidromic spikes superimposed on the psp's (Obara and Bennett, 1972).

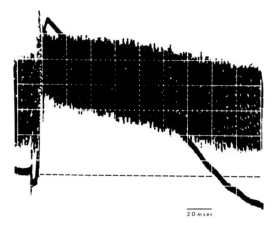

20 msec

FIG. 13. A conductance increase accompanies the psp. The wide fuzzy line is the partially balanced output of an AC bridge with a 1,500 Hz stimulating frequency and a high pass filter. The other trace is the unfiltered output of the bridge, showing the waveform of the psp that is filtered to give the high gain record. Note a decrease in width of the fuzzy line during the psp, which with this bridge setting indicated a conductance increase of less than 1 kΩ (or about .3% imbalance).

D. The psp Is Blocked by Mg

Mg at any concentration had the effect of raising threshold (Fig. 14, Table 1). If Ca was also raised, threshold could be partially maintained. The threshold for direct stimulation of nerve spikes, tested with a brief large inward current stimulus, remained nearly constant (Fig. 14). The apparent antagonism of Ca and Mg had a limited range. Mg above 10 mM increased psp threshold and reduced maximum amplitude, and this effect could not be antagonized by raised Ca concentration. At 20 to 30 mM Mg, psp's were reduced to less than 10% initial amplitude (Table 1). The small response sometimes remaining had a brief duration, regardless of stimulus strength, and a brief latency (Fig. 15). It only occurred following strong stimulation that produced a regenerative presynaptic response. More Mg, or less Ca, did not progressively affect this residual psp. It may be an electrically transmitted potential, although the delay (about 5 msec) seems

TABLE 1. *Effect of divalent ions on threshold and maximum psp amplitude (ampulla of Lorenzini)*

		Ca = 4.0 mM		Ca = 8.0 mM	
	Mg	T(mV)	PSP(μV)	T(mV)	PSP(μV)
A.	0	1.3	110		
	1	2.1	110		
	4	2.6	60	2.2	80
	8	4.0	10		
	20	7.1	8	4.9	8
	40	7.0	7		

		Mg = 1.0 mM	
B.	Ca	T(mV)	PSP(μV)
	EGTA	—	0
	0	6.1	30
	1	3.2	70
	8	3.0	80
	20	4.0	40

T = threshold in mV for 5 msec duration outward current pulse. PSP = maximum amplitude of psp (in μV) measured 15 msec after onset of 3 to 5 × T stimulus. In both experiments, amplitude and threshold values are interpolated using first and last records in the same solution, to correct for deterioration. A. Effect of Mg at two different Ca concentrations. Deterioration not more than 30% of initial response. B. Effect of Ca. Deterioration not more than 20% of initial response.

too long. Since Mg-resistant, synaptically evoked responses were observed in teleost electroreceptors, it is possible that a component of transmission in this system is also Mg insensitive. Alternatively, the Ca required for transmission at a very low level may already be inside receptor cells. The lack of a progressive effect of Mg on the residual psp argues against the possibility that Mg substitutes for Ca as a facilitator of transmission.

In three experiments, lanthanum (La) was added to the saline. In all respects La seemed to act similarly to Mg, but 1 mM La was about as effective as 8 mM Mg.

E. The psp Requires Ca

Reduction of Ca in the external saline produced an increase in threshold and a decrease in maximum psp amplitude. If TTX was not present, transmission (measured as threshold for excitation of a postsynaptic spike) often decreased in threshold, because threshold for direct excitability of

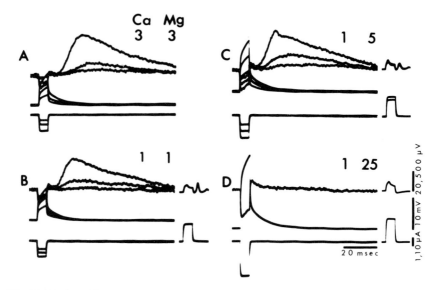

FIG. 14. Mg ions block transmission. Each set of records is arranged similarly to Fig. 11 (positive outward current down). The insets at the ends of records in B–D show nerve spikes directly evoked by large stimuli (lower voltage and current gains). The nerve responses occur at the beginning of the pulses; the responses after the pulses are synaptically evoked. The concentrations of Ca and Mg are shown by numbers above and to the right of each set of records. Increasing Mg raised the threshold of and then blocked the psp, but the threshold of the nerve to direct stimulation was increased only slightly.

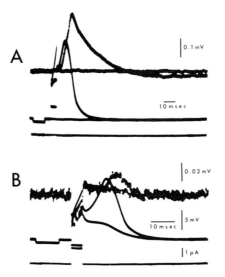

FIG. 15. There is a small residual psp after going to high Mg. Records are similar to Fig. 12. (A) Psp and regenerative presynaptic response in saline with Ca 3mM, Mg 1 mM. (B) Residual psp and presynaptic response in saline with Ca O and Mg 15 mM. (Note the more rapid sweep speed.) The residual psp was not progressively affected by more concentrated Mg, nor by addition of L-glutamic acid (see text).

the nerve decreased, as in Mormyrid electroreceptors (Steinbach and Bennett, 1971). In healthy preparations psp's were not eliminated simply by removing Ca from the saline. A saline with 0 Ca, normal or elevated Mg, and 5 mM EGTA completely eliminated psp's. During the early phases of this treatment, direct excitation thresholds of the nerve were decreased only slightly, but this gave way to a general depression, and recovery of the preparation was poor (often nonexistent). Lowering Ca from 5 to 1 mM only slightly increased threshold of the psp; threshold also increased somewhat with increasing Ca (Fig. 16). Above 5 mM, addition of Ca tended to prolong both threshold and suprathreshold psp's, although not in every experiment (Fig. 16). If left in the bath for more than a few minutes, such solutions irreversibly depressed psp amplitude (Table 1). The cause of this effect is not clear, but it may relate to the marginal viability of the preparation and to the small size of the cells involved.

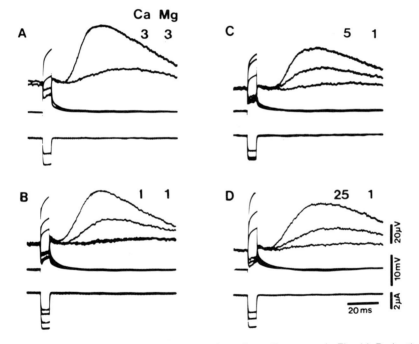

FIG. 16. Ca ions facilitate transmission. Records and notation are as in Fig. 14. Reduction of Ca below 3 mM increases threshold slightly. Increase of Ca above 3 mM also increases threshold slightly.

F. Lithium Substitutes for Na Postsynaptically

In several experiments Li was substituted for 10 to 100% of Na in the saline. If the presynaptic cell layer was not subjected to a DC inward "holding" current, Li initially increased psp amplitude by 10 to 20% in rough proportion to the amount substituted, and then eliminated presynaptic regenerative responses and psp's irreversibly. In experiments where a holding current was used, only the enhancement occurred. These results are consistent with the hypothesis that Li can substitute for Na as a charge carrier of the postsynaptic current producing the psp, but that Li is detrimental to the function of the receptor cells, perhaps because it leaks into the cells and is not pumped out. Monitoring of the receptor cell membrane potential would be required to test this hypothesis.

G. L-*Form Dicarboxylic Amino Acids Mimic Transmitter Action*

In most preparations the smallest psp that could be evoked by receptor stimulation was about 10 μV in amplitude. Depolarizations of greater amplitude but much slower time course could be evoked by the addition of 10^{-5} L-glutamic acid to the saline (Fig. 17). Using a DC recording system, such depolarizations were found to be of long duration, and could be at least partially reversed by removal of L-glutamic acid. In three experiments the mean depolarization produced was increased by 10 to 30% when psp's had been blocked by 30 mM Mg. The increase may not have been

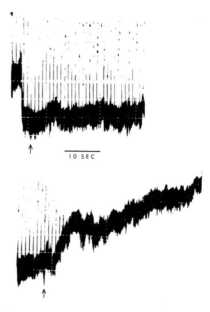

FIG. 17. L-Glutamic acid causes postsynaptic depolarization. In each record the thick trace is a high gain DC recording from the nerve bundle; a 50-μV calibration pulse is shown at the beginning of the upper record. The brief upward strokes are psp's. In the upper record, 10^{-3}M alpha ketoglutaric acid was added at the arrow and produced no effect. In the lower record, 10^{-5}M L-glutamic acid was added (arrow) which caused a depolarization and elimination of the psp's (responses to a larger stimulus could still be elicited, but are not shown). Drift in the recording system makes it difficult to quantify such results.

significant, but it is interesting that L-glutamic acid depolarized postsynaptic elements after synaptic transmission was blocked. L-Aspartic and homocysteic acid in comparable concentrations also produced depolarization of nerve terminals. L-Aspartic acid was about $1/3$ as effective as L-glutamic acid. The relative effectiveness of homocysteic acid was not determined accurately. D-glutamic acid was not observed to cause depolarization at concentrations up to 10^{-4} M. At concentrations above 10^{-4} M, both D- and L-glutamic acid reversibly eliminated psp's (Fig. 18) leaving only the small residual psp mentioned earlier (Fig. 15). In the range 5×10^{-6} to 10^{-5} M, both D and L forms altered psp amplitude and waveform. L-Glutamic acid depressed the prolonged phase of the psp more than D-glutamic acid at the same concentration. Both slight increases and slight decreases in threshold were recorded. DOPA at 5×10^{-4} M caused a slight transient increase in psp amplitude, but did not cause depolarization. Alpha ketoglutaric acid (Fig. 17), gamma amino butyric acid, glycine, acetylcholine, gallamine (Flaxedil®), atropine, and noradrenaline had no reproducible effects at 1 to 2×10^{-3} M.

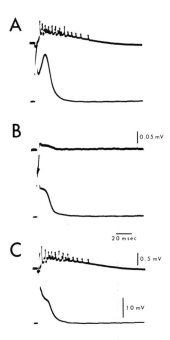

FIG. 18. L-Glutamic acid can reversibly block transmission. In this experiment (A) a preparation giving a psp (upper trace) and regenerative presynaptic response (lower trace) in response to above threshold stimulation (current amplitude not shown) was treated with 0.5 mM L-glutamic acid which eliminated the psp (B). It was then returned to saline without L-glutamic acid. Transmission recovered in about 4 min (C). Note the progressive deterioration in the presynaptic regenerative response without effect on the psp. Postsynaptic gain is higher in B.

Direct evidence for a conductance increase was not obtained, but in experiments where L-glutamic acid was added to preparations showing a tonic spike activity (Fig. 19), spike amplitudes were decreased during the onset of L-glutamic acid action. Direct evidence for a desensitization of the depolarizing effect of L-glutamate (i.e., a decrease in depolarization during continued application of the chemical) was not obtained which is ascribable to instability of the recording system. In preparations where evoked psp's were largely eliminated by L-glutamate, threshold for electrical excitation of the nerve terminal was initially increased, and later returned to near normal. This provides indirect evidence that desensitization occurs.

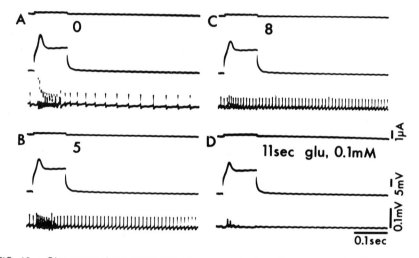

FIG. 19. L-Glutamate alters tonic spike frequency in the afferent nerve. In these records, stimulating current is monitored in the top trace, presynaptic voltage in the middle trace, and postsynaptic activity in the bottom trace for each group. The number beginning with 0 in A refers to time after addition of 10^{-4}M L-glutamic acid to the bath. In this preparation tonic activity was increased in frequency and finally eliminated (as was the psp) by the treatment. The decreasing amplitude of the spikes suggests that postsynaptic membrane conductance was shunted by the action of L-glutamic acid.

H. Discussion of Results

Synaptic transmission in ampullae of Lorenzini of the skate is chemically mediated. Synaptic delays can be made as short as 1 msec by strong stimuli (Obara and Bennett, 1972); they are usually as long as 10 msec because of the complexity of the events leading to presynaptic release. Psp's evoked by two to three times threshold stimuli have an initial transient and later prolonged phase. The transient may not be a physiologically significant event, since brief strong stimuli that synchronize all receptor cells probably do not occur *in vivo*, due to the filtering effect of the ampullary canal impedance (see discussion by Bennett, 1971a). However, the fact that a transient phase can be produced suggests that the release mechanism may be complex. At low temperature, threshold psp's appear to be composed of long latency, asynchronous, but brief "lumps" of depolarization (Fig. 12). Threshold is lowered. Since Sands's 1938 paper it has been known that lowering temperature produced an increase in afferent spike frequency (see Murray, 1965a,b). The effect is probably presynaptic, and almost undoubtedly on the receptor outer face, since the thresholds for psp's evoked by strong inward current did not seem to be decreased. The noise in the threshold responses may represent the contributions of single receptor cells, but there is no obvious reason why they should be larger at low temperature. Stronger stimuli at low temperature have the effect of synchronizing the psp into a transient. The time course and amplitude of this transient closely resemble those of the early phase of the psp at room temperature (Fig. 12). Thus with strong stimuli, release appears to be dominated by a process that is relatively temperature insensitive. Perhaps low temperature enhances outer face sensitivity and slows down the release process (thus producing the asynchronous threshold psp) and also decreases the amount of transmitter available (thus the effect of a strong stimulus that synchronizes release is to release all available transmitter in a brief transient; there is none left to produce a prolonged phase). How strong stimuli manage to override the hypothetical slowdown in release is not clear. The transient phase, both at room and cold temperatures, might be the result of a large influx of Ca presynaptically (Katz and Miledi, 1969). Perhaps examination of the morphology of synapses fixed in the cold may give some clue to what is happening.

The chemically mediated transmission in skate ampullae requires Ca and is depressed by Mg. The divalent ion effects are probably presynaptic in locus because Ca and Mg in the range used do not greatly alter nerve excitability, and Mg does not depress postsynaptic depolarization by L-glutamate. Ca in excess of 1 to 3 mM does not appear to further enhance transmission. There is no evidence that Mg can facilitate synaptic transmission, although a small component of transmission may be Mg insensitive.

The chemically mediated transmission in skate ampullae is probably mediated by a transmitter chemically related to L-glutamic acid. This chemical applied exogenously alters psp's, and can produce postsynaptic depolarization even when transmission is blocked presynaptically by high Mg. The concentration range (about 10^{-5} M) required for these effects is comparable to the concentration of glutamic or aspartic acids in skate CSF or plasma, as determined by amino acid analysis of these fluids (E. Kaneshiro and A. Steinbach, *unpublished results*). Preliminary studies indicate that skate ampullae can take up exogenous glutamic acid (M. Dowdall and A. Steinbach, *unpublished*). The effects of L-glutamic acid are specific in the sense that the D-form can alter psp's but does not seem to cause depolarization, and in that a range of other chemicals known to alter synaptic transmission in other systems do not have comparable effects. The effect is nonspecific in the sense that L-aspartic and homocysteic acids produce effects comparable to L-glutamic acid. Further studies may be able to identify the various components of a mechanism for handling a dicarboxylic amino acid transmitter, and may lead to an identification of the physiological transmitter chemical(s).

III. THE GENERAL PHYSIOLOGY OF RECEPTOR-NERVE SYNAPSES

At least in the acoustico-lateralis-electroreceptor systems, there is good evidence for chemically mediated afferent synaptic transmission. Synaptic delays of 0.5 msec or greater are the rule. In fish S1 nerves, which are afferent from hair cells in the saccular macula, there is a low-amplitude potential that is presumably the result of a primitive form of electrical transmission across extracellular space; this phenomenon is probably not important for *in vivo* function (Ishii et al., 1971a,b). In contrast to this example of relatively weak electrical transmission, the major mode of synaptic coupling between "large" electroreceptors in Mormyrids and sensory nerves appears to be electrically mediated (Steinbach and Bennett, 1971; Bennett, 1971a). The relatively large area of contact (the chalice synapses) between afferent nerves and receptors in the bottle type vestibular receptors of birds and mammals may also facilitate electrical transmission (Wersäll et al., 1965).

In all receptor afferent nerve synapses of the acoustico-lateralis-electroreceptor system, a presynaptic dense body lies in the receptor cell near the synapse. The function of this element is obscure (see Dowling, *This Volume*). The presynaptic dense body is not a consequence of tonic transmitter-release requirements, since it occurs in phasic electroreceptors (Bennett, 1971a) and nontonic vestibular hair cells of fish (Hama, 1969). It may be useful in prolonged or repetitive synaptic activation. Perhaps further studies of such structures in "fatigued" preparations may be helpful.

Evidence for quantal transmission in sensory synapses is not yet very good (see Bennett, 1971a). Psp's in the goldfish S1 nerves fluctuate in amplitude, and the fluctuation is most extreme for low-amplitude stimuli (Ishii et al., 1971a). Analysis of the fluctuation according to the hypothesis that a "quantal" Poisson process is involved gives somewhat ambiguous results; the analysis correctly predicts the data in some cases and does not in others (Ishii et al., 1971a). Since many receptor cells synapse with a single S1 nerve (Hama, 1969), the quanta observed may represent single synapses rather than single release events (see below).

In both medium electroreceptors of Mormyrids and ampullae of Lorenzini, transmission is at least largely blocked by high Mg, and in the skate preparation, a requirement for Ca has been demonstrated. Comparable experiments are needed in other preparations. Efferent control in *Xenopus* lateral line receptors requires Ca (Russell, 1968). The fact that removal of Ca did not abolish afferent spikes is not necessarily surprising, since there is a component of transmitter release in motor synapses that seems not to require Ca (Katz, 1969).

Not much can be said about release mechanisms in sensory synapses. Psp's in fish S1 nerves are very brief. Psp's in the ampullae of Lorenzini of skate can be very long lasting. Synapses contribute to adaptation to long-lasting stimuli in taste systems (Uzeki, 1971; Sato, 1971) but it is not known whether this reflects adaptation in release or in the various postsynaptic mechanisms.

Receptor cells are very sensitive to effective stimuli (see, for example, Bennett's review, 1971*a*). Much of this sensitivity is a result of the way in which stimuli are relayed to the receptor cells. For example, although electric fish can detect 10-μV gradients in external voltage, the voltage changes across receptors are more likely to be in millivolts (see Bennett, 1971*a*). Very small receptor potentials have been recorded intracellularly from *Necturus* lateral line receptor cells (Harris et al., 1970). However, cell damage is likely, and the receptor potentials in intact cells may be larger. Weak electric stimuli appear to act as receptor potentials in *Kryptop-terus* electroreceptors as well as other tonic electroreceptors (Bennett, 1971*a,b*). Although external recording makes this unlikely, damage during intracellular recording possibly obscures an active response that makes the actual presynaptic potential larger. At the moment, there is no accurate estimate of the exact relationship between a change in receptor cell potential and the change in postsynaptic nerve terminal potential.

Considering the general input-output relationships at sensory synapses (usually this means stimulus strength versus spike frequency; psp amplitudes have been measured accurately in fish S1 nerves and less accurately in ampullae of Lorenzini), there is a general finding of linearity over a certain range (Murray, 1965*a,b;* Harris and Milne, 1966; Bennett, 1971*a,b;* Ishii et al., 1971*b*). The relationship of input to output over a wider range is not linear in taste systems (see Beidler, 1962; Kimura and Beidler, 1961), but the relationship is the same whether nerve spikes or receptor potentials are considered to be output, and thus this finding does not relate to the function of afferent synapses. Input-output over a wider range of stimuli are also nonlinear in electroreceptors (Murray, 1965*a,b;* Bennett, 1971*a,b*), and it is not known whether this involves the synapse.

Motor synapses do not exhibit such linearity starting from what seems to be a normal presynaptic potential (Kusano, 1970). A depolarization of 10 to 30 mV is required before any evoked release occurs, and then the relationship is only linear in the middle range of a general sigmoidal rela-tionship between pre- and postsynaptic potential. In the linear range, however, motor synapses are quite sensitive – a 12-mV presynaptic change causes a 10-fold change in postsynaptic potential (Kusano, 1970). If one imagines a motor synapse presynaptically biased so that the normal pre-synaptic potential is held in the middle of the general sigmoidal relation-ship, the situation might closely resemble that at sensory synapses.

Presynaptic biasing may help to achieve input-output linearity, but can also serve other functions. Some electroreceptors of electric fish are tuned to respond to the discharge of the fish's electric organ. They are thus part of an active system (Bennett, 1971a) and often have a relatively high threshold *and* a roughly linear and very sensitive input-output relation above threshold. In passive systems there may be no output in the absence of stimulation (e.g., fish vestibular system; Ishii et al., 1971b) or consid-erable output (e.g., tonic electroreceptors; Bennett, 1971a; Murray, 1965a,b), and in both cases sensitivity can still be high.

As a consequence of presynaptic biasing, one might expect some tonic release of transmitter, and thus tonic depolarization postsynaptically and tonic afferent spikes. This may occur in many receptor systems, e.g., tonic electroreceptors of teleosts (Bennett, 1971a,b). In the ampullae of Loren-zini, tonic release probably occurs, but it appears to be a consequence of asynchronous regenerative activity in single receptor cells (Obara and Ben-nett, 1972). The linearity of input-output relationships in this system thus may reflect a "linear-with-voltage" frequence of outer face activity; the ex-treme convergence of receptor cells to sensory fibers allows frequency of firing of nerves and single receptor cells to be quite different. The relation of stimulus to psp amplitude in fish S1 nerves is approximately linear, and there is no tonic postsynaptic spike activity. There are, however, spon-taneous quantal postsynaptic psp's. These quanta could be either single release packets or single synapses releasing several packets. A gaussian distribution in amplitude of the spontaneous events suggests the former, un-less each receptor cell has either a small invariant number or a large number of packets to release for each stimulus at each synapse. This, in turn, would imply that each receptor cell-nerve input-output relationship would amount to a step function; nothing below a certain stimulus, and all above that (as might be obtained if the receptor cells had a regenerative response as do many phasic electroreceptors). The fact that this kind of conjecture is still possible in a well-studied example of sensory synaptic transmission indicates the amount of work that needs to be done. To sum up, it is not yet clear whether the observed linearity of input-output relationships in sensory systems reflects a comparable linearity of input-output at a single synapse, and whether the range of linearity in terms of presynaptic membrane po-tential is such that the motor and the sensory synapse are truly different in this respect.

The chemical transmitter in sensory synapses probably causes an increase in postsynaptic membrane conductance. This is the case in the ampullae of Lorenzini. Because psp's must depolarize to elicit spikes, there are a limited number of ion species that could be charge carriers for a (alternative) conductance decrease that could produce depolarization, and clever experimentation might be able to rule out this mechanism, as well as alternative "nonconductance change" methods of depolarization.

Depolarization of receptor cells results in release of transmitter. Depolarizing receptor potentials have been recorded from phasic electroreceptors (Bennett, 1971a), lateral line organs (Harris et al., 1970), and taste cells (Ozeki, 1971; Sato, 1969). *Necturus* taste cells are probably large, and might reward study. Decisive results from other systems will be difficult, because cells are small (Fig. 1). Indirect methods of monitoring electrical potential (such as changes in optical properties) might be attempted. At least one taste-stimulating chemical (quinine) causes receptor cell depolarization by means of a conductance decrease, and this may occur in other sensory cells as well.

In the two electroreceptor systems that I have studied, there is bad pharmacological evidence that a dicarboxylic amino acid may be the transmitter. In skate electroreceptors, the evidence is getting better: direct depolarization of the postsynaptic element during high Mg block of transmission, relatively low concentrations for observed effects, and preliminary studies that show a mechanism for glutamate uptake. Glutamate is said not to affect the fish vestibular receptor system (Furukawa, *personal communication*). In the frog taste cells, vesicles are dense cored, and said to be depleted by reserpine (DeHan and Graziadei, 1971), although some investigators have reported effects of cholinergic compounds (see Landgren, Liljestrand, and Zotterman, 1954; Duncan, 1964; Steiner, 1971). The pharmacological work so far is not very convincing. In the acoustic system of mammals, there is now considerable evidence that a cholinergic transmission mechanism is involved in efferent control (see Lehrer, Maliner, and Gioia, 1966; Bobbin and Konishi, 1972). D-Tubocurarine blocks efferent modulation of afferent discharges in *Xenopus* lateral line nerves (Russell, 1968). The occurrence of glutamate in sensory nerve pathways has been reviewed (e.g., Duggan and Johnson, 1970). Even in well-studied, invertebrate motor systems, it has been difficult to positively identify glutamate as a transmitter.

The skate electroreceptor system seems a good system for further biochemical studies, because there are a large number of receptor cells and not much else, and because the ampullary canal provides a way of separating inner and outer membranes of the receptor cells.

Sensory Synapses Are Like Motor Synapses

Presynaptic depolarization (Bennett, 1971a,b; Ozeki, 1971; Harris et al., 1970; Sato, 1969) causes increased release probability (Ishii et al., 1971a). Transmission requires Ca and is inhibited by Mg (Steinbach and Bennett, 1971). Transmitter chemical is released from vesicles (conjecture based on morphology and weak evidence for quantal psp's) and depolarizes the postsynaptic nerve terminal (Furukawa and Ishii, 1967; Obara and Bennett, 1972; Nomura and Sakada, 1969) by means of a conductance decrease. Psp's are not TTX sensitive. Similar observations have been made in the retina (Dowling, *This Volume*).

Sensory Synapses Are Unlike Motor Synapses

They probably are, but the question remains as to where the differences in mechanism occur. The presence or absence of presynaptic dense bodies may reflect the duty cycle of a synapse, but may be involved in something else entirely. In taste systems synaptic morphology is complex, and may imply a mode of cell-cell transmission that is very different from that of the motor synapse. But as yet there is no evidence that any of the basic mechanisms involved in sensory synaptic transmission requires major modifications of the generalized hypothesis of neurochemical transmission generally attributed to Katz (1969).

ACKNOWLEDGMENTS

I would like to thank Marilyn Steinbach for inspiration and support. The work on skates would not have been possible without the generous loan of equipment by Dr. Harry Grundfest, nor without the guidance and interest of my teacher and friend Michael V. L. Bennett. Several of the authors cited discussed their work with me, and I thank them for this courtesy. This chapter is not intended to be a comprehensive review, but I would like to apologize to any investigators who may feel ill-used by my selection or presentation of material. I would like to thank Walter Phillips for technical assistance.

REFERENCES

Barets, A., and Szabo, T. (1962): Appareil synaptique des cellules sensorielles de l'ampoule de Lorenzini chez la torpille, *Torpedo marmorata. J. Micr.*, 1:47–54.
Beidler, L. M. (1962): Taste receptor stimulation. *Prog. Biochem. Biophys. Chem.*, 12:109–151.
Beidler, L. M. (1965): Comparison of gustatory receptors, olfactory receptors, and free nerve endings. *Cold Spring Harbor Symp. Quant. Biol.*, 30:191–200.
Bennett, M. V. L., (1967): Mechanisms of electroreception. In: *Lateral Line Detectors*, edited by P. Cahn, pp. 313–393. Indiana University Press, Bloomington.
Bennett, M. V. L. (1971a): Electroreception. In: *Fish Physiology*, Vol. 5, pp. 493–574. Academic Press, New York.
Bennett, M. V. L. (1971b): Electrolocation in fish. *Ann. N.Y. Acad. Sci.*, 188:242–269.
Biscoe, T. J. (1971) Carotid body: Structure and function. *Physiol. Rev.*, 51:437–495.
Biscoe, T. J., and Pallot, D. (1972): Serial reconstructions with the electron microscope of carotid body tissue: The type I cell nerve supply. *Experientia*, 28:33–34.
Bobbin, R. P., and Konishi, T. (1972): ACh mimics crossed olivocochlear bundle stimulation. *Nature New Biology*, 231:222–223.
DeHan, R., and Graziadei, P. P. C. (1971): Functional anatomy of frog's taste organs. *Experientia*, 27:823–826.

Duggan, A. W., and Johnson, G. A. R. (1970): Glutamates and related amino acids in cat spinal roots, dorsal root ganglia, and peripheral nerves. *J. Neurochem.*, 17:1205–1208.

Duncan, C. J. (1964): Synaptic transmission at taste buds. *Nature*, 203:875–877.

Eyzaguirre, C., Leitner, L. M., Nishi, K., and Fidone, S. (1970): Depolarization of chemosensory nerve endings in carotid body of the cat. *J. Neurophysiol.*, 33:685–695.

Fishman, I. Y. (1957): Single fiber gustatory impulses in rat and hamster. *J. Cell. Comp. Physiol.*, 49:319–334.

Fjällbrant, N., and Iggo, A. (1961): The effect of histamine, 5-HT and ACh on cutaneous afferent fibres. *J. Physiol.*, 156:578–590.

Flock, A., and Wersäll, J. (1962a): Synaptic structures in the lateral line canal organ of the teleost fish *Lota vulgaris*. *J. Cell Biol.*, 13:337–343.

Flock, A., and Wersäll, J. (1962b): A study of the orientation of the sensory hairs of the receptor cells in the lateral line organs of fish, with special reference to the function of the receptors. *J. Cell Biol.*, 15:19–27.

Flock, A., and Wersäll, J. (1963): Polarization and orientation of the hair cells in the sensory epithelium of the labyrinth and the lateral line organs. *J. Ultrastruct. Res.*, 8:193–194.

Fugimoto, S., and Murray, R. G. (1970): Fine structure of degeneration and regeneration in denervated rabbit vallate taste buds. *Anat. Rec.*, 168:393–413.

Furukawa, T., and Ishii, Y. (1967): Neurophysiological studies on hearing in goldfish. *J. Neurophysiol.*, 30:1377–1403.

Goodman, N. W., and McCloskey, D. I. (1972): Intracellular potential in the carotid body. *Brain Res.*, 39:501–504.

Graziadei, P. P. C. (1969): The ultrastructure of vertebrate taste buds. In; *Olfaction and Taste III*, edited by C. Pfaffman, pp. 315–330. Rockefeller University Press, New York.

Graziadei, P. P. C., and DeHan, R. S. (1971): The ultrastructure of frog's taste organs. *Acta Anat.*, 80:563–603.

Hama, K. (1965): Some observations on the fine structure of the lateral line organ of the Japanese sea eel *Lyncozymba nyshomi*. *J. Cell Biol.*, 24:193–210.

Hama, K. (1969): A study on the fine structure of the saccular macula of the goldfish. *Z. Zellforsch.*, 94:155–171.

Harris, G. G., and Milne, D. C. (1966): Input-output characteristics of the lateral line sense organs of *Xenopus laevis*. *J. Accoust. Soc. Am.*, 40:32–42.

Harris, G. G., Frishkopf, L. S., and Flöck, A. (1970): Receptor potentials from hair cells of the lateral line. *Science*, 167:76–79.

Iggo, A., and Muir, A. R. (1969): The structure and function of a slowly adapting touch corpuscle in hairy skin. *J. Physiol.*, 200:763–796.

Ishii, Y., Matsuura, S., and Furukawa, T. (1971a): Quantal nature of transmission at the synapse between hair cells and eighth nerve fibers. *Jap. J. Physiol.*, 21:79–89.

Ishii, Y., Matsuura, S., and Furukawa, T. (1971b): An input-output relation at the synapse between hair cells and eighth nerve fibers in goldfish. *Jap. J. Physiol.*, 21:91–98.

Jande, S. S. (1966): Fine structure of lateral-line organs of frog developing. *J. Ultrastruct. Res.*, 15:496–509.

Johnson, J. L. (1972): Glutamic acid as a synaptic transmitter in the nervous system. A review. *Brain Res.*, 37:1–19.

Katsuki, Y., Hashimoto, T., and Kendall, J. I. (1971): The chemoreception in the lateral line organs of teleosts. *Jap. J. Physiol.*, 21:99–118.

Katz, B. (1969): *The Release of Neural Transmitter Substances. Sherrington Lectures X.* Liverpool University Press, Liverpool.

Katz, B., and Miledi, R. (1969): Spontaneous and evoked activity of motor nerve endings in calcium Ringer. *J. Physiol.*, 203:689–706.

Kimura, K., and Beidler, L. M. (1961): Microelectrode study of taste reception of rat and hamster. *J. Cell. Comp. Physiol.*, 58:131–140.

Kusano, K. (1970): Influence of ionic environment on the relationship between pre- and postsynaptic potentials. *J. Neurobiol.*, 1:435–457.

Landgren, S., Liljestrand, G., and Zotterman, Y. (1954): Chemical transmission in taste fiber endings. *Acta Physiol. Scand.*, 30:105–114.

Lehrer, G. M., Maliner, R., and Gioia, M. (1966): The electron microscope localization of acetylcholinesterase in the guinea pig organ of Corti. *J. Histochem. Cytochem.*, 14:816A.

Miller, I. J. (1971): Peripheral interactions among single papilla inputs to gustatory nerve fibers. *J. Gen. Physiol.*, 57:1–25.

Mills, E., and Jöbsis, F. F. (1972): Mitochondrial respiratory chain of carotid body and chemoreceptor response to change in oxygen tension. *J. Neurophysiol.*, 35:405–427.

Murray, R. W. (1965a): Electroreceptor mechanisms: The relation of impulse frequency to stimulus strength and responses to pulsed stimuli in the ampullae of Lorenzini of elasmobranchs. *J. Physiol.*, 180:592–606.

Murray, R. W. (1965b): Receptor mechanisms in the ampullae of Lorenzini of elasmobranch fishes. *Cold Spring Harbor Symp. Quant. Biol.*, 30:233–244.

Murray, R. G. (1969): Cell types in rabbit taste buds. In: *Olfaction and Taste III*, edited by C. Pfaffman, pp. 331–344. Rockefeller University Press, New York.

Murray, R. G., and Murray, A. (1960): The fine structure of the taste buds of rhesus and cynomalgous monkeys. *Anat. Rec.*, 138:211–219.

Nomura, H., and Sakada, S. (1969): Local potential changes at sensory nerve fiber terminals of the frog tongue. In: *Olfaction and Taste III*, edited by C. Pfaffman, pp. 345–351. Rockefeller University Press, New York.

Obara, S., and Bennett, M. V. L. (1972): Mode of operation of ampullae of Lorenzini of the skate *Raja*. *J. Gen. Physiol.*, 60:534–557.

Ozeki, M. (1971): Conductance change associated with receptor potentials of gustatory cells in rat. *J. Gen. Physiol.*, 58:688–699.

Rapuzzi, G., and Casella, C. (1965): Innervation of the fungiform papillae in the frog tongue. *J. Neurophysiol.*, 28:154–165.

Robbins, N. (1967): The role of the nerve in maintenance of frog taste buds. *Exp. Neurol.*, 17:364–380.

Russell, R. J. (1968): Influence of efferent fibers on a receptor. *Nature*, 219:177–178.

Sato, T. (1969): The response of frog taste cells *(Rana nigromaculata* and *Rana catesbiana)*. *Experientia*, 25:709–710.

Sato, T. (1971): Site of gustatory neural adaptation. *Brain Res.*, 34:385–388.

Smith, C. A., and Sjöstrand, F. S. (1961): Structure of the nerve endings on the external hair cells of the guinea pig cochlea by serial sections. *J. Ultrastruct. Res.*, 5:523–556.

Spoendlin, H. (1972): Innervation densities of the cochlea. *Acta Otolaryng.*, 73:235–248.

Steinbach, A. B., and Bennett, M. V. L. (1971): Effects of divalent ions and drugs on synaptic transmission in phasic electroreceptors in a Mormyrid fish. *J. Gen. Physiol.*, 58:580–598.

Steiner, J. E. (1971): Transmitter mechanism responsible for initiation of sweet and bitter signals in the glossopharyngeal nerve of frogs. *J. Dent. Res.*, 50:651–652.

Szabo, T., and Wersäll, J. (1970): Ultrastructure of an electroreceptor (mormyromast) in a mormyrid fish, *Gnathonemus petersii*. *J. Ultrastruct. Res.*, 30:473–490.

Szamier, R. B., and Wachtel, A. W. (1969): Special cutaneous receptor organs of fish: The ampullary organs of *Eigenmannia*. *J. Morph.*, 128:261–290.

Szamier, R. B., and Wachtel, A. W. (1970): Special cutaneous receptor organs of fish: VI ampullary and tuberous organs of *Hypopomus*. *J. Ultra. Res.*, 30:450–471.

Uga, S. (1966): The fine structure of gustatory receptors and their synapses in frog's tongue. *Sym. Cell. Chem.*, 16:75–86.

Uga, S., and Hama, K. (1967): Electron microscopic studies on the synaptic region of the taste organ of carps and frogs. *J. Electron Microsc.*, 16:269–277.

Wachtel, A. W., and Szamier, R. B. (1966): Special cutaneous receptor organs of fish: The tuberous organs of *Eigenmannia*. *J. Morph.*, 119:51–80.

Wachtel, A. W., and Szamier, R. B. (1969): Special cutaneous receptor organs of fish: III ampullary organs of nonelectric catfish, *Kryptopterus*. *J. Morph.*, 128:291–308.

Waltman, B. (1968): Electrical excitability of the ampullae of Lorenzini in the ray. *Acta Physiol. Scand.*, 74:29A–30A.

Wersäll, J., Flöck, A., and Lundquist, P. G. (1965): Structural basis for directional sensitivity in cochlear and vestibular sensory receptors. *Cold Spring Harbor Symp. Quant. Biol.*, 30:115–132.

Synaptic Transmission and Neuronal Interaction
Raven Press, New York 1974

Synaptic Potentials Resulting from Conductance Decreases

Forrest F. Weight

Laboratory of Neuropharmacology, National Institute of Mental Health, St Elizabeths Hospital, Washington, D.C. 20032

Postsynaptic potentials are generated by an increased permeability of postsynaptic membrane to certain ions at virtually all chemically mediated synaptic junctions that have been investigated (see Eccles, 1964; Ginsborg, 1967; Weight, 1971). Recent studies in sympathetic ganglia, however, have presented evidence that synaptic potentials can also be generated by decreases in membrane permeability (Weight and Votava, 1970; Weight and Padjen, 1973a). In this chapter the generation of synaptic potentials by conductance decreases is discussed, but first we briefly review the generation of the conventional type of synaptic potential and the organization of the sympathetic ganglion.

The Xth sympathetic ganglion of frog is particularly well suited for investigating the mechanism of generation of synaptic potentials for several reasons. First, the transmitter of preganglionic fibers innervating sympathetic ganglion cells is known to be acetylcholine (ACh) (Blackman et al., 1963; Nishi et al., 1967), and the transmitter of postganglionic fibers of ganglion cells is epinephrine (Norberg and McIsaac, 1967). Second, frog sympathetic ganglion cells do not have dendrites, and most preganglionic synapses on ganglion cells are axosomatic (Grillo, 1966), thus avoiding the problem of interpreting conductance changes of remote axodendritic synapses (see Smith et al., 1967). Third, most ganglion cells are innervated by a single preganglionic fiber (Blackman et al., 1963), so that repetitive presynaptic stimulation will not activate different presynaptic fibers. Fourth, there are two cell types in the Xth ganglion that can be identified by the antidromic conduction velocity of their axon—cells with axons of B fiber conduction velocity termed B cells and cells with axons of C fiber conduction velocity termed C cells (Nishi et al., 1965). The two cell types receive separate preganglionic input through different pathways: B cells are innervated by preganglionic B fibers in the sympathetic chain, and C cells are innervated by C fibers in the VIIIth spinal nerve (Tosaka et al., 1968). In addition, different types of slow synaptic potentials are generated in the two cell types: a slow excitatory postsynaptic potential (EPSP) is generated in B cells and a slow inhibitory postsynaptic potential (IPSP) in C cells (Tosaka et al., 1968).

I. GENERATION OF SYNAPTIC POTENTIALS BY
CONDUCTANCE INCREASES

The mechanism of generation of postsynaptic excitation at most synaptic junctions can be illustrated by the fast EPSP in frog sympathetic ganglion cells. When recording intracellularly in ganglion cells, a single stimulus to preganglionic nerve fibers generates an EPSP as shown in Fig. 1A. The time course of the EPSP is in the millisecond range, in contrast to slow synaptic potentials which last many seconds. The fast EPSP is mimicked by the iontophoretic application of ACh and is antagonized by nicotinic blocking agents such as d-tubocurarine (Blackman et al., 1963), indicating that it is generated by cholinergic activation of nicotinic membrane receptors. When an antidromic spike is elicited during the fast EPSP, the spike amplitude is decreased, indicating that the membrane resistance is shunted by the EPSP (Nishi and Koketsu, 1960; Blackman et al., 1963). This increased conductance during the fast EPSP is due to the increased permeability of postsynaptic membrane to certain ions. If the increased conductance were only to Na, the synaptic current (I_{Na}) would be given by

$$I_{Na} = \Delta g_{Na}(E_m - E_{Na})$$

where Δg_{Na} = sodium conductance, E_m = membrane potential, and E_{Na} = $RT/F \; ln \; ([Na]_o/[Na]_i)$. From this equation it can be seen that as E_m approaches E_{Na}, I_{Na} approaches 0. It is also apparent that when E_m becomes more positive than E_{Na}, the sign of I_{Na} will reverse. Thus, the reversal potential for a synaptic potential generated only by a sodium current will be the sodium equilibrium potential E_{Na}. In most nerve cells, E_{Na} is approximately 50 to 60 mV (Hodgkin, 1964; Katz, 1966). With electrical polarization of sympathetic ganglion cells, it has been found that the reversal potential for the fast EPSP (Fig. 1A) is approximately -14 mV (Nishi and Koketsu, 1960; Blackman et al., 1963). Since this value is less than E_{Na}, the fast EPSP cannot be accounted for by an increase in Na conductance alone, and it has been proposed that the fast EPSP is generated by an increased conductance to both Na and K, as at the neuromuscular junction (Takeuchi and Takeuchi, 1960). Recent experiments changing $[Na]_o$ and $[K]_o$ have provided data consistent with the hypothesis that the fast EPSP is generated by an increase in both Na and K conductances (Koketsu, 1969).

The generation of the fast EPSP by an increase in membrane conductance can be represented schematically by an electrical circuit diagram. In Fig. 2C, activation of nicotinic membrane receptors (N) is illustrated as increasing the postsynaptic membrane conductance, which would shift the membrane potential toward the series electromotive force (e.m.f.) for the fast EPSP. The generation of most synaptic potentials can be explained by this type of model (Ginsborg, 1967; Weight, 1971). Although the ions involved may differ somewhat at different excitatory junctions, the general model for an EPSP generated by an increased conductance to certain ions

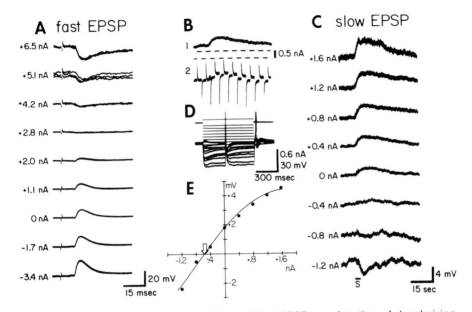

FIG. 1. Fast and slow EPSPs. (A) Amplitude of fast EPSP as a function of depolarizing
(+) and hyperpolarizing (−) current. Polarizing current is indicated in nanoamperes. B
fibers were stimulated with a single, 0.5-msec stimulus to generate the fast EPSP in
a type B ganglion cell. (B) and (C) Slow EPSP in a type B ganglion cell. The fast EPSP
was blocked by nicotine (5 μg/ml). B fibers were stimulated repetitively at a frequency
of 100/sec for 2 sec. Stimulation began 10 sec after the beginning of each record. The
period of stimulation is indicated by the line labeled S under the bottom record in C.
(B₁) Slow EPSP at resting membrane potentials. (B₂) *Upper record,* hyperpolarizing
constant current pulses of −0.5 nA; *lower record,* bridge balanced before stimulation
such that current pulses produced no voltage deflection. Note that during EPSP the
−0.5-nA current pulses produced a hyperpolarizing voltage deflection of 1 mV, indicating
that the membrane resistance had increased by 2 MΩ. Time and voltage calibration for
(B) is the same as for (C). (C) Amplitude of slow EPSP as a function of depolarizing
(+) and hyperpolarizing (−) current. Note that the slow EPSP reversed with hyperpolarizing
current, the opposite of fast EPSP in (A). (D) Amplitude of antidromic spike after-hyperpolarization as a function of membrane potential. The same cell as (B) and (C). Upper
record monitors current; note that the larger hyperpolarizing current traces are superimposed on voltage records. Lower record shows antidromic spike superimposed at
various levels of membrane potential; top of spike was cut off by limitation of oscilloscope
excursion. Note that the after-hyperpolarization reverses with hyperpolarizing current
between −0.5 and −0.6 nA. (E) Graphic relationship of amplitude of slow EPSP [in (C)]
to current. The reversal potential of slow EPSP is the point at which the curve crosses
the abscissa. Arrow indicates the reversal potential of antidromic spike after-hyperpolarization shown in (D). Note that the reversal potential of after-hyperpolarization
(arrow) coincides with the reversal potential of slow EPSP (curve intercept). From Weight
and Votava (1970).

usually obtains. Such a model can also be used to explain the generation
of IPSPs, except that the battery is reversed and the specific ions involved
will differ (Ginsborg, 1967; Weight, 1971). Nevertheless, the general
mechanism is similar in that most IPSPs are generated by an increased
conductance of postsynaptic membrane to ions.

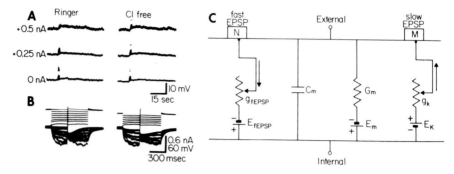

FIG. 2. (A) Effect of removing extracellular Cl⁻ on slow EPSP. *Left,* potentiation of small slow EPSP by depolarizing current; *right,* effect of removing extracellular Cl⁻ on potentiation of slow EPSP by depolarizing current. (B) Effect of removing extracellular Cl⁻ on reversal of antidromic spike after-hyperpolarization. *Left,* upper record monitors current, and lower record shows antidromic spike superimposed at various levels of membrane potential; *right,* similar to *left* but after removal of extracellular Cl⁻. Note that data taken when Cl⁻ was removed were recorded over a more limited current range than were control data. (C) Schematic electrical circuit diagram of sympathetic ganglion B cell membrane representing the fast EPSP *(left)* and the slow EPSP *(right).* See text for further discussion. From Weight and Votava (1970).

Such a model for increased postsynaptic conductance does not explain, however, the generation of slow synaptic potentials in sympathetic ganglia. The slow EPSP and slow IPSP have been found to have properties that differ from most synaptic potentials (Koketsu, 1969; Libet, 1971). Recent investigations on the slow PSPs have presented evidence consistent with the hypothesis that they are generated by decreases in membrane conductance. We will now discuss these recent studies.

II. SLOW SYNAPTIC EXCITATION IN SYMPATHETIC GANGLION CELLS

In addition to the fast EPSP in frog sympathetic ganglia, repetitive stimulation of preganglionic B fibers also generates a slow depolarization of B cells—the slow EPSP. In contrast to the fast EPSP (Fig. 1A), the slow EPSP reaches its peak in several seconds and lasts for approximately a minute (Fig. 1B). The slow EPSP is generated in the presence of nicotinic antagonists and is blocked by atropine, indicating that it is produced by the cholinergic activation of muscarinic receptors (Koketsu, 1969; Libet, 1970). In order to investigate the properties of the slow EPSP, without contamination by the fast EPSP, experiments on the slow EPSP are usually performed in the presence of nicotinic blocking agents.

As shown in Fig. 1B, when membrane resistance is tested during the slow EPSP, it is usually increased (Kobayashi and Libet, 1970; Weight and

Votava, 1970). This contrasts with the change of resistance during the fast EPSP and most other EPSPs in that membrane resistance is usually decreased. Since conductance is defined as the reciprocal of resistance, this observation indicates that conductance is decreased during the slow EPSP. As discussed previously, the reversal potential of a conductance change can give an index of the ion(s) involved. Therefore, membrane polarization was used to study the effect on the slow EPSP (Weight and Votava, 1970).

As shown in Fig. 1C, progressive depolarization of the sympathetic ganglion cell membrane resulted in a progressive increase in the amplitude of the slow EPSP. On the other hand, moderate hyperpolarizing current decreased the amplitude of the slow EPSP. Stronger hyperpolarizing current abolished and then reversed the slow EPSP to a hyperpolarizing potential (Fig. 1C). To obtain an index of the reversal potential for the slow EPSP, the reversal of the antidromic spike after-hyperpolarization was used (Fig. 1D). As shown in Fig. 1E, the reversal potential for the slow EPSP was near the reversal potential for the spike after-hyperpolarization. Since the reversal potential of the after-hyperpolarization is usually near the potassium equilibrium potential (E_K), these data suggested that the conductance that is decreased during the slow EPSP is g_K.

The equilibrium potential for g_{Cl} is not known for sympathetic ganglion cells, and thus the above data did not exclude the possibility of a decrease in g_{Cl}. This was tested by removing extracellular chloride. As shown in Fig. 2A, 0 Cl did not significantly affect the slow EPSP, indicating that an inactivation of g_{Cl} does not play a significant role in the generation of the slow EPSP. If the slow EPSP is generated by a decrease in g_K, then reducing the potassium gradient $([K]_o/[K]_i)$ should reduce the reversal potential for the slow EPSP. In recent experiments (Weight, *unpublished observations*), increasing $[K]_o$ has been found to reduce the reversal potential for the slow ACh depolarization, providing further support for the hypothesis that the slow EPSP is generated by a decrease in g_K.

The hypothesis that the slow EPSP is generated by a decrease or inactivation of resting potassium conductance (Weight and Votava, 1970) can be represented by an electrical circuit diagram. In Fig. 2C, activation of muscarinic receptors (M) is illustrated decreasing resting potassium conductance (g_K). This would shift the membrane potential away from E_K and toward the equilibrium potential of the other resting conductances (G_m). There are data that frog sympathetic ganglion cells have little or no resting g_{Cl} (Blackman et al., 1963), so that the predominant resting conductance other than g_K would be g_{Na}. Thus, inactivation of g_K would result in an increase in membrane resistance and a depolarization of the membrane. The depolarization would be potential dependent, being increased in amplitude by depolarizing current, decreased by hyperpolarizing current, and reversing at E_K.

III. SLOW SYNAPTIC INHIBITION IN SYMPATHETIC GANGLION CELLS

In addition to the slow EPSP generated in B cells by stimulation of the sympathetic chain, a slow IPSP is generated in C cells by repetitive stimulation of the VIIIth nerve (Tosaka et al., 1968; Weight and Padjen, 1973a). The slow IPSP reaches its peak in 1 to 3 sec and lasts for approximately 10 to 20 sec (Fig. 3B1). Like the slow EPSP, the slow IPSP is generated in the presence of nicotinic antagonists and is blocked by atropine (Libet et al., 1968; Nishi and Koketsu, 1968). Experiments on the slow IPSP are usually performed in the presence of nicotinic antagonists to prevent contamination by the fast EPSP.

It will be recalled that synaptic inhibition at most synaptic junctions is produced by an increased conductance of postsynaptic membrane. By contrast, when membrane resistance was tested during the slow IPSP (Weight and Padjen, 1973a), it was found that membrane resistance increased markedly (Fig. 3B2).

To study the conductance that was decreased during the slow IPSP, the membrane of C cells was electrically polarized (Weight and Padjen, 1973a). As shown in Fig. 3C, moderate hyperpolarizing current increased the amplitude of the slow IPSP, whereas progressive depolarizing current decreased and then abolished the slow IPSP. Further, very strong depolarizing current either resulted in unstable recording or damaged the membrane. In Fig. 3D, the amplitude of the slow IPSP and the antidromic spike recorded during the same polarizing current are plotted on the same graph as a function of polarizing current. Since the peak of the antidromic spike is a point of high sodium conductance, the parallelism between the amplitudes of the antidromic spike and slow IPSP suggests that the predominant conductance that decreased is g_{Na}.[1]

---

[1] The C cells in frog sympathetic ganglion were too small to insert two electrodes so that polarizing current was passed through the recording electrode using a bridge circuit. When stronger depolarizing currents were used, bridge balance position became uncertain and it could not be assumed that the electrode resistance did not change with increasing current. Therefore, the spike-height method (Frank and Fuortes, 1956) was used to estimate membrane potential during polarization, the assumption being that the spike height will give a relatively good reflection of the change in membrane potential during polarization because of the high g_{Na} at the peak of the spike.

This method will be subject to the limitation that if the strong depolarizing current produces some inactivation of the spike sodium conductance, the null point for the antidromic spike will be less than the sodium equilibrium potential. However, it is not known whether or to what extent this occurs in frog sympathetic ganglion cells. If it does occur, the null point for the antidromic spike would still be decidedly positive to 0, which is consistent with the suggestion that the predominant conductance change is a change in g_{Na}; it would not, however, exclude the possibility of a small contribution by another ion.

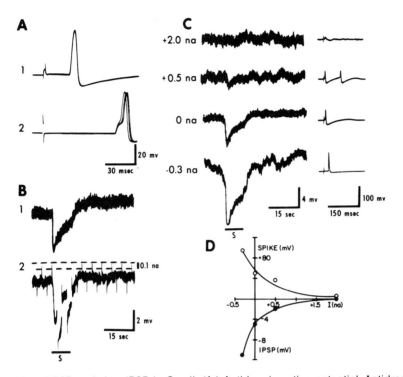

FIG. 3. Fast EPSP and slow IPSP in C cell. (A_1) Antidromic action potential. Antidromic conduction velocity of 0.24 M/sec identifies neuron as C cell. (A_2) Fast EPSP generated by stimulation of preganglionic C fibers in VIIIth spinal nerve. (B_1) Slow IPSP generated in same C cell, after nicotinic blockade (nicotine, 5 μg/ml), by stimulation of preganglionic C fibers in the VIIIth spinal nerve at a frequency of 50/sec. Period of stimulation indicated by line labeled S under record in B_2. (B_2) *Upper record*, hyperpolarizing constant current pulses of −0.1 nA; *lower record*, resistance change during slow IPSP. Bridge balanced before stimulation such that current pulses produced no voltage deflection. Note that during the slow IPSP the −0.1-nA current pulse produced a maximal hyperpolarizing voltage deflection of 2 mV, indicating that membrane resistance increased by 20 MΩ. Resting input resistance of this cell, determined from I-V curves, was 78 MΩ. (C) *Left,* amplitude of slow IPSP as a function of depolarizing (+) and hyperpolarizing (−) current; *right,* amplitude of antidromic spike recorded during the same polarizing current. (D) Amplitudes of slow IPSP (filled circles) and antidromic spike (open circles) in (C), represented graphically as a function of polarizing current. From Weight and Padjen (1973a).

The hypothesis that the slow IPSP is generated by a decrease or inactivation of g_{Na} can be tested by reducing the sodium gradient ($[Na]_o/[Na]_i$). One way to reduce the sodium gradient is by increasing intracellular sodium.

It is not clear from the data if the apparent decrease in resting sodium conductance associated with the slow IPSP would also involve the sodium conductance in spike generation. Further experiments with tetrodotoxin might clarify that question.

Ouabain inhibits the electrogenic sodium pump in nerve cells and can lead
to an accumulation of intracellular sodium (Thomas, 1972). The administration of ouabain (10^{-6} M) has been found to reduce or abolish the slow IPSP
after 30 min (Nishi and Koketsu, 1967). The effect of ouabain was interpreted as evidence that the slow IPSP is generated by activation of the
electrogenic sodium pump (Nishi and Koketsu, 1967). This hypothesis
does not explain, however, the decreased conductance and potential dependence of the slow IPSP, since in most tissues the sodium pump does
not exhibit these properties (Thomas, 1972). On the other hand, the decrease
in the slow IPSP could be accounted for by an increase in intracellular
sodium. However, ouabain might also reduce transmitter release (Libet,
1970), thus making the reduction of the slow IPSP by ouabain difficult to
interpret.

   The sodium inactivation hypothesis can be tested more directly by reducing extracellular sodium. Removal of extracellular sodium would abolish
the sodium gradient and would be expected to abolish the response. Sodium-
free Ringer's, however, also abolishes nerve conduction so that 0Na cannot
be tested on the synaptic response. The iontophoretic administration of
ACh to C cells has been found (Weight and Padjen, 1973b) to produce a
hyperpolarization of C cells with a time course similar to the time course
of the slow IPSP (Fig. 4).

   The properties of the ACh hyperpolarization were similar to the properties of the slow IPSP in that membrane resistance increased during the

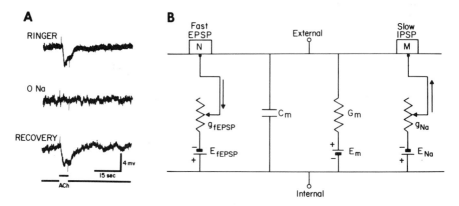

FIG. 4. (A) Effect of removing extracellular Na$^+$ on slow ACh hyperpolarization. ACh ad-
ministered extracellularly to C cell by iontophoresis during period indicated by bottom
line. *Top*, control ACh hyperpolarization in Ringer's solution; *middle*, administration of
ACh 30 min after removal of extracellular Na$^+$ (NaCl replaced by isotonic sucrose); *bottom*, recovery of ACh hyperpolarization 30 min after return to Ringer's solution with
normal Na$^+$. (B) Schematic electrical circuit diagram of sympathetic ganglion C cell
membrane representing the fast EPSP *(left)* and the slow IPSP *(right)*. See text for further
discussion. From Weight and Padjen (1973a).

ACh hyperpolarization (Fig. 5) and hyperpolarizing current increased the amplitude of the ACh response whereas depolarizing current decreased the ACh response (Fig. 6). Since stimulation of cholinergic afferents that make monosynaptic connection with C cells elicits the slow IPSP and atropine antagonizes the slow IPSP, the effect of ACh on C cells suggests that the slow IPSP may be mediated by ACh. The iontophoretic adminis-tration of ACh to C cells was therefore used to test the effect of sodium removal on the generation of the hyperpolarizing response (Weight and Padjen, 1973a). In sodium-free Ringer's (NaCl was replaced by isotonic sucrose), the membrane potential of C cells increased by 25 to 40 mV. Although electrical hyperpolarization of the membrane increased the amplitude of the slow ACh response, sodium-free Ringer's solution reduced and then abolished the slow ACh hyperpolarization (Fig. 4A). The effect was reversible; return to Ringer's solution with normal sodium repolarized the membrane and restored the generation of the hyperpolarization (Fig. 4A). These data provide strong support for the proposal that the slow IPSP is generated by a decrease in g_{Na}.

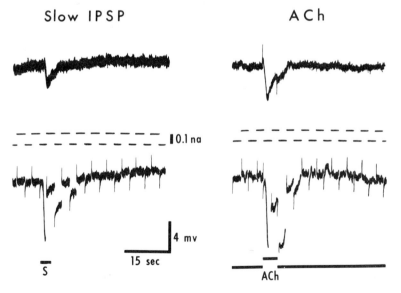

FIG. 5. Resistance change during slow IPSP and ACh hyperpolarization. *Top left,* slow IPSP generated by stimulation of preganglionic C fibers in the VIIIth spinal nerve at a frequency of 50/sec for period indicated by line labeled S under lower record. *Top right,* hyperpolarization produced by the iontophoretic administration of ACh for period indi-cated by bottom line. *Bottom,* hyperpolarizing constant current pulse of −0.1 nA during slow IPSP *(left)* and ACh hyperpolarization *(right).* Bridge balanced before stimulation such that current pulses produced no voltage deflection. Note that the hyperpolarizing current pulses produced hyperpolarizing voltage deflections during the slow IPSP and the ACh hyperpolarization. From Weight and Padjen (1973b).

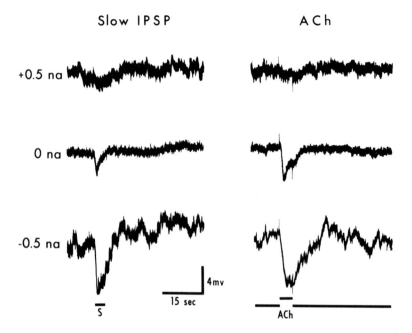

FIG. 6. Effect of polarization of slow IPSP and ACh hyperpolarization. *Middle,* amplitude
of control slow IPSP *(left)* and ACh hyperpolarization *(right); top,* effect of depolarizing
current of +0.5 nA on slow IPSP *(left)* and ACh hyperpolarization *(right); bottom,* effect
of hyperpolarizing current of −0.5 nA on slow IPSP *(left)* and ACh hyperpolarization
(right). From Weight and Padjen (1973b).

The hypothesis that the slow IPSP is generated by an inactivation of g_{Na}
(Weight and Padjen, 1973a) can be represented schematically by an electrical circuit diagram. In Fig. 4B, activation of membrane receptors (M)
is illustrated as decreasing resting sodium conductance (g_{Na}). This would
shift the membrane potential away from E_{Na} and toward the equilibrium
potential for the other resting conductances (G_m). In this case the other
resting conductances would be predominantly g_K, so that inactivation of
g_{Na} would result in a hyperpolarization with an increase in resistance. The
hyperpolarization would be potential dependent, being increased by hyperpolarizing current, decreased by depolarizing current, and abolished at
E_{Na}.

IV CONCLUSIONS

Although synaptic potentials with the properties of the slow PSPs have
not been reported at other synaptic junctions, there are several recent
reports of other responses that have properties similar to the slow PSPs.
With regard to the inactivation of g_K, an ACh depolarization of cortical
neurons with an increase in membrane resistance has recently been pro-

posed to be generated by an inactivation of g_K (Krnjevic et al., 1971). Similarly, Bulbring (1972) recently suggested that a depolarization of smooth muscle with an increase in membrane resistance may be generated by a decrease in resting g_K. With respect to the inactivation of g_{Na}, the hyperpolarizing response of vertebrate photoreceptors to light has properties very similar to the slow IPSP in sympathetic ganglion cells, and it has been proposed that the photoreceptor response is generated by an inactivation of g_{Na} (Baylor and Fuortes, 1970; Tomita, 1970). It has also been recently reported that the response of cerebellar Purkinje cells (Siggins et al., 1971) and spinal motoneurons (Engberg and Marshall, 1971) to norepinephrine (NE) is a hyperpolarization with an increase in membrane resistance. Although further work is necessary to establish the mechanism of generation of some of these responses, these studies suggest that the generation of membrane potentials by decreasing membrane conductance may be more common than had previously been recognized.

In conclusion, it appears that in addition to the conventional generation of synaptic potentials by increased conductance mechanisms, synaptic potentials may also be generated by decreases in membrane conductance. Although at present synaptic potentials with conductance decreases have only been reported in sympathetic ganglion cells, it is possible that generation of synaptic potentials by conductance decreases may be a more general mechanism in the synaptic control of neuronal function.

REFERENCES

Baylor, D. A., and Fuortes, M. G. F. (1970): Electrical responses of single cones in the retina of the turtle. *J. Physiol.*, 207:77–92.

Blackman, J. C., Ginsborg, B. L., and Ray, C. (1963): Synaptic transmission in the sympathetic ganglion of the frog. *J. Physiol.*, 167:355–373.

Bulbring, E. and Kuriyama, H. (1973): The actions of catecholamines on guinea-pig taenia coli. *Phil. Trans. Roy. Soc. Lond. B*, 265:115–121.

Eccles, J. C. (1964): *The Physiology of Synapses.* Academic Press, Inc., New York.

Eccles, R. M., and Libet, B. (1961): Origin and blockade of the synaptic responses of curarized sympathetic ganglia. *J. Physiol.*, 157:484–503.

Engberg, I., and Marshall, K. C. (1971): Mechanism of noradrenaline hyperpolarization in spinal cord motoneurones of the cat. *Acta Physiol. Scand.*, 83:142–144.

Frank, K., and Fuortes, M. G. F. (1956): *J. Physiol.*, 134:451–470.

Ginsborg, B. L. (1967): Ion movements in junctional transmission. *Pharm. Rev.*, 19:289–316.

Grillo, M. A. (1966): Electron microscopy of sympathetic tissues. *Pharm. Rev.*, 18:387–399.

Hodgkin, A. L. (1964): *The Conduction of the Nervous Impulse.* Charles C Thomas, Publ., Springfield, Ill.

Katz, B. (1966): *Nerve, Muscle and Synapse.* McGraw Hill Co., New York.

Kobayashi, H., and Libet, B. (1970): Actions of noradrenaline and acetylcholine on sympathetic ganglion cells. *J. Physiol.*, 208:353–372.

Koketsu, K. (1969): Cholinergic synaptic potentials and the underlying ionic mechanisms. *Fed. Proc.*, 28:101–112.

Krnjevic, K., Pumain, R., and Renaud, L. (1971): The mechanism of excitation by acetylcholine in the cerebral cortex. *J. Physiol.*, 215:247–268.

Libet, B. (1970): Generation of slow inhibitory and excitatory postsynaptic potentials. *Fed. Proc.*, 29:1945–1956.

Libet. B., Chichibu, S., and Tosaka, T. (1968): Slow synaptic responses and excitability in sympathetic ganglia of the bullfrog. *J. Neurophysiol.,* 31:383–395.

Nishi, S., and Koketsu, K. (1960): Electrical properties and activities of single sympathetic neurons in frogs. *J. Cell. Comp. Physiol.,* 55:15–30.

Nishi, S., and Koketsu, K. (1967): Origin of ganglionic inhibitory postsynaptic potential. *Life Sci.,* 6:2049–2055.

Nishi, S., and Koketsu, K. (1968): Early and late afterdischarges of amphibian sympathetic ganglion cells. *J. Neurophysiol.,* 31:109–121.

Nishi, S., Soeda, H., and Koketsu, K. (1965): Studies on sympathetic B and C neurons and patterns of preganglionic innervation. *J. Cell. Comp. Physiol.,* 66:19–32.

Nishi, S., Soeda, H., and Koketsu, K. (1967): Release of acetylcholine from sympathetic preganglionic nerve terminals. *J. Neurophysiol.,* 30:114–134.

Norberg, K.-A., and McIsaac, R. J. (1967): Cellular location of adrenergic amines in frog sympathetic ganglia. *Experientia,* 23:1052.

Siggins, G. R., Oliver, A. P., Hoffer, B. J., and Bloom, F. E. (1971): Cyclic adenosine monophosphate and norepinephrine: Effects on transmembrane properties of cerebellar Purkinje cells. *Science,* 171:192–194.

Smith, T. G., Wuerker, R. B., and Frank, K. (1967): Membrane impedance changes during synaptic transmission in cat spinal motoneurons. *J. Neurophysiol.,* 30:1072–1096.

Takeuchi, A., and Takeuchi, N. (1960): On the permeability of end-plate membrane during the action of transmitter. *J. Physiol.,* 154:52–67.

Thomas, R. C. (1972): Electrogenic sodium pump in nerve and muscle cells. *Physiol. Rev.,* 52:563–594.

Tomita, T. (1970): Electrical activity of vertebrate photoreceptors. *Quart. Rev. Biophys.,* 3:179–222.

Tosaka, T., Chichibu, S., and Libet, B. (1968): Intracellular analysis of slow inhibitory and excitatory postsynaptic potentials in sympathetic ganglia of the frog. *J. Neurophysiol.,* 31:396–409.

Weight, F. F. (1971): Mechanisms of synaptic transmission. *Neurosci. Res.,* 4:1–27.

Weight, F. F., and Padjen, A. (1973*a*): Slow synaptic inhibition in sympathetic ganglion cells: Evidence for synaptic inactivation of sodium conductance. *Brain Res.,* 55:219–224.

Weight, F. F., and Padjen, A. (1973*b*): Acetylcholine and slow synaptic inhibition in frog sympathetic ganglion. *Brain Res.,* 55:225–228.

Weight, F. F., and Votava, J. (1970): Slow synaptic excitation in sympathetic ganglion cells: Evidence for synaptic inactivation of potassium conductance. *Science,* 170:755–758.

Synaptic Transmission and Neuronal Interaction
Raven Press, New York 1974

Flexibility and Rigidity in Electrotonically Coupled Systems

M. V. L. Bennett

*Rose F. Kennedy Center for Research in Mental Retardation and Human Development,
Department of Anatomy, Albert Einstein College of Medicine, New York, New York 10461
and Marine Biological Laboratory Woods Hole, Massachusetts 02543*

INTRODUCTION

The incidence of electrical and chemical transmission in various systems can to some extent be understood in terms of functional differences between the two modes of transmission (Bennett, 1972*a,b*). Electrical transmission is clearly better where speed is important. Chemical transmission is clearly better for inhibition unless speed is very important. At chemical synapses, activity is often followed by changes in postsynaptic potential (PSP) amplitude, whereas changes in junctional resistance produced by activity are unknown at electrical synapses. A possible but less obvious difference is in respect to reciprocal and linear transmission which appears simpler electrically. Unidirectional action can be achieved at electrical synapses in several ways, but may be somewhat simpler chemically.

In these functional arguments one generally assumes that the organism has a choice of which mode of transmission it will have at a particular synapse. Molecular biology gives some support to this assumption in that every organism from the coelenterates up has both electrical and chemical synapses, and thus the DNA of every cell can be expected to contain the required genetic plans for both kinds of synapses.

In the present chapter I briefly review the occurrence of electrical transmission in synchronously responding systems in which the behavior is essentially rigid. Then I discuss more recent findings on two systems in which the degree of electrical interaction between cells is under physiological control. The latter systems involve spatial localization of inputs that adapts the neurons to operate synchronously and asynchronously under appropriate physiological conditions.

In all the examples I discuss here the electrical synapse behaves like a simple resistance connecting the cell interiors. Because the electrical behavior is essentially the same as in electrotonic spread along a core conductor, these may be termed electrotonic synapses. Examples of electrical coupling across extracellular space and of rectifying junctional membrane are known, but will not be considered here (see Auerbach and Bennett, 1969; Bennett, 1973*a,b*). The morphological substrate of the electrotonic synapse is quite well established as the gap junction. A variety of indirect evidence indicates that these junctions contain small intercellular bridges each with a central hydrophilic channel that connects the cytoplasms of the coupled cells (see Payton et al., 1969; Bennett, 1973*a,b*).

ELECTROTONIC COUPLING IN SYNCHRONIZATION

The role of electrotonic coupling in controlling highly synchronized activity has been established in many systems (Bennett, 1966, 1972*a,b*). The speed of electrotonic transmission allows neurons to interact very rapidly and to achieve a degree of synchrony that could not be mediated by chemically transmitting synapses with their characteristic delay.

In order for a group of cells to initiate a highly synchronous volley they must be rather close together, close enough that propagation delays between them are not significant. Although electrotonic propagation along a core conductor from one point of view proceeds at the speed of light, the component that propagates infinitely fast is infinitely small. A similar consideration applies to transmission across electrotonic synapses. Although current starts to flow across the synapse without delay, it must charge up the postsynaptic capacity to a level where a PSP is detectable. Depending on time constants, coupling resistances, and detection thresholds, PSPs at electrical synapses can exhibit significant delays, comparable in magnitude to those associated with chemical mediation (Bennett, 1966). Another aspect of neuronal togetherness is electrotonic spread of subthreshold potentials. Where a synchronous volley is to be initiated by a gradually rising depolarization, synchrony is better if all the cells arrive near threshold at the same time. Spread of subthreshold potentials between cells favors this uniformity of potential. As has been pointed out previously, the action of electrotonic synapses that couple a compact group of cells is both excitatory and inhibitory. A more depolarized cell depolarizes its less depolarized neighbors and, simultaneously, is made less depolarized by them. Rephrased, the depolarized cell transmits depolarization to its neighbors, and simultaneously the neighbors transmit hyperpolarization to the depolarized cell. The action can also be viewed as mediation of positive feedback between cells.

Coupling of neuron somata can be mediated by direct dendrodendritic synapses or there can be presynaptic axons that form electrotonic synapses on two or more neurons and thus mediate coupling indirectly (Pappas and Bennett, 1966; Bennett et al., 1967*d;* Meszler et al., 1972). In terms of the postsynaptic cells there seems to be little difference, but coupling by way of prefibers sometimes allows antidromic invasion into the prefibers from the postsynaptic cells. Antidromic propagation of this kind may be functionally important, or it may never occur because the impulses always proceed in the same direction. Similarly, axons may normally carry impulses in either direction, or the impulse may always arise in the same place and conduction can be unidirectional under normal conditions.

Some of the actions of electrotonic synapses in synchronization are illustrated in Fig. 1. The electric organ of the electric catfish is innervated by only two axons, one on each side of the body (Bennett et al., 1967c). These axons arise from two giant neurons in the rostral spinal cord. When one records from them simultaneously and stimulates fibers afferent to them by means of electrodes on the nearby spinal cord, one obtains graded PSPs as stimulus strength and the number of excited afferent fibers is changed. Although PSP amplitude is quite smoothly graded, one can never obtain a stimulus strength at which only one of the two neurons is excited. This behavior, which is quite different from what one would obtain with ordinary motoneurons, can be explained very simply. The cells are closely coupled electrotonically (by way of presynaptic fibers) and an impulse in one cell excites the other cell. Thus, whichever cell fires first, the other cell must then also fire. Obviously this characteristic is of advantage to the catfish for it thereby achieves maximum voltage and current output from its electric organ.

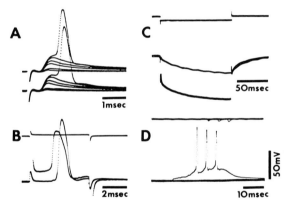

FIG. 1. Properties of the giant electromotor neurons of the electric catfish. *A:* Upper and lower traces, recording from right and left cells, respectively. Brief stimuli of gradually increasing strength are applied to the nearby medulla (several superimposed sweeps, the stimulus artifact occurs near the beginning of the sweep). Depolarizations of successively increasing amplitude are evoked until in one sweep both cells generate spikes. *B:* Two electrodes in the right cell, one for passing current (shown on the upper trace) and one for recording; one recording electrode in the left cell. The traces from the recording electrodes are the lower ones starting from the same base line. When an impulse is evoked in the right cell by a depolarizing pulse, the left cell also generates a spike after a short delay. *C:* When a hyperpolarizing current is passed in the right cell, the left cell also becomes hyperpolarized, but more slowly and to a lesser degree (display as in *B*). *D:* When organ discharge is evoked by irritating the skin, a depolarization gradually rises up to the threshold of the giant cell and initiates a burst of three spikes (lower traces, base line indicated by superimposed sweeps). Each spike produces a response in the organ (upper trace, recorded at high gain and greatly reduced in amplitude because curare is used to prevent movement). Modified from Bennett et al. (1967c).

The two giant neurons appear to be the "command nucleus" that controls organ discharge, for a physiological stimulus to the skin produces graded PSPs that gradually rise up to the threshold of the giant cells (Fig. 1D). The two cells integrate sensory inputs and, depending on whether threshold is reached, "decide" whether or not an organ discharge will occur. In the Sherringtonian sense, the cells are the final common path for organ discharge, the only extension of the concept being that two closely coupled neurons are involved rather than a single motoneuron.

There is significant attenuation and slowing of hyperpolarization in spreading from cell to cell, and when a spike is evoked by a strong depolarizing pulse in one cell, the second cell fires with a delay of about 0.5 msec. This degree of synchrony might well be achieved chemically. However, when the cells are depolarized by synaptic inputs, there are comparable degrees of depolarization in each cell and the cells fire much more synchronously. As is quite reasonable, the propagation of an impulse between them is more rapid when the coupling pathway is depolarized. The synchronization is better than could be achieved by mutually excitatory chemically transmitting synapses with the synaptic delays that have been demonstrated in other systems.

The control system for electric organ discharge in the gymnotids illustrates several additional points (see Bennett et al., 1967d; Bennett, 1968). In this group of fishes the electric organ runs for much of the body length and is innervated segmentally by spinal neurons. The spinal neurons are innervated by a medullary nucleus which is in turn innervated by a higher level medullary nucleus. Recordings from cells of the two medullary nuclei are shown in Fig. 2. What we have termed pacemaker cells (A and B) have a gradually rising potential between spikes; these cells appear to be spontaneously active. In contrast, the potential in the other cells, medullary relay cells, is essentially level between spikes. These cells clearly are activated from somewhere else. Stimulation in a single pacemaker cell produces a small PSP in the relay cells, and hyperpolarization reveals a large PSP underlying the abruptly rising relay-cell spike. Thus, it can be concluded that the PSP is generated by synchronous activity of the pacemaker cells. (As illustrated below, an abruptly rising spike can also arise in dendrites, but the recording of PSPs in the relay cells indicates that this is not the case here.)

Direct evidence by recording from two pacemaker cells in a closely related species suggests that the pacemaker cells are electrically coupled in this species as well. A different kind of experiment confirms electrical coupling as well as indicates that the pacemaker cells are the highest level of the command system, that is, that they are where the frequency of organ discharge is set. If a hyperpolarizing pulse is applied to a single cell, its next impulse is delayed and each subsequent impulse is delayed by a similar amount (Fig. 3B, D). Furthermore, the command signal going down the

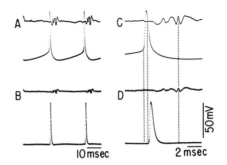

FIG. 2. Responses of pacemaker and relay cells in a weakly electric gymnotid *Gymnotus*. *Upper traces:* Activity in the spinal cord and peripheral nerves leading to the electric organ (recorded by needle electrodes at high gain in a curarized animal). *Lower traces:* Intracellular recordings in pacemaker *(A, C)* and relay *(B, D)* neurons. Faster sweep in C and D where the dotted lines indicate the times of firing of the cells in relation to the descending activity. From Bennett et al. (1967*d*).

spinal cord is also delayed and it is not desynchronized or altered in time course. Clearly the hyperpolarization has spread to the other pacemaker cells and reset the phase of firing of the entire nucleus. Because hyperpolarization spreads from cell to cell, the transmission is presumably electrotonic, although transmission of subthreshold potentials across chemical synapses is also possible (Bennett, 1972*b*). (The next spike in the polarized cell is delayed and its apparent firing level is also increased: probably it is being

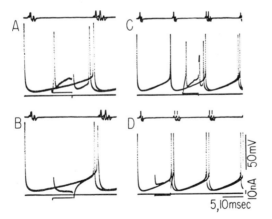

FIG. 3. Effect of polarization in a single pacemaker cell of a weakly electric gymnotid *Gymnotus*. Recording as in Fig. 2 except that current applied through the recording electrode is indicated on the lower trace. Two superimposed sweeps in each record, one with and one without applied current. The sweeps are triggered by the spike of the pacemaker cell. Faster sweep in *A* and *B*. *A, C:* A depolarizing pulse that evokes a spike advances the next and subsequent spikes but does not desynchronize or itself cause any descending activity. *B, D:* A hyperpolarizing pulse retards the next and subsequent spikes but does not desynchronize the descending activity. From Bennett et al. (1967*d*).

fired by its neighbors in the unconditioned case; perhaps its threshold is higher as a result of injury.)

When a single pacemaker cell is stimulated by a depolarizing pulse midway through the cycle, the spike does not propagate into the other cells for there is no discharge recorded in the spinal cord (Fig. 3A, C). And, as shown in other experiments, only a small PSP is recorded in a relay cell. Thus, the pacemaker cells are relatively loosely coupled in contrast to the catfish electromotor neurons. The depolarization does spread to adjacent neurons and does advance their firing, for the command volley in the spinal cord is advanced, again without desynchronization. Although the polarized cell is made relatively refractory following its spike, it is driven to generate a nearly full-sized spike earlier than normal by the surrounding synchronously firing neurons that are coupled to it. An impulse will not spread between cells midway during the pacemaker cycle, but as they near threshold late in the cycle, a small potential spread from one cell should become able to excite neighboring cells. In fact the cells do fire highly synchronously, which indicates that whichever cell or cells fire before the others, this activity spreads very quickly to excite still inactive cells.

In a pacemaker nucleus where cells are continuously active, it is essential that they be coupled if they are to stay in synchrony, for even a tiny frequency difference would soon get them to firing out of phase. Similarly in a command nucleus that receives smoothly graded inputs, such as that controlling organ discharge in the electric catfish, coupling is essential if all cells are to fire at the same time. In a relay nucleus, however, such as that in the medulla of gymnotids, coupling is not obligatory. A large and synchronous volley from a higher level nucleus will produce synchronous firing whether or not the cells are electrotonically coupled to each other. It turns out that many relay nuclei in electric organ control systems are electrotonically coupled, but at least one is not. Those in which coupling is found are in the more precisely synchronized systems, and presumably the coupling helps to resynchronize activity at that level if any asynchrony is present in the descending volley. In the one case where relay cells are known not to be coupled, the electric organ discharge is relatively long lasting and low frequency, and the requirement for synchrony is much less.

As noted above, the precision of synchronization by means of electrotonic coupling must be limited by the size of nucleus involved. A nucleus can initiate a synchronous volley within the limitation of the time required for an impulse to propagate between the cells when all of them are depolarized to near threshold. Synchronous commands perforce arise in small nuclei. The spinal electromotor nucleus of gymnotids, which runs most of the length of the body, is far too long for it to operate synchronously just by interconnections between the neurons (and coupling between these cells can only increase synchrony at a quite local level). The spinal nucleus must be driven by a synchronous volley, and this requirement accounts for occurrence of the pacemaker or command nuclei at a higher level. To return to the Sherringtonian concept, the final common path for organ discharge extends three nuclei back into the nervous system, each nucleus consisting of a number of synchronously firing neurons.

At this point one might ask why there should not be, instead of nuclei, single command cells such as are known in a number of invertebrate systems. [Electrotonically coupled command or pacemaker nuclei are also known in invertebrates (e.g., Willows et al., 1973).] Indeed the electric catfish has but two neurons that innervate some millions of electrocytes. And even in vertebrates there is the Mauthner cell which is a single cell controlling a tail flip to the contralateral side (Diamond, 1971). To explain the multicell and multilevel structure of the gymnotid control system, as well as of those in several other electric fish, one can appeal to biochemical and developmental factors, as well as to considerations of protection against cell loss. For example, there might be an upper limit to the amount of synaptic area that a single neuron can supply. In the catfish, with two command neurons, there is only a tiny synaptic area on each electrocyte, whereas in the electric eel, with thousands of spinal relay neurons, the total synaptic area supplied is much larger. Furthermore, the catfish electric organ apparently arises from a muscle in the pectoral girdle region that could be innervated by neurons in a single segment. The gymnotid organs are derived from axial musculature innervated all along the spinal cord, and developmental mechanisms for extrasegmental innervation by spinal or medullary neurons may not exist. In any case, the precision of firing in the electrotonically coupled nuclei is sufficient for the effector organs controlled.

Another relevant question is how widely separated effector cells fire synchronously when conduction time from the pacemaker would be expected to differ, as, for example, in rostral and caudal electrocytes controlled by a medullary nucleus. An answer has been obtained for the electric eel: there are compensatory delays in presynaptic terminals of the bulbospinal fibers to the more anterior electromotor neurons, and the time from ventral root to electrocyte activation is greater in more anterior regions. These two added delays just compensate for the additional conduction time for the medullary volley to reach the caudal electrocytes. Other mechanisms are known to aid in synchronous activation of widely separated effector cells by a synchronous volley arising in a compact group of controlling cells. Control fibers may proceed more deviously to the nearer cells, thus tending to equalize conduction distance (Bennett, 1968) or fibers going directly to the nearer cells may be of lower conduction velocity (e.g., Pumphrey and Young, 1938). Compensatory delays in synaptic transmission could be another mechanism for synchronization of widely separated effector organs. This possibility is not operative in the electric eel, in which transmission from descending fibers to spinal neurons is electrotonic with a rapidly rising

PSP that allows of little delay. In many systems these mechanisms of getting the signal to all the effector cells simultaneously may be more important than synchronization of the command volley in limiting the final degree of synchronization of effector activity.

The functional significance of electrotonic coupling in the control of highly synchronous effector organs is clear; interaction between controlling cells can be extremely rapid and the observed precision of synchronization requires electrotonic coupling. A few relatively poorly synchronized systems are known to be electrically coupled. An example is shown in Fig. 4. The supramedullary neurons of the puffer (fish) comprise a nucleus of about

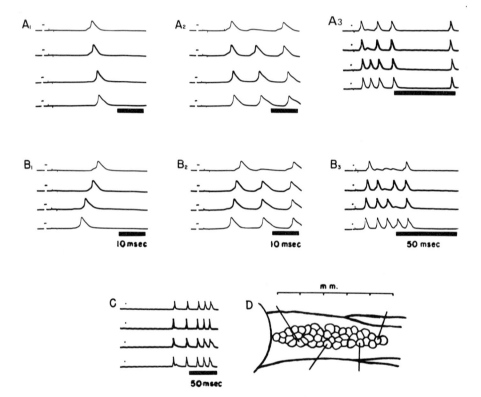

FIG. 4. Synchronous activity of the supramedullary neurons of the puffer. Four cells are recorded from as indicated in the diagram in *D*. Rostral to the left in *D* and uppermost in the recordings. Stimuli of increasing strength are applied by electrodes on the trigeminal and facial nerves (A_1–A_3) and the cauda equina (B_1–B_3). Near-threshold stimuli (A_1, B_1) evoke a single impulse in each cell or no impulses in any cell. The latencies at opposite ends of the cluster can differ by as much as 5 msec under these conditions. Stronger stimuli evoked multiple discharges. Although later impulses may fail to invade the cell bodies because of refractoriness, each axon generates the same number of impulses. Tactile stimuli also evoke synchronous firing *(C)*. A calibration pulse (50 mV, 1 msec) is followed by the stimulus artifact (except C) at the beginning of the sweep. From Bennett et al. (1959).

50 cells that are electrotonically coupled (Bennett et al., 1959, 1967a). They are effector cells that are synaptically activated by cutaneous inputs and that carry efferent impulses in cutaneous nerves. Their function is still unknown, but for whatever they do, they appear to comprise the command nucleus in that they respond synchronously to gradually rising inputs. When responding, every cell generates the same number of impulses, but the dispersion of firing times for different cells can be at least 5 msec, which would allow chemical transmission across a number of synapses. In this example it appears that electrotonic transmission allows a simpler reciprocal action, although reciprocal, excitatory, chemically transmitting synapses conceivably could achieve the same result. As yet, very few systems with this low precision of synchronization have been investigated, and one cannot make an inductive argument for a functional advantage of electrotonic coupling in slow reciprocal excitation.

The foregoing examples are all systems which could be characterized as rigid; generally all the cells fire together. In a few coupled systems there is some effect of stimulus strength on number of cells becoming active, but the systems are very nearly all or none. The concept of the final common path is only a little stretched to cover chains of synchronously firing nuclei. There are a few additional complexities known. There are bilateral command nuclei that therefore cannot be part of the final common path (Bennett, 1968). In the electromotor system of mormyrids, the number of impulses per unit representing a command for one organ discharge changes at each relay (Bennett et al., 1967b; Bennett, 1968). In the electric eel, the frequency of activity in the same controlling neurons determines whether all the electric organs are discharged or whether only the weakly electric organ becomes active for electrolocation (Bennett, 1968) or communication (Bullock, 1970). These minor variations are interesting, but are not yet known to be of much general relevance. There remain the two common observations: synchronization by electrotonic coupling and initiation of synchronous volleys in small nuclei.

SYNCHRONY AND ASYNCHRONY IN ACTIVITY OF OCULOMOTOR NEURONS

In efforts to extend the observations on synchronization and electrotonic transmission to more ordinary motor systems, we found several additional adaptations. A different functional problem arises in the control of muscles which contract quite synchronously for one kind of movement and quite asynchronously for another. We have studied two such systems and have found two different but related modifications that allow for flexibility of control.

The speed of contraction of eye muscles made the oculomotor system an obvious candidate for study of synchronization. Continuing with fish for the sake of experimental convenience, we soon found that the oculo-motor neurons are indeed electrotonically coupled (Kriebel et al., 1969). The coupling is specifically between motoneurons that innervate each single muscle (except that we did not check the abducens neurons). This spec-ificity permits coupling to have a role in directional movements of the eye, rather than merely to increase synchronization in the less interesting act of eye withdrawal.

Another characteristic of the oculomotor neurons soon became apparent and the remaining discussion will concern itself with neurons innervating the medial rectus muscle which we have studied most extensively). If the ipsilateral 8th nerve or the nerve to the horizontal semicircular canal is stimulated, the impulses arise from a nearly level baseline (Fig. 5A$_1$–A$_3$). Very little preceding PSP is seen. In contrast, if the ophthalmic nerve is stimulated, there are large PSPs that rise gradually toward an apparent firing level that is close to that measured by direct stimulation through the recording electrode (Fig. 5B$_1$–B$_3$). The electrode is in or close to the neuron somata because the recordings are obtained just below the ventricular surface where the somata are found. We presumed that the impulses evoked by ipsilateral 8th nerve stimulation are arising out in the dendrites, whereas impulses evoked by ophthalmic nerve stimulation are arising near the cell body, probably in the initial segment. The different origins of the impulses are confirmed by hyperpolarizing in the cell body. A hyperpolarizing pulse easily blocks impulses evoked by ophthalmic nerve stimulation revealing

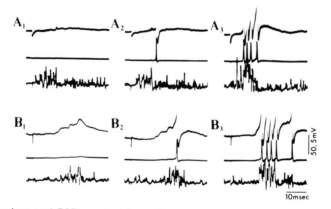

FIG. 5. Impulses and PSPs evoked in oculomotor neurons by ipsilateral 8th nerve and ophthalmic nerve stimulation. *Upper and middle traces:* Intracellular recording at high and low gain from a medial rectus oculomotor neuron. *Lower traces:* Efferent activity in the medial rectus nerve. A$_1$, A$_2$: Threshold stimulation of the ipsilateral 8th nerve. Little PSP is seen whether or not an abruptly rising spike occurs. A$_3$: A stronger stimulus evokes a multispike discharge. The first two spikes arise abruptly. The last two are preceded by some PSP. B$_1$–B$_2$: Threshold stimulation of the ipsilateral ophthalmic nerve. Large slow PSPs appear to initiate the spike. B$_3$: A stronger stimulus evokes a more rapidly rising PSP and multiple spikes.

a large underlying PSP (Fig. 6A$_1$, A$_2$). A similar hyperpolarizing pulse only delays the first spike and reduces the number of spikes evoked by ipsilateral 8th nerve stimulation (Fig. 6B$_1$, B$_2$). At the time when the first spikes arise in the absence of hyperpolarization (arrows), little PSP is seen in the cell body. These data clearly demonstrate that the impulses evoked by ipsilateral 8th nerve stimulation arise distant from the soma. Other experiments show that if these impulses are blocked just before invading the soma, no activity goes out the axon, thus indicating a dendritic site of origin (Korn and Bennett, *unpublished*).

At this point we formulated a hypothesis to explain our results (Fig. 7). For ocular movements of graded amplitude, as are required to stabilize the retinal image during head movements, the impulses arise in the dendrites. The neurons are presumed not to be coupled in the dendritic region, so that a volley can be initiated that is smoothly graded in terms of number of active cells. Very little PSP spreads from dendrites to the somata, as is shown directly. Furthermore, the coupling between cell bodies is sufficiently weak that impulses propagating through the cell bodies do not excite any inactive neurons to which the active cells are coupled. (This last property is established by antidromic stimulation as is described below.) For rapid synchronous movements, such as eye withdrawal evoked by ophthalmic nerve stimulation, large PSPs are generated in the cell bodies and impulses arise in this region. The electrotonic coupling between cell bodies, although

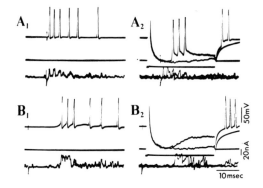

FIG. 6. Differential effects of hyperpolarizing current on impulses arising close to and far from the soma. *Upper trace:* Intracellular recording from a medial rectus oculomotor neuron. *Middle trace:* Current passed through the recording microelectrode using a bridge circuit. *Lower trace:* Efferent activity in the medial rectus nerve. *A$_1$:* Spikes arise abruptly from a level baseline in response to stimulation of the ipsilateral 8th nerve. *A$_2$:* When the same stimulus is given during a hyperpolarizing current pulse, the first response is delayed and the number of spikes is reduced, but little PSP is recorded at the times that the first and second spikes arise in *A$_1$* (two superimposed sweeps with and without nerve stimulation). *B$_1$:* PSPs precede the initial spikes evoked by ipsilateral ophthalmic nerve stimulation. *B$_2$:* When the same stimulus is given during a hyperpolarizing pulse, spikes are blocked revealing a large PSP. (Two superimposed sweeps, with and without nerve stimulation.) From Kriebel et al. (1969).

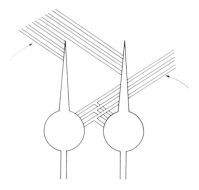

FIG. 7. Diagram of somatic and dendritic inputs to medial rectus oculomotor neurons. The dendritic inputs (left arrow) are activated by stimulation of the ipsilateral 8th nerve. There is no coupling, and movements are smoothly graded in amplitude. The somatic inputs (right arrow) are activated by stimulation of the ophthalmic nerve or contralateral 8th nerve. There is weak coupling between the cell bodies (by way of the presynaptic fibers) and some increase in synchronization of firing results.

weak, provides a significant synchronizing influence since many of the cells are near threshold because of the somatic PSPs.

We could strengthen our hypothesis if we showed that other synchronous and graded movements were controlled by impulses arising in cell bodies and dendrites, respectively, and to date we have extended our studies to vestibular nystagmus (Korn and Bennett, 1971, 1972). Mechanical or repeated electrical stimulation of one horizontal semicircular canal induces slow conjugate movements of the eyes away from the side of stimulation followed by quick movements back toward the stimulated side (Fig. 8B). In the medial rectus muscle, the slow-phase contractions are evoked by ipsilateral stimulation and fast-phase contractions by contralateral stimulation. In the intact animal, the speed of the slow phase is controlled in a graded fashion by the rate of head rotation. Our hypothesis predicts that the slow-phase impulses should arise in the dendrites, and in confirmation we observed that these impulses arise from a level baseline (Fig. 8C$_2$). This is, of course, only a minor extension of our observation of dendritic impulse initiation in response to single shock stimulation of the ipsilateral 8th nerve.

The fast phase is a sudden, convulsive movement, and our hypothesis predicts that the mediating impulses should arise in the cell bodies. In fact, the impulses arise from large PSPs indicating somatic origin (Fig. 8C$_1$). Here the impulses would to some extent be synchronized by the electrotonic coupling between cells.

We have obtained some verification for synchronization of impulses arising in the somata and lack of interaction between impulses arising in the dendrites. If we antidromically stimulate the medial rectus nerve, we usually find that the cell we are recording from is not that with the lowest threshold

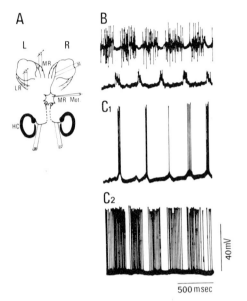

FIG. 8. Different sites of impulse initiation in vestibular nystagmus. *A:* Diagram of recording and stimulating electrodes. LR, lateral rectus; MR, medial rectus; HC, horizontal semicircular canal. *B:* EMG recordings from the left medial rectus muscle *(upper trace)* and left lateral rectus muscle *(lower trace)*. Nystagmus is evoked by a train of brief electrical stimuli to the left horizontal canal. Brief fast phases in the lateral rectus alternate with longer lasting slow phases in the medial rectus. *C:* Intracellular recording from a right medial rectus motoneuron. Stimulation as in *B* evokes brief bursts of spikes corresponding to the fast phases. The impulses arise from large PSPs indicating somatic origin. Similar stimulation of the right horizontal canal evokes longer lasting trains of spikes separated by brief silent periods corresponding to the fast phases in *B*. These impulses rise abruptly, indicating dendritic origin. From Korn and Bennett *(unpublished)*.

axon. Thus graded antidromic stimulation subthreshold for the penetrated cell's axon produces graded depolarizations that represent electrotonic potentials from spike activity of stimulated neighboring cells to which the penetrated cell is coupled. Because the coupling is weak, these graded depolarizations never reach the threshold of the resting penetrated cell (which is how we know the coupling is weak). If, however, we stimulate the contralateral horizontal semicircular canal to evoke a subthreshold PSP in the soma of the penetrated cell, then the graded antidromic depolarizations can summate with the vestibular PSP to fire the cell (Fig. 9). This demonstrates a significant synchronizing effect of the coupling, i.e., if the cells are depolarized by somatic PSPs and some of the cells fire, their activity can spread to excite other cells that would otherwise not fire. In the case of Fig. $9B_3$, the synchronization is fairly precise; the penetrated cell fires near the peak of the antidromic depolarization which is only shortly after the other cells have fired. Synchronization need not be so precise. The penetrated cell can be made to fire quite a long time after the antidromic

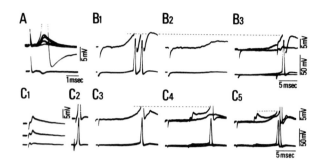

FIG. 9. Synchronization mediated by electrotonic coupling between somata of oculomotor neurons: interaction of somatic inputs with responses to antidromic stimulation. *A, upper trace:* Graded depolarizations produced in a medial rectus motoneuron by graded antidromic stimulation. Five superimposed traces. As stimulus strength is increased, an increasing depolarization is recorded which reaches a maximum amplitude of about 4 mV before the axon of the impaled cell is excited. *A, lower trace:* Potential later recorded just outside the cell with an antidromic stimulus near threshold for the cell. *B:* A different motoneuron, higher gain on upper trace. B_1: A relatively strong stimulus to the contralateral horizontal semicircular canal evokes two spikes preceded by a large, slowly rising PSP. The firing level of the cell for somatic inputs may be taken as the point at which the rapid rise of the spike begins (dashed line). B_2: A weaker vestibular stimulus evokes only a subthreshold PSP. B_3: Two superimposed sweeps, one with an antidromic stimulus just subthreshold for the impaled cell, one with the antidromic stimulus preceded by vestibular stimulation as in B_2. The antidromic stimulus evokes a depolarization that summates with the vestibular PSP to excite the cell at the firing level for somatic inputs. *C:* A different motoneuron. Higher gain on upper trace in all but C_1. C_1: Two sizes of the antidromic depolarization in this cell *(upper two traces)* and extracellular antidromic potential recorded later *(lower trace)*. C_2: Antidromic spike evoked by a stronger stimulus. C_3: Stimulation of the nerve to the contralateral horizontal semicircular canal adequate to evoke a spike; the dotted line indicates the firing level. C_4: Two superimposed sweeps, one with a weaker vestibular stimulus that evokes only a PSP and one with this vestibular stimulus followed by an antidromic stimulus. The antidromic stimulus evokes a depolarization that summates with the PSP to excite the cell when the firing level is reached. C_5: As in C_4 but with vestibular stimulation adequate to excite the cell. Summation of PSP and preceding antidromic depolarization advanced firing of the cell by causing it to reach the firing level sooner. (The firing level and the spike amplitude are decreased slightly, presumably due to injury.)

depolarization (Fig. $9C_4$), or its impulse which occurs anyway can be slightly advanced in time by a preceding antidromic depolarization (Fig. $9C_5$). The latter result represents a small improvement in synchronization rather than recruitment of unexcited cells.

Although we have not recorded from the dendrites, we can infer from experiments similar to those just described that there is no significant coupling between dendrites. We have interacted antidromic stimuli with ipsilateral 8th nerve stimuli. We have never observed antidromic stimulation of neighboring cells to summate with a dendritic input to excite otherwise unexcited cells or to generate additional spikes in those which were already excited. To conclude that there is no coupling between dendrites we need to know that the antidromic impulse propagates out the dendrites to the impulse-initiating site or sites. We can show that it does by the effect of an antidromic spike on dendritic responses. If the impulse propagates out to the impulse-initiating site in the dendrite, it should leave that region refractory. A large dendritic PSP would be able to evoke an impulse sooner in the relative refractory period after the antidromic spike than a small dendritic PSP. In fact we observe that a strong stimulus to the ipsilateral 8th nerve will evoke a dendritic impulse sooner after an antidromic stimulus than will a weak ipsilateral 8th nerve stimulus. Thus we conclude that antidromic impulses propagate far enough into the dendrite that they should reveal any coupling that was present.

To recapitulate our theory, for movements smoothly graded in amplitude, impulses arise in the dendrites where there is no interaction between the cells; for movements which are convulsive and involve large contractions, impulses arise in the cell bodies where electrotonic coupling provides a significant synchronizing influence. The electrotonic separation between dendritic and somatic sites of impulse initiation is so great that there is little spread of PSPs between them (which we know directly for dendrosomatic spread, and can infer for somatodendritic spread from lack of effect of antidromic graded depolarizations in the somata on dendritic inputs). The coupling between cell bodies is sufficiently weak that significant interaction between impulses in the cell bodies does not occur unless the cells are depolarized by PSPs. Finally, one should not confuse coupling between dendrites with electrotonic transmission to them; that is, short latency of response and degree of synchronization are not the same. Image-stabilizing movements of the eye should occur with the shortest possible latency, which could involve electrical transmission from vestibular fibers, but these movements should be smoothly graded in amplitude, which implies absence of coupling between the dendrites on which the vestibular fibers synapse.

We have demonstrated dendritic impulse initiation for the slow phase of nystagmus and for single stimuli to the 8th nerve which would correspond to the compensatory movements for sudden head rotations. We have demonstrated somatic impulse initiation for the fast phase of nystagmus and for ophthalmic nerve stimulation which evokes eye withdrawal. We plan to extend these investigations to optokinetic nystagmus where we expect slow- and fast-phase movements to be mediated by impulses arising in dendrites and somata, respectively.

Our present data indicate that the oculomotor neurons are relay cells for the fast phase of nystagmus in the sense discussed previously in respect to electric organ control in gymnotids. The neurons in between fast phases are not depolarized; there is a PSP that arises fairly suddenly when the fast phase is about to begin. Thus these neurons are not integrating during the slow phase to reach a group threshold which then initiates the fast phase. Similarly, cells that are active during the slow phase presumably are responding as individual cells to vestibular inputs relayed in the vestibular nuclei. Each motoneuron is, of course, the final common path for its motor unit, but one would not apply the concepts of command and relay nuclei to a smoothly graded evoked response of a population such as that mediating the slow phase of nystagmus.

If the failure to observe axon collaterals morphologically can be relied upon, then activity of the oculomotor neurons does not participate in the triggering of convulsive movements in any way and a higher level nucleus or nuclei must be considered responsible. Thus, because oculomotor neurons only relay the fast-phase command signal, coupling between them is not required; it can only be considered an aid to synchronization. This allows us to retain a hypothetical role for electrotonic coupling in control of eye movements in mammals, in which the oculomotor neurons apparently are not coupled (Baker and Precht, 1972; Korn and Bennett, *unpublished*). We hypothesize that there is coupling between neurons of the command nucleus that initiates fast-phase movements (and perhaps eye withdrawal where it occurs).

Saccadic eye movements allow for some interesting speculation. These movements are brief and rapid and occur either spontaneously or in response to gradually increasing displacement of retinal images. These characteristics suggest that there would be coupling between a group of neurons initiating a command for a saccadic movement. However, the amplitude of a saccadic movement is smoothly graded, which implies a lack of interaction between controlling neurons. A way out is provided by a system analogous to a square-wave stimulator in which positive feedback is responsible for initiating a rapidly rising all-or-nothing pulse that is then fed through an independently controlled attenuator that determines amplitude. In the biological case, there could be a command nucleus of coupled cells that initiates a synchronous volley. Then this volley could pass through a relay nucleus in which the excitability of the cells is varied by inhibitory or excitatory inputs. Thus, an all-or-nothing volley from the command nucleus could be attenuated to a controlled degree, and, assuming that the PSP produced by the command volley rose rapidly to its peak, there would be very little desynchronization as a result of attenuation. A possible example is provided by motoneurons controlling the sonic muscle of the toadfish (Bennett, 1966; Pappas and Bennett, 1966a,b). These cells are subject to a large, slow hyperpolarization before abruptly rising PSPs excite them. The inhibition may represent an amplitude control of the type suggested. There is also some support for this kind of mechanism in the oculomotor system of monkeys (R. Llinás, *personal communication*). The responses of certain cerebellar Purkinje neurons are inversely related in terms of number of impulses to the amplitude of spontaneous saccadic eye movements. These neurons are presumably inhibitory and could be projecting to a relay for volleys initiating saccadic movements.

COUPLING AND DECOUPLING IN THE BUCCAL GANGLION
OF *NAVANAX*

A different mechanism whereby the same group of neurons can control both synchronous and asynchronous movements is provided by the opistho-branch mollusc *Navanax*. This organism exhibits very unusual behavior for a mollusc. It eats other molluscs including *Aplysia* and *Navanax* and pursues them by following their mucous trails. Upon encountering a prey organism, it convulsively expands its pharynx and sucks the hapless victim in with a speed that is truly remarkable for this otherwise sluggish (indeed) creature (Paine, 1965). (*Navanax* will sometimes make passes at an animal too big to swallow; if the oversized prey is another *Navanax*, they then will mate.)

Neurons controlling the radial musculature of the pharynx are found in the buccal ganglia (Spira and Bennett, 1972). It is these muscles that mediate pharyngeal expansion. Their contraction thins the pharyngeal wall and thereby enlarges the lumen; these muscles apparently push sideways as well as pull lengthwise. Several large and identifiable neurons are involved (Fig. 10). It is not clear whether these cells constitute a command nucleus or whether they relay a command volley from a higher level, but under ordinary circumstances they are electrotonically coupled (Levitan et al., 1970; Spira and Bennett, 1972). Coupling is not particularly close, but if each of a pair of neurons is depolarized by current applied in it, a moderate degree of synchronous firing can result (Fig. 11). Widespread depolarizating PSPs is what one would expect these cells to receive if they did constitute the command nucleus for convulsive pharyngeal expansion, but more work is required to establish the pathways of the feeding response.

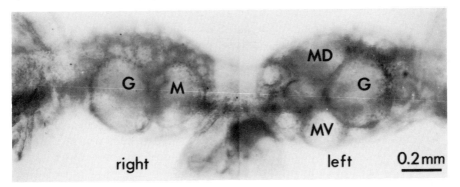

FIG. 10. The buccal ganglia of *Navanax inermis* viewed from the anterior side. The giant (G) cells and medium-sized (M) cells are labeled. There are dorsal and ventral M cells on the left side (MD and MV). The two sides are connected by a commissure from which a nerve runs anteriorly (out of the plane of focus of the picture). Pharyngeal nerves and connectives to the cerebral ganglia leave the ganglia at their lateral margins. The preparation is unstained and the sheath is intact. From Spira and Bennett (1971).

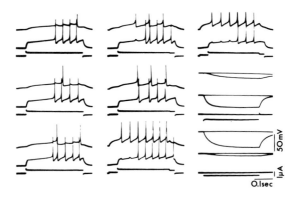

FIG. 11. Electrotonic coupling and synchronization of G and M cells in *Navanax. Upper traces:* Recording from an M cell, the spike of which goes off screen. *Middle traces:* Recording from an ipsilateral G cell. *Lower traces:* Current applied in the two cells. For the left and center columns a constant depolarizing pulse is passed in the G cell, while increasing pulses are applied in the M cell. Greater degrees of synchronization are observed when the M cell is depolarized. With appropriate currents a spike in either cell can initiate a spike in the other. The right column shows another record with depolarizing current in both cells and records with hyperpolarization applied in one cell at a time. From Spira and Bennett *(unpublished).*

Although we had begun to study these cells in order to look at biophysical properties of the coupling, an unexpected and surprising behavior spotted by my collaborator Micha Spira led us into the area I am now describing. This peculiar observation was that the degree of coupling between cells could suddenly and spontaneously decrease for a short period. After having checked for all the obvious artifacts, we became convinced that the phenomenon was real; we also observed that it was associated with increased synaptic activity. We then found that the effect could be produced by a brief train of stimuli to the pharyngeal nerve as is illustrated in Fig. 12.

The decoupling for slow electrotonic potentials is dramatic and virtually complete. It is associated with a fairly large decrease in input resistance, which drops to a half or a third of its resting value. The decrease in input resistance is due to activation of inhibitory synapses, for the inhibitory PSP (IPSP) reversal potential is very close to the resting potential. To some extent the decoupling can be explained in terms of a simple equivalent circuit for coupling in which the resistances of the two cells and the coupling pathway are each represented by a single resistor (Fig. 13A). The coupling coefficients in the two directions are given by:

$$\frac{V_2}{V_1} = \frac{r_2}{r_c + r_2} \qquad \text{(potential generated in cell 1 and spread to cell 2)}$$

$$\frac{V_1}{V_2} = \frac{r_1}{r_c + r_1} \qquad \text{(potential generated in cell 2 and spread to cell 1)}$$

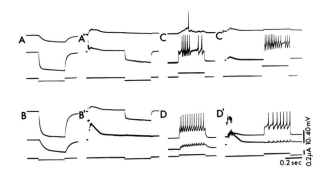

FIG. 12. Synaptic control of electrotonic coupling of G and M cells. *Upper traces:* Recording from an M cell. *Middle traces:* Recording from an ipsilateral G cell (higher gain in row of *B,B', D,D'*). *Lower traces:* Polarizing current applied in G cell for upper records and in M cell for lower records. Primed letters indicate that a decoupling train of stimuli is applied to the large ipsilateral pharyngeal nerve at the beginning of the sweep. *A, B:* Electrotonic spread of hyperpolarization. *C, D:* Spread of depolarization. Spikes in the polarized cells produce small, somewhat slowed, depolarizing components in the unpolarized cell. These relatively brief potentials are superimposed on a slow depolarization. The irregularity of firing in *C* is due to activation of an inhibitory interneuron by stimulation in the G cell. *A', B':* Electrotonic spread of hyperpolarization is practically eliminated after decoupling stimuli. The input resistance of the cells is reduced to about half. During hyperpolarization small oscillations become visible which represent variations in the synaptic activity responsible for the decoupling. These oscillations are much smaller at the resting potential because their equilibrium (or, better, reversal) potential is near this point. *C', D':* Electrotonic spread of depolarization is greatly reduced after decoupling stimuli. Reduction in spread of maintained depolarization is greater than reduction in spread of spikes. Stimulation in the G cell no longer can excite the M cell. The M cell can still be excited by stimuli applied in its own soma, although its excitability is reduced *(D')*. From Spira and Bennett (1971).

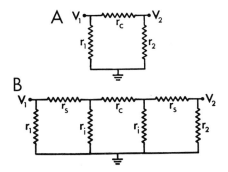

FIG. 13. Equivalent circuits for electrotonic coupling and synaptic decoupling. *A:* The simplest equivalent. Each cell and the coupling pathway are represented by a single resistor (r_1, r_2, and r_c, respectively). *B:* A more complicated circuit where r_s represents the series resistance of collaterals that constitute the coupling pathway and r_i represents the resistance of inhibitory synapses at the site of coupling. From Spira and Bennett *(unpublished)*.

A decrease in the cell resistances without change in the coupling resistance will decrease the coupling coefficients. The observed decreases in input resistances are insufficient to explain the decrease in coupling by this simple model, and it is necessary to invoke additional factors. A simple and reasonable possibility is that there are inhibitory synapses distributed or localized along the coupling pathway. With suitable parameters such a placement could lead to a given reduction of electrotonic spread between cells with much less change in input resistance than required by the simple model. This point may be seen by inspection of the more complex equivalent circuit in Fig. 13B. Here r_1 and r_2 represent the cell resistances exclusive of the coupling pathway; r_s represents the series resistance of collaterals that are presumed to mediate coupling of the cells; r_c represents the junctional resistance; and r_i represents the resistance of inhibitory synapses localized at the site of coupling. It is obvious, if r_i goes to zero, that the cells will be completely decoupled but that the input resistances will remain finite. Simple calculations show that the values of coupling coefficients and input resistances at rest and during decoupling are consistent with this circuit. A possibility which is quite unconventional is that the junctional resistance itself changes. While there are a few known instances of reversible changes in coupling resistance, none of these involves synaptic control (Asada and Bennett, 1971; Rose and Loewenstein, 1971; Socolar and Politoff, 1971). Although it is possible that strategically placed synapses could affect gap junctions by means involving a chemical transmitter, we will not consider such mechanisms seriously until we have much more data.

Transmission of spikes is less reduced by the synaptically controlled decoupling than is transmission of slow potentials. At least two factors may contribute to this difference. The spikes probably propagate part of the way along the coupling pathway and are thereby less reduced, and some of the spike contributions recorded during decoupling may be transmitted across the extracellular space of the large area of apposition between the cells that we were studying. If the latter mechanism contributes, differential recording across the cell wall should reduce it. Moreover, in terms of synchronization with the observed degree of imprecision, transmission of slow potentials may be as important as transmission of spikes. These qualifications become of less concern given the indications of physiological significance discussed below.

Of course, two explanations of the decoupling quickly come to mind. One is that it is just a simple side effect that accompanies the observed inhibition and that it has no function. The other relates to the control of synchronous movements of prey capture and asynchronous movements such as peristalsis. Perhaps the decoupling allows the cells to fire asynchronously when they are mediating the latter kind of movement, and indeed we had observed the cells to fire asynchronously following a stimulus that evoked decoupling.

Support for the latter function of decoupling is provided by the following experiments. The isolated pharynx with buccal ganglia attached but disconnected from the remainder of the nervous system often exhibits a certain amount of spontaneous movement. If one inflates a small balloon in the pharynx, peristalsis is evoked that causes the balloon to be passed out of the pharynx into the esophagus (Fig. 14). If the same inflationary stimulus is given and the balloon is kept in the pharynx, periodic activity ensues (Fig. 15). In an M cell which controls expansion of about one-quarter of the pharynx, there are bursts of impulses alternating with large apparently unitary IPSPs (which are depolarizing). Before each burst of impulses the cell is markedly decoupled from the G cell which causes expansion over the entire pharynx. Most important, these data demonstrate that decoupling can be evoked by physiological stimuli. The balloon we have used is, after all, a good deal smaller than the snails that *Navanax* can swallow. We require further information on patterns of motor activity and coupling during the peristalsis, but the present observations certainly suggest that decoupling is allowing cells to act independently under appropriate conditions.

The flexibility of coupling in *Navanax* differs from the mechanism in teleost oculomotor neurons in that it is mediated by inhibitory synapses. The inhibitory synapses appear to be appropriately localized along the coupling pathway, just as localization of specific inputs is basic to the oculomotor mechanism.

The control of coupling by inhibition may be of much wider importance. For example, lumbar motoneurons of the frog apparently are coupled

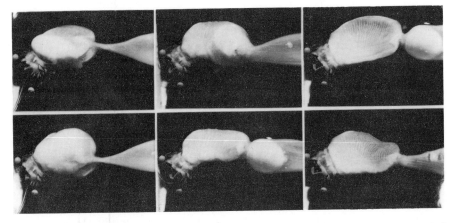

FIG. 14. Pharyngeal peristalsis controlled by the buccal ganglion. A balloon connected to a small tube is inserted into the pharynx. *Upper left,* prior to inflation. *Lower left,* immediately after inflation. *Upper middle,* the balloon is at the posterior end of the pharynx. *Lower middle,* the balloon has been pushed into the esophagus. *Upper right,* the pharynx is more or less relaxed again. *Lower right,* the balloon has been moved further down the esophagus. The pharynx is about 3 cm long. From Spira and Bennett *(unpublished).*

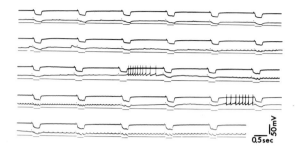

FIG. 15. Decoupling evoked by physiological stimulation. The preparation is a pharynx with buccal ganglia attached. *Upper traces:* Recording from a G cell in which a hyperpolarizing current pulse was passed every 1.7 sec. *Middle traces:* Recording from an adjacent M cell. *Lower traces:* Polarizing current. A continuous recording from top to bottom. A balloon was inflated in the pharynx (see Fig. 14) near the beginning of the second line. Two bursts of spikes appear in the M cell which are preceded by decoupling from the G cell. The bursts of spikes alternate with trains of depolarizing inhibitory PSPs. A 10-mV calibration pulse precedes each current pulse. From Spira and Bennett *(unpublished).*

electrotonically, probably out in the dendritic regions (Grinnell, 1970). The coupling may help to synchronize the convulsive act of jumping. In this response virtually all the hind-leg muscles are involved, for most are an extensor of one joint and a flexor of another. The frog also moves about more sedately, and his hind leg can be used to scratch his back or belly in response to local irritations. Under these circumstances, coupling might well be decreased by inhibitory inputs to the dendrites. The sensory neurons of the mesencephalic nucleus of the fifth cranial nerve are coupled in rodents, if not in other mammals (Baker and Llinás, 1971). Chemical synapses that occur on the cell bodies may be inhibitory and control the spread of impulses between the sensory fibers. Dendrodentric electrotonic synapses have recently been found (morphologically) in the olfactory bulb (Pinching and Powell, 1971), sensory motor cortex (Sloper, 1972), cerebellar cortex (Sotelo and Llinás, 1972), and inferior olive of mammals (Sotelo and Llinás, *personal communication*). Again inhibitory inputs to the dendrites could control the degree of coupling between cells.

SUMMARY AND CONCLUSIONS

Initially in this chapter I discussed how a number of neurons can act together to operate effector organs in which all the effector cells respond together. For very precise synchronization of a command nucleus, which is often observed, electrical transmission is required. At the least, electrical transmission allows a number of cells to act together as a single unit, obviating the necessity of single-celled command elements. For less precise synchronization, the reciprocal property of electrotonic synapses and transmission of subthreshold signals may be important. Certainly electrical transmission is found in several systems where the precision of synchronization is not very great and where one might anticipate that the delay of chemical transmission would not be prohibitive. Moreover, although the number of slow systems studied is small, there are no nuclei in which synchronization is known to be mediated by mutually excitatory, chemically transmitting synapses.

Sherrington's concept of the final common path was extended from the single motoneuron to two or more synchronously firing cells controlling an organ to a chain of nuclei, the highest level comprising the command or pacemaker nucleus and successive lower level nuclei comprising relays. It was noted how mutual excitation by electrotonic synapses worked rather well over short distances, but that effector organs—such as electric organs—had difficulty in getting the signal to all the right places simultaneously. The solution was the introduction of compensatory delays in various ways, always involving impulse conduction time as far as has yet been determined.

A number of complications were considered, such as bifurcation of the controlling pathway where either of two command nuclei can activate the lower common relay nuclei. Another complication was control by frequency in the common pathway that runs to different sections of the electric organ of the electric eel.

The basic theme to this point was how mutually excitatory interaction or positive feedback between cells leads to synchronization. I then turned to a different set of problems, namely, how a set of effectors could be activated synchronously under some conditions and asynchronously under others. Coupling between cells was found to be under physiological control in two examples. In the first instance, teleost oculomotor neurons, the cells are weakly coupled in the region of the somata and apparently not coupled at all in the dendrites. Large PSPs generated on or near the somata initiate impulses apparently in the initial segment of the axon, and the coupling provides significant feedback and sharpening of the input-output relation. These impulses mediate the convulsive movements of eye withdrawal and the quick phase of vestibular nystagmus. In contrast, graded movements of the eye associated with image stabilization and evoked by vestibular stimulation arise in the dendrites where no interaction between neighboring cells can be demonstrated. These impulses of dendritic origin propagate through the cell bodies where the coupling is too weak to mediate interaction in the absence of any synaptic depolarization. Thus spatial segregation of inputs allows mutual excitation with one set of inputs and independence with another. The problem of amplitude control of a synchronous act was considered, and a possible mechanism was proposed. A synchronous and all-or-none volley could arise in a coupled nucleus and then be attenuated (in terms of number of active elements) by passage through a relay nucleus that was inhibited to a variable degree. Appropriate neural circuitry apparently exists in the control system of the sonic muscle in the toadfish, and there is some evidence for this mechanism in the oculomotor system of mammals.

The neurons controlling pharyngeal expansion in *Navanax* provide a different kind of mechanism in which control of coupling is provided by inhibitory synapses, apparently also strategically placed. The neurons are coupled ordinarily, and increased synchronization of firing presumably occurs when the cells fire to control the sudden pharyngeal expansion for prey capture. When the neurons are involved in peristalsis, they fire asynchronously, and under these conditions inhibitory inputs reduce their input resistances and decrease electrotonic spread between them. The changes of input resistance and of degree of coupling are such as to suggest that the inhibitory synapses are strategically located along the pathway coupling the cells. This mechanism of controlling spread between cells by inhibitory synapses along the coupling pathway is one that appears applicable to a number of systems in higher vertebrates in which coupling has been observed.

Finally one may ask whether the concepts of command nucleus, relay nucleus, and final common path have any relevance to higher level decision problems. Does positive feedback, electrically mediated or not, act to mobilize large numbers of cells in the threshold decisions of "is a signal present" or of "approach versus avoidance?" Certainly, if coupling between cells can be modulated, cells can have different functions under different conditions, and the simple notions of command and relay break down; yet the extension required to cover such cases does not seem too large. To go back to the simplest case, the command to discharge the electric organ of the electric catfish can be considered to be two neurons reaching threshold, or it can be considered the activity of any set of inputs to the cells that will excite them.

The first idea is simple and perhaps useful; the second idea requires so complete a knowledge as to be virtually useless, although it does represent a much more nearly complete description. It would seem best to press on in the analysis of specific systems, using our terminology to design experiments, but also using our results to modify our terminology.

ACKNOWLEDGMENTS

I am indebted to my colleagues Mahlon Kriebel, Henri Korn, and Micha Spira for permission to use hitherto unpublished figures and ideas that are of collaborative origin. This work was supported in part by U.S. Public Health Service grants NB-07512 and HD-04248 from the National Institutes of Health and by a grant from the Alfred P. Sloan Foundation.

REFERENCES

Asada, Y., and Bennett, M. V. L. (1971): Experimental alteration of coupling resistance at an electrotonic synapse. *J. Cell Biol.* 49:159–172.

Auerbach, A. A., and Bennett, M. V. L. (1969): A rectifying synapse in the central nervous system of a vertebrate. *J. Gen. Physiol.* 53:211–237.

Baker, R., and Llinás, R. (1971): Electrotonic coupling between neurons in the rat mesencephalic nucleus. *J. Physiol.*, 212:45–63.

Baker, R., and Precht, W. (1972): Electrophysiological properties of trochlear motoneurons as revealed by VIth nerve stimulation. *Exp. Brain Res.* 14:125–157.

Bennett, M. V. L. (1966): Physiology of electrotonic junctions. *Ann. N.Y. Acad. Sci.* 137:509–539.

Bennett, M. V. L. (1968): Neural control of electric organs. In: *The Central Nervous System and Fish Behavior*, edited by D. Ingle, pp. 147–169. Univ. of Chicago Press, Chicago.

Bennett, M. V. L. (1972a): Electrical versus chemical neurotransmission. In: *Research Publication of the A.R.N.M.D.*, Vol. 50: *Neurotransmitters*, pp. 58–89. Williams & Wilkins, Baltimore.

Bennett, M. V. L. (1972b): A comparison of electrically and chemically mediated transmission. In: *Structure and Function of Synapses*, edited by G. D. Pappas and D. P. Purpura, pp. 221–256. Raven Press, New York.

Bennett, M. V. L. (1973a): Function of electrotonic junctions in embryonic and adult tissues. *Fed. Proc.* 32:65–75.

Bennett, M. V. L. (1973b): Permeability and structure of electrotonic junctions and intercellular movement of tracers. In: *Intracellular Staining in Neurobiology*, edited by S. D. Kater and C. Nicholson, pp. 115–133. Elsevier, New York.

Bennett, M. V. L., Crain, S. M., and Grundfest, H. (1959): Electrophysiology of supramedullary neurons in *Spheroides maculatus*. III. Organization of the supramedullary neurons. *J. Gen. Physiol.* 43:221–250.

Bennett, M. V. L., Nakajima, Y., and Pappas, G. D. (1967a): Physiology and ultrastructure of electrotonic junctions. I. Supramedullary neurons. *J. Neurophysiol.* 30:161–179.

Bennett, M. V. L., Pappas, G. D., Aljure, E., and Nakajima, Y. (1967b): Physiology and ultrastructure of electrotonic junctions. II. Spinal and medullary electromotor nuclei in Mormyrid fish. *J. Neurophysiol.* 30:180–208.

Bennett, M. V. L., Nakajima, Y., and Pappas, G. D. (1967c): Physiology and ultrastructure of electrotonic junctions. III. Giant electromotor neurons of *Malapterurus electricus*. *J. Neurophysiol.* 30:209–235.

Bennett, M. V. L., Pappas, G. D., Giménez, M., and Nakajima, Y. (1967d): Physiology and ultrastructure of electrotonic junctions. IV. Medullary electromotor nuclei in gymnotid fish. *J. Neurophysiol.* 30:236–301.

Bullock, T. H. (1970): Species differences in effect of electroreceptor input on electric organ pacemakers and other aspects of behavior in electric fish. *Brain, Behav. Evol.* 2:85–118.

Diamond, J. (1971): The Mauthner cell. In: *Fish Physiology*, Vol. 5, edited by W. S. Hoar and D. J. Randall, pp. 265–346. Academic Press, New York.

Grinnell, A. D. (1970): Electrical interaction between antidromically stimulated frog motoneurons and dorsal root afferents: Enhancement by gallamine and TEA. *J. Physiol.* 210:17–43.

Korn, H., and Bennett, M. V. L. (1971): Dendritic and somatic impulse initiation in fish oculomotor neurons during vestibular nystagmus. *Brain Res.* 27:169–175.

Korn, H., and Bennett, M. V. L. (1972): Electrotonic coupling between teleost oculomotor neurons: restriction to somatic regions and function of somatic and dendritic sites of impulse initiation. *Brain Res.* 38:433–439.

Kriebel, M. E., Bennett, M. V. L., Waxman, S. G., and Pappas, G. D. (1969): Oculomotor neurons in fish: Electrotonic coupling and multiple sites of impulse initiation. *Science* 166:520–524.

Levitan, H., Tauc, L., and Segundo, J. P. (1970): Electrical transmission among neurons in the buccal ganglion of a mollusc, *Navanax inermis*. *J. Gen. Physiol.* 55:484–496.

Meszler, R. M., Pappas, G. D., and Bennett, M. V. L. (1972): Morphological demonstration of electrotonic coupling of neurons by way of presynaptic fibers. *Brain Res.* 37:412–415.

Paine, R. T. (1963): Food recognition and predation on opisthobranchs by *Navanax inermis*. *Veliger* 6:1–9.

Pappas, G. D., and Bennett, M. V. L. (1966a): Specialized junctions involved in electrical transmission between neurons. *Ann. N.Y. Acad. Sci.* 137:495–508.

Pappas, G. D., and Bennett, M. V. L. (1966b): Fine structure of two transmission systems operating toadfish motoneurons. Sixth Int. Cong. for Electron Microscopy, Kyoto. pp. 429–430.

Payton, B. W., Bennett, M. V. L., and Pappas, G. D. (1969): Permeability and structure of junctional membranes at an electrotonic synapse. *Science* 166:1641–1643.

Pinching, A. J., and Powell, T. P. S. (1971): The neuropil of the glomeruli of the olfactory bulb. *J. Cell. Sci.* 9:347–377.

Pumphrey, R. J., and Young, J. Z. (1938): The rates of conduction of nerve fibers of various diameters in cephalopods. *J. Ext. Viol.*, 15:453–466.

Rose, B., and Loewenstein, W. R. (1971): Junctional membrane permeability. Depression by substitution of Li for extracellular Na, and by long-term lack of Ca and Mg; restoration by cell repolarization. *J. Membrane Biol.* 5:20–50.

Sloper, J. J. (1972): Gap junctions between dendrites in the primate neocortex. *Brain Res.* 44:641–646.

Socolar, S. J., and Politoff, A. L. (1971): Uncoupling cell junctions in a glandular epithelium by depolarizing current. *Science* 172:492–494.

Sotelo, C., and Llinás, R. (1972): Specialized membrane junctions between neurons in the vertebrate cerebellar cortex. *J. Cell Biol.* 53:271–289.

Spira, M. E., and Bennett, M. V. L. (1972): Synaptic control of electrotonic coupling between neurons. *Brain Res.* 37:294–300.

Willows, A. O. D., Dorsett, D. A., and Hoyle, G. (1973): The neuronal basis of behavior in *Tritonia*. III. Neuronal mechanism of a fixed action pattern. *J. Neurobiol.* 4:255–285.

Synaptic Transmission and Neuronal Interaction
Raven Press, New York 1974

The Nicotinic Acetylcholine Receptor: Characterization and Properties of a Macromolecule Isolated from *Electrophorus electricus*

R. P. Klett, B. W. Fulpius, D. Cooper, and E. Reich

Rockefeller University, New York, New York 10021

I. INTRODUCTION

The chemical theory of synaptic transmission is based on two main elements: the chemical transmitter that is released at the nerve ending upon arrival of a nerve impulse and the specific receptor that initiates a change in ionic permeability of the postsynaptic membrane following interaction with transmitter. Although the transfer of excitation at the neuromuscular junction is the most thoroughly studied example of chemical transmission in the nervous system, the molecular events at the postsynaptic membrane are still poorly understood. In spite of numerous attempts, no molecule that exhibits all the properties expected of the acetylcholine receptor has been isolated and fully characterized. This failure has been due in part to the lack of a specific reagent for the detection of such molecules; cholinergic ligands which have been used in the past proved unsatisfactory, since they do not possess the necessary binding specificity. These limitations appear to have been relieved by the work of Chang and Lee (1963), who first demonstrated the curare-like effect of neurotoxins isolated from elapid venoms; electrophysiological evidence suggests that the block in neuromuscular transmission is caused by binding of the toxins directly to the acetylcholine receptor, thereby preventing the depolarizing action of acetylcholine. In contrast to curare, neurotoxin binding to receptor sites on intact tissue is practically irreversible. On the other hand, toxin binding is also decreased in presence of cholinergic drugs. These toxins thus act as specific and powerful affinity reagents for detecting cholinergic receptor molecules, and they are being used for this purpose in several laboratories.

II. NEUROTOXIN

The commercially available venom of the Siamese cobra—*Naja naja siamensis*—is a particularly rich and relatively inexpensive source of neurotoxin. After chromatography of venom on phosphocellulose, Sephadex G 50 M, and carboxymethylcellulose, a protein is isolated that is homogeneous on polyacrylamide gel electrophoresis (Cooper and Reich, 1972). This protein accounts for approximately 20% of the total protein and more than 80% of the original toxicity of the crude venom.

Radioactively labeled neurotoxin is prepared by reaction with pyridoxal phosphate followed by reduction with tritiated sodium borohydride (Cooper and Reich, 1972). The reaction product, when subjected to chromatography on phosphocellulose, yields two derivatized, radioactive toxins, and the unreacted nonradioactive starting material. The two derivatives are the mono- and disubstituted toxins as shown by the specific radioactivity and by the fluorescence of the reduced pyridoxal phosphate residues. Both of these derivatives retain the characteristic pharmacological properties of the parent, unsubstituted toxin. The specific radioactivity obtained in this way (2 to 5 C/mmole) is convenient for measuring receptor amounts in the pmole range.

III. ASSAY FOR NICOTINIC RECEPTOR

Two assays have been developed for detection and quantitation of receptor activity. The first, which can be used only with crude preparations of receptor, is based on the fact that potent rabbit antisera directed against the neurotoxin quantitatively precipitate free toxin but not the toxin-receptor complex. When the receptor has been partially purified, the toxin-receptor complexes coprecipitate with free toxin.

The second, and more generally useful assay, is based on the fact that the toxin is small and strongly cationic, and therefore does not adsorb to anion-exchange resins, such as DEAE-cellulose, at neutral pH. This is in contrast to the receptor, which is strongly anionic and thus strongly bound to anion-exchange resins. Moreover, since the receptor is much larger than the toxin, the chromatographic behavior of the complex is dominated by the properties of the receptor; consequently, the adsorption of radioactive toxin to filter paper discs of DEAE-cellulose can be employed routinely for assaying the receptor content of preparations, and for monitoring the results of purification steps. The formation of complexes is independent of the presence of divalent cations and is unaffected by pH in the range pH 6 to 8. The rapidity of this procedure allows it to be used for kinetic and equilibrium studies of toxin binding. The sensitivity of the test obviously depends on the specific radioactivity of the toxin; with the preparations used in our experiments, 0.1 pmole of receptor can be detected. The sensitivity could easily be increased by a factor of 10 by using more highly radioactive toxin, such as can be prepared by labeling with radioiodine instead of tritium.

IV. RECEPTOR PURIFICATION

As starting material for the isolation of receptor we have selected the electric organ of the eel, *Electrophorus electricus*. This source is convenient because (1) it is commercially available, and (2) its high concentration of homogeneous cholinergic junctions provides a level of receptor that is practical for isolation procedures. Moreover, observations on isolated receptor can ultimately be related to the extensive information already derived from electrophysiological studies of the electroplaque.

Purification of receptor is begun by large-scale isolation of membrane fragments according to the procedure outlined by Changeux, Meunier, and Huchet (1971). To obtain the receptor in a form suitable for fractionation, these fragments are solubilized in any one of a number of nonionic detergents (Triton X-100; Emulphogen BC-720; Tween 20, 40, 60, or 80). We have routinely used a 1% (w/v) aqueous solution of Tween 80. The insoluble material is removed by high speed ($100,000 \times g$) centrifugation at 4°C for 30 min. The supernatant solution, which contains most of the binding activity for cobra toxin, is then concentrated under vacuum dialysis to a final concentration of 20 mg/ml of protein. At this stage, the receptor has been purified 225-fold compared with the starting material (Table 1).

Gel permeation chromatography on Sepharose 6B (Fig. 1) yields a further threefold purification, and removes most of the cholinesterase in the

TABLE 1. *Purification of nicotinic receptor. Receptor activity and protein content were measured as described in Fig. 1. Tween 80 (0.5% or 1%) was present throughout.*

Purification step	Protein content (mg)	Binding capacity (pmole)	Specific activity (pmole/mg)	Fold Purification
Electric organ (660 gm)	$5.25 \cdot 10^4$	[*]$2.3 \cdot 10^4$	.440	—
Membrane fragments solubilized in Tween 80	105	$1.05 \cdot 10^4$	100	228
Sepharose 6B	10	$2.96 \cdot 10^3$	296	675
Affinity chromatography + Hydroxylapatite	$2.55 \cdot 10^{-1}$	$4.80 \cdot 10^2$	1880	4290
DEAE-cellulose	$3.24 \cdot 10^{-2}$	90	2780	6350

[*]Assuming 35 pmoles bound per gr of wet tissue [Raftery et al.]

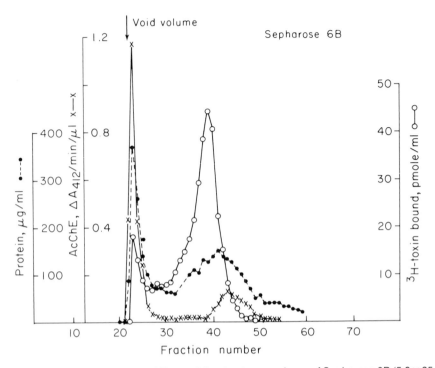

FIG. 1. Chromatography of 25 ml Tween-80 extract on a column of Sepharose 6B (5.0 × 85 cm) at 4°C. Eluent is 100 mM NaCl, 20 mM Tris HCl (pH 7.4), 0.5% Tween 80. Fraction size is 24 ml. Binding activity was assayed by the DEAE-paper method *(see text)* using 0.1 ml aliquots. Acetylcholinesterase activity was tested by the method of Ellman et al. (1961). The protein content was measured by the method of Lowry et al. (1951) with bovine serum albumin as standard. Due to the presence of Tween-80, the samples were centrifuged before reading the absorbance at 750 nm.

preparation. In this procedure the receptor emerges from the gel column very slightly ahead both of apoferritin (molecular weight 480,000) and of a minor peak of cholinesterase. However, this behavior of the receptor cannot be taken as an accurate indication of its molecular weight because we do not know to what extent the individual protein species, including the marker apoferritin, bind the detergent molecules that are present in all of the solutions.

The peak tubes obtained from the Sepharose column, containing the highest specific receptor activity, are pooled and the receptor purified further by a combination of affinity and ion-exchange chromatography (Fig. 2). The affinity column (I) is composed of Sepharose 4B to which cobra neurotoxin is covalently attached following activation of the matrix by reaction with cyanogen bromide (Axen, Porath, and Ernback, 1967). The affinity column is first loaded with receptor and washed free of unbound protein; it is then coupled to a second column (II) containing hydroxylapa-

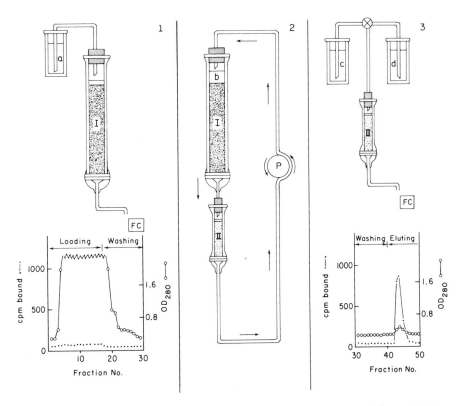

FIG. 2. Purification of nicotinic receptor by affinity chromatography (I) followed by ion-exchange on hydroxylapatite (II). Details of the procedure are given in the text.

tite. The entire system is filled with a buffer solution containing hexa-methonium chloride (10 mM) which is continuously recycled overnight. Under these conditions the receptor is eluted from the affinity column and adsorbed onto the hydroxylapatite. The hydroxylapatite column is then de-tached, washed with potassium phosphate buffer (5×10^{-3} M, pH 7.4, containing Tween 80, 0.5%), and the receptor is eluted with a similar buffer of higher molarity (5×10^{-2} M). The peak tubes, corresponding to the highest content of receptor are pooled, dialyzed against potassium phosphate buffer (10^{-3} M, pH 7.0), and adsorbed onto a column of DEAE-cellulose, previ-ously equilibrated with the same buffer. The DEAE column is first washed with phosphate buffer (0.1 M, pH 7.0, containing Tween 80, 1%), and the bulk of the receptor is eluted with 0.5 M phosphate buffer, pH 7.0 (also containing Tween 80, 1%).

The results of this purification procedure are summarized in Table 1. The final fraction, 6,000-fold purified in relation to the starting material, binds 2.8 pmoles of cobra toxin per mg of protein (i.e., one molecule of toxin per 360,000 g of receptor protein).

V. SOME CHARACTERISTICS OF THE RECEPTOR-TOXIN
INTERACTION

We have observed that cholinergic ligands inhibit binding of cobra toxin to the receptor, and the spectrum of competing ligands shows the nicotinic specificity expected of a postsynaptic receptor from the electric organ. We have characterized the binding specificity of the receptor at every stage of purification and have established (Klett, Fulpius, Cooper, Possani, Smith, and Reich, 1973) that the nicotinic pattern is retained throughout. In addition, we have defined the kinetic and thermodynamic constants for the formation of complexes between the toxin and the receptor.

Owing to the limiting quantities of pure receptor available, these studies have been performed on material purified by gel permeation chromatography. It is estimated that the purity of these fractions is in the range of 0.5 to 10% for different preparations, and their binding activity for cobra toxin is stable for 2 months at 4°C but is lost on freezing and thawing. The time course of binding of tritiated cobra toxin to the partially purified receptor has been measured at concentrations of 3.0×10^{-8} M and 1.2×10^{-9} M for toxin and receptor, respectively; it is determined at 25°C, using the DEAE-paper assay (Fig. 3). This gives a half-time of association of 140 sec which yields a k_1 of 1.67×10^5 M^{-1}sec^{-1}. The rate constant for the reverse reaction, i.e., toxin-receptor complex dissociation, is presented in Fig. 4 and is measured as follows: the fraction containing partially purified receptor is preincubated with the tritiated toxin for 1 hr at 25°C, a condition in which free toxin, free receptor, and complex remain stable and retain full activity. Then a 3,000-fold excess of cold toxin is added and the concentration of the residual tritiated toxin-receptor complex is measured as a function of time using the DEAE-paper assay. Under these conditions the complex does not dissociate completely even after 2 days of incubation. There are two components in the dissociation curve, a relatively rapid and a much slower one. The relatively fast component, which accounts for 65% of the dissociation, has a half-time of 160 min which yields a k_2 of 7.25×10^{-5}sec^{-1} at 25°C. The dissociation constant calculated from the ratio of the rate constants k_2/k_1 is 4.3×10^{-10} M.

The dissociation constant has also been derived by direct measurement of the toxin binding at equilibrium. As expected, the specific binding of tritiated cobra toxin to partially purified receptor is a function of the toxin concentration. The pattern is that of a typical, reversible equilibrium which is attained after 15 min under the conditions of our experiments. The values given in Fig. 5 have been obtained after 80 min of incubation. When the data are plotted according to Scatchard (1949), the straight-line relationship indicates that a single class of binding sites is being observed. The method of double reciprocal plotting gives a value for the dissociation constant K_D of 1.00×10^{-9} M at 25°C for impure receptor. The material

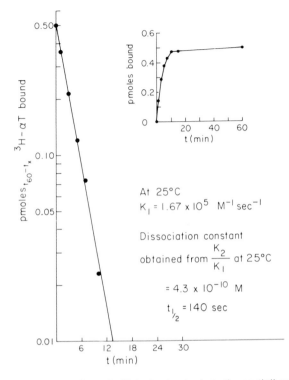

FIG. 3. Time course of the binding of tritiated cobra toxin to the partially purified receptor. At various times, specific binding was assayed by the DEAE-paper method *(see text)*.

eluted from the affinity column and further purified on ion-exchange chromatography gives a dissociation constant K_D of 1.25×10^{-9} M, which is identical with that derived from the less pure material. This value is also close to that (4.3×10^{-10} M) calculated from the ratio of the rate constants k_2/k_1.

The equilibrium of the reaction has been determined throughout the temperature range 10 to 34°C (Fulpius, Cha, Klett, and Reich, 1972), and the affinity of the receptor for ^{3}H-toxin is decreased with increasing temperature. From the equilibrium constant at 25°C, $\Delta G° = -12.3$ kcal/mole. From the dependence of the equilibrium constant on temperature $\Delta H° = 9.7$ kcal/mole. The entropy change at 25°C is 74 e.u.

VI. PHARMACOLOGICAL PROPERTIES OF THE NICOTINIC RECEPTOR

As noted above, some cholinergic ligands compete with cobra toxin for receptor binding and the specificity of effective competing ligands is typically that anticipated from a nicotinic receptor: neither muscarinic ligands nor cholinesterase inhibitors block toxin binding. On the other hand, the action

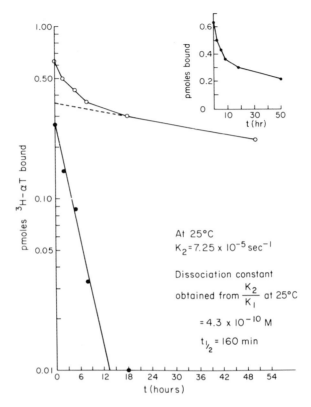

FIG. 4. Time course of the dissociation of the complex consisting of receptor and tritiated toxin *(see text).*

of the nicotinic agents is not uniform, and kinetic and equilibrium studies reveal that these fall into two classes. One class is defined by the behavior of the well-known nicotinic antagonist O,O'-dimethyl-d-tubocurarine. A detailed analysis of the effects of this compound on binding of cobra toxin shows a pattern of "hyperbolic competitive inhibition" as defined by Cleland for enzymes (1970). This means that both the curare and the cobra toxin can be bound to the receptor simultaneously; the formation of a complex between the receptor and either one of these does not exclude complex formation with the second ligand. The effect of binding both ligands is simply to decrease the affinity of the receptor for each. The behavior of L-nicotine, alloferine, and tetramethylammonium is identical with that of curare.

The second class of nicotinic agents is defined by the action of the "*bis*-onium" compounds decamethonium and hexamethonium. Both of these compounds give a pattern of "linear competitive inhibition" (Chang and Lee, 1963) when complexing of cobra toxin to receptor is measured in their

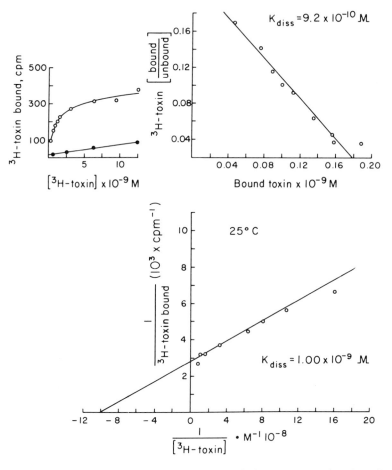

FIG. 5. Binding of tritiated cobra toxin to partially purified receptor as a function of toxin concentration. The reaction is performed in 4-ml final volume containing NaCl 130 mM, Tris HCl 20 mM (pH 7.4), Tween 80 1%, receptor 2.5 × 10⁻¹⁰ M; bound toxin is determined after 80 min of incubation at 25°C, using the DEAE-paper assay *(see text). Small frame upper left:* raw data. The closed circles show the background values obtained with in-activated receptor (5 min, 100°C) and the open circles give the values for specific binding. *Small frame upper right:* values for specific binding plotted according to Scatchard (1949). *Bottom:* Reciprocal plot of the specific binding. The ordinate shows the reciprocal of the ³H-toxin bound to the receptor; the abscissa the reciprocal of the ³H-toxin concentration.

presence. The implication of this pattern of inhibition is that the binding of the "*bis*-onium" compounds and cobra toxin to receptor are mutually exclusive, so that both ligands cannot simultaneously reside on the surface of the receptor. These observations are presented in detail elsewhere (Fulpius, Klett, Cooper, and Reich, 1973), and suggest the schematic representation of the binding modes of the various ligands given in Fig. 6.

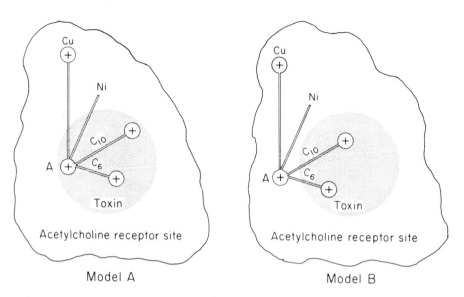

Model A   Model B

FIG. 6. Schematic model for relationship of binding sites of cobra toxin *(stippled area)*, dimethyltubocurarine (Cu), nicotine (Ni), hexamethonium (C$_6$) and decamethonium (C$_{10}$). The site indicated A ⊕ is visualized as the cation-binding site common to all nicotinic cholinergic ligands. The observation that curare and nicotine decrease the affinity of the receptor for cobra toxin but do not prevent toxin binding can be visualized as the result of one of two mechanisms. In one mechanism, Model A, the toxin-binding site is considered to overlap the cation-binding site A ⊕ ; thus the presence of a cholinergic ligand would decrease the toxin-receptor interaction energy either by reducing the total number of specific interactions or by slightly distorting the binding site and thereby the excellence of "fit." In a second mechanism, Model B, the same consequences are visualized as the result from the proximity of the sites that mediate cation and toxin binding. In this case the reciprocal changes in affinity would be due to modifications transmitted in the protein structure. The ligands illustrated here are considered to interact with the receptor at two sites. On the assumption that the cation-binding site A ⊕ is common to all, the second sites for curare (Cu) and nicotine (Ni) are represented as remote from the toxin-binding region, thereby permitting these molecules to attach to the receptor simultaneously with the toxin. In contrast, the second sites for hexa- (C$_6$) and decamethonium (C$_{10}$) are shown as completely overlapping the toxin-binding region; this would render binding of toxin and "*bis*-onium" compounds mutually exclusive.

VII. DISCUSSION

Although the current status of knowledge of the nicotinic receptor isolated from electric organs is still quite rudimentary, the effort that is being devoted to this problem in a number of laboratories ensures that rapid progress will be made within the next few years.

The purification protocol summarized here and described in full elsewhere (Klett et al., 1973) is reliable and reproducible, and yields a purified macromolecule that is either fully homogeneous, or nearly so. It is a realistic method for the isolation of small quantities of receptor that could be used for a variety of biochemical, biophysical, and pharmacological studies. However, the low yields make this procedure impractical for large-scale preparations that could permit detailed application of the methods of protein chemistry. For this purpose the yields would require significant improvement, and a better starting material—presumably the electric organ of *Torpedo*—would allow the purification of larger amounts of material. Even so, the preparation of even 1 micromole of pure receptor will present difficulties.

It seems clear that the receptor molecule as isolated by our procedure is a protein. Although our purest preparations do not contain any detectable noncovalently bound lipid phosphorus, we have not yet rigorously excluded the presence of covalently bound lipid or other prosthetic groups such as carbohydrates, sialic acid, or glycolipids. Nevertheless, the bulk of the material is protein, as indicated by the absorption spectrum, color and staining reactions, heat lability, amphoteric character, and susceptibility to denaturing agents (urea and guanidinium) and to proteolytic digestion. The solubility properties, i.e., the requirement for detergent to retain aqueous solubility, and the tendency to aggregation are consistent with the behavior of other membrane proteins.

The molecular weight of the receptor remains uncertain for the present. Although it has been reported that purified preparations complexed with cobra toxin yield a single band in SDS-polyacrylamide gel electrophoresis whose mobility corresponds to a molecular weight of approximately 45,000, there is no evidence that this structure retains the properties of the native molecule or that it can form complexes with cholinergic ligands (Meunier, Olsen, Menez, Fromageot, Boquet, and Changeux, 1972). Likewise, the behavior of the receptor on gel permeation chromatography does not provide a reliable basis for molecular weight estimations since the nonionic detergents, whose presence is required to maintain the solubility of the receptor, may be bound differentially by the receptor and by the marker proteins used to calibrate the gel. For the present, the estimate of 360,000, drawn from the data in Table 1, appears more reasonable than the 480,000 indicated by gel permeation, but either or both of these estimates may be in error.

Apart from its ability to bind cobra toxin and cholinergic ligands, the receptor is a membrane protein, with biological activity that can be assayed, at least in part, in free solution. Thus the study of this protein may be expected to yield some insights into physical and chemical properties that may be common to other proteins normally involved in membrane structure and function. It remains to be seen whether the molecule we have isolated can be incorporated into artificial lipid membranes and, if so, whether the complexing of cholinergic ligands will suffice to produce changes in membrane permeability.

REFERENCES

Axen, R., Porath, J., and Ernback, S. (1967): Chemical coupling of peptides and proteins to polysaccharides by means of cyanogen halides. *Nature*, 214:1302–1304.

Chang, C. C., and Lee, C. Y. (1963): Isolation of neurotoxins from the venom of *Bungarus multicinctus* and their modes of neuromuscular blocking action. *Arch. Intern. Pharmacodyn.*, 144:241–257.

Changeux, J. P., Meunier, J. C., and Huchet, M. (1971): Studies on the cholinergic receptor protein of *Electrophorus electricus*. *Mol. Pharmacol.*, 7:538–553.

Cleland, W. W. (1970): In: *The Enzymes*, Vol. 2, edited by P. D. Boyer, p. 1. Academic Press, New York.

Cooper, D., and Reich, E. (1972): Neurotoxin from venom of the cobra, *Naja naja siamensis*. *J. Biol. Chem.*, 247:3008–3013.

Ellman, G. L., et al. (1961): A new and rapid colorimetric determination of acetylcholinesterase activity. *Biochem. Pharmacol.*, 7:88–95.

Fulpius, B., Cha, S., Klett, R., and Reich, E. (1972): Properties of the nicotine acetylcholine receptor macromolecule of *Electrophorus electricus*. *FEBS Letters*, 24:323–326.

Fulpius, B., Klett, R., Cooper, D., and Reich, E. (1973): The nicotinic acetylcholine receptor. In: *Proc. Intern. Cong. Pharm.*, Vol. 5, pp. 68–80. San Francisco.

Klett, R., Fulpius, B., Cooper, D., Possani, L., Smith, M., and Reich, E. (1973): The acetylcholine receptor. *J. Biol. Chem.*, 248:6841–6853.

Lowry, O. H., et al. (1951): Protein measurement with the folin phenol reagent. *J. Biol. Chem.*, 193:265–275.

Meunier, J. C., Olsen, R. W., Menez, A., Fromageot, P., Boquet, P., and Changeux, J. P. (1972): Some physical properties of the cholinergic receptor protein from *Electrophorus electricus* revealed by a tritiated-toxin from *Naja nigricollis* venom. *Biochemistry*, 11:1200–1210.

Scatchard, G. (1949): The attractions of proteins for small molecules and ions. *Ann. N.Y. Acad. Sci.*, 51:660–672.

Synaptic Transmission and Neuronal Interaction
Raven Press, New York 1974

Purification of the Acetylcholine Receptor by Affinity Chromatography

Jon Lindstrom[a] and Jim Patrick[b]

Salk Institute for Biological Studies, San Diego, California 92112

I. INTRODUCTION

For many years acetylcholine receptors were studied as hypothetical entities characterized only by the responses of the cells containing them to a spectrum of agonists and antagonists. Study of the molecular biology of receptors required the development of special techniques. In order to localize and quantitate receptors cytologically, methods were required for labeling receptors *in situ;* and, in order to study the structural basis of receptor ligand binding specificities or the mechanism by which receptors controlled membrane permeability, methods were required for their purification. Although acetylcholine receptors were thought to be present in extremely low concentrations in most tissues, electric organ provided a relatively rich source of receptor that has greatly facilitated biochemical studies. Since receptors lacked any known enzymatic activity which could be used for their identification during solubilization from the membrane and purification, identification had to be based in some way on the only biochemical property which could be attributed to them with certainty — the binding of cholinergic ligands. Recently three types of study, all taking advantage of the binding specificities of the acetylcholine receptors of electric organs, have made substantial progress toward the goals of labeling and/or purifying receptors. One approach, directed at labeling receptors and identifying their component macromolecules, has been to attach covalently a radioactive affinity labeling reagent to the receptor in the intact cell and to then identify the polypeptide chain to which it is bound (19). Another approach, directed at purification of active receptors, has been to study the readily reversible binding of radioactive ligands to membrane fragments and detergent extracts of these fragments by equilibrium dialysis (7). A third approach has employed radioactively labeled snake venom toxins. Investigators in several laboratories have shown that a class of protein

[a] Supported by a Muscular Dystrophy Association Postdoctoral Fellowship.
[b] Supported in part by National Institutes of Health grant No. NS–10297–01 and in part by a grant from the Damon Runyon Foundation to David Schubert.

toxins found in the venom of elapid snakes, the α-neurotoxins, bind specifically and virtually irreversibly to the acetylcholine binding site of acetylcholine receptors (1–3, 8, 14–18). These toxins can be used rather like affinity labeling reagents to tag receptors *in situ* or in mild detergent extracts. But as this chapter will show, toxin binds to receptors by a high-affinity, reversible mechanism. Thus, toxin can also be used actively in the purification of solubilized receptors by employing a toxin-agarose conjugate as an adsorbent for affinity chromatography from which active receptors can be specifically eluted by receptor ligands.

II. METHODS

α-Neurotoxin was purified from the venom of the cobra *Naja naja siamensis* as described elsewhere (17). The toxin was purified by methods similar to those used by Karlsson, Eaker, and Porath (9) and labeled with ^{125}I to specific activities of 1 to 3 C/mmole using chloramine-T. Native toxin was conjugated to Bio-Gel A50 M by the method of Cuatrecasas (5).

A membrane fraction containing vesicles was prepared at 4°C. An eel (*Electrophorus electricus*, Paramount Aquarium, New York) was killed by decapitation and dissected. The main electric organ was sliced into 1 cm³ pieces. In a 250-ml vessel of a Virtis homogenizer 68 g batches of organ were homogenized with 115 ml of Ringer's solution (163 mM NaCl, 5 mM KCl, 2 mM CaCl$_2$, 2 mM MgCl$_2$, 1.5 mM Na phosphate buffer pH 7.4) for 90 sec at 75% of maximum speed. The homogenate was then centrifuged for 20 min at 5,090 × g in the SS 34 head of a Sorvall RC2B centrifuge. The pellet was discarded and the supernatant centrifuged for 30 min at 105,000 × g. This pellet was resuspended in 23 ml of Ringer's solution, using a motor driven tube and pestle homogenizer to give a "crude vesicle fraction" which was then centrifuged 10 min at 17,300 × g to remove large membrane fragments not in the form of vesicles. The supernatant was diluted twofold in Ringer's solution and centrifuged 30 min at 105,000 × g. The supernatant was discarded and the pellet resuspended overnight in 4.6 ml of Ringer's solution. Aggregated material was then removed by centrifugation for 5 min at 17,300 × g. A typical supernatant "vesicle containing fraction" contained 4 mg protein/ml, 6 nmole receptor sites/g protein (by specifically protectable labeling with ^{125}I-toxin), 13 nmole acetylcholine esterase sites/g protein (by specifically protectable labeling with ^{3}H-diisopropyl fluorophosphate), and its *in vitro* receptor activity was unaltered for nearly a week. Addition of 1 mM NaN$_3$ increased the time that the preparation could be kept.

A total membrane fraction was prepared at 4°C by homogenizing electric organ with an equal volume of Ringer's solution for 60 sec at 75% maximum speed in the Virtis homogenizer, and then centrifuging the homogenate 30 min at 105,000 × g. The pellet was homogenized again for 30 sec with 4 volumes of 1 M NaCl and pelleted a second time for 60 min at 105,000 × g. Receptor was solubilized from this pellet by stirring the pellet overnight with 4 volumes 3% Triton X-100, 0.1 M NaCl, 3 mM Tris pH 7.4. Unsolubilized material was removed by centrifugation for 60 min at 105,000 × g leaving the "solubilized receptor containing fraction" in the supernatant, which was decanted through glass wool to remove large aggregations of lipid which collected at the surface during centrifugation. Addition of 1 mM NaN₃ had no effect on the ¹²⁵I-toxin binding activity of the solubilized receptor fraction and reduced bacterial contamination so that a preparation could be used for several weeks. The extract was usually sonicated for 30 sec before being applied to affinity columns in order to reduce the size of particles (probably of lipid) which were not sufficiently dense or cohesive to pellet well, but which were otherwise trapped in the matrix of the column. Particles trapped on the column were removed by stirring the column bed several times during washing, and any particles in the specific eluate of the column were removed by Millipore filtration of the eluate. Columns were washed and eluted with a "Triton buffer" solution, containing 0.5% Triton X-100 (or occasionally 0.1%), 0.1 M NaCl, 1 mM Tris pH 7.4, and this buffer was used for dialysis of eluates from the columns.

Assay of acetylcholine receptor activity *in vitro* was accomplished by a slight modification of the method of Kasai and Changeux (10) which measured the effect of carbamylcholine on the passive efflux of sodium from vesicles at 0°C. Vesicles were "loaded" with ²²Na⁺ by mixing 1 volume of vesicles with 0.1 volume of 0.1 M ²²Na⁺ phosphate pH 7.0 (0.29 mC/ml diluted from carrier-free ²²Na⁺, New England Nuclear) and incubating overnight to allow the ²²Na⁺ concentration inside and outside the vesicles to equilibrate. At the start of the assay, 0.1 ml of ²²Na⁺ loaded vesicles was rapidly diluted into 10 ml of vigorously stirred Ringer's solution in an ice bath. At intervals, 1-ml aliquots were collected on 2.5 cm, 0.45 μm Millipore filters and quickly washed three times with 3 ml of ice cold Ringer's solution. The filters were dried and the radioactivity contained in the vesicles trapped on the filter determined in a liquid scintillation counter. The ²²Na⁺ nonspecifically bound to the filters was determined by incubating an aliquot of each assay mix 1 hr at room temperature before filtering to allow equilibration of the concentration of ²²Na⁺ inside and outside the vesicles.

Binding of ¹²⁵I-toxin to membrane fractions was determined by adding ¹²⁵I-toxin to suspensions of the membrane fragments (usually 0.5 ml at 1-mg protein/ml) contained in screw top tubes for the #40 rotor of a Spinco Model L ultracentrifuge. To eliminate all the specific binding of ¹²⁵I-toxin by competition, protectors of the acetylcholine binding site (usually 10^{-3} M decamethonium or 10^{-4} M benzoquinonium) were added to the suspension before ¹²⁵I-toxin. After 1 or 2 hr at room temperature, the tubes were centrifuged for 20 min at 40,000 rpm at 24°C (for Scatchard plot experiments) or 4°C (for all other experiments). The radioactivity in the supernatant and/or the radioactivity in the pellet resuspended in an equal volume of 2% sodium dodecyl sulfate (SDS) was then determined in a liquid scintillation counter.

Binding of ^{125}I-toxin to solubilized receptor was determined by velocity sedimentation of ^{125}I-toxin-receptor complexes on linear gradients of sucrose or glycerol in a Beckman Spinco Model L or L-2 ultracentrifuge using an SW39 or, most often, an SW50.1 rotor. Gradients consisted of 4.9 ml of 10 to 30% glycerol or (most often) 5 to 20% (weight to volume) sucrose in a solution containing 0.5% (weight to volume) Triton X-100, 0.1 M NaCl, 1 mM Tris pH 7.4. Samples consisting of 0.1 ml of solubilized receptor incubated with ^{125}I-toxin for several hours at 4°C or ^{125}I-toxin-receptor complexes solubilized from membranes were layered on the gradients which were then centrifuged at 2°C. Further purification of receptor purified by affinity chromatography was achieved by sedimentation of 0.3-ml aliquots on 10.5-ml 5 to 20% sucrose gradients in the SW41 rotor for 22 hr at 37,000 rpm.

SDS acrylamide gel electrophoresis using a Tris-glycine buffer system and 10% acrylamide in the running gel was conducted essentially according to the method of Laemmli (11). However, fixing and staining were performed simultaneously by a 2-hr incubation in freshly prepared 0.2% Coomasie Blue in 50% methanol, 7% acetic acid. All samples were prepared in the presence of β-mercaptoethanol.

Protein was assayed by the method of Lowry, Rosebrough, Farr, and Randall (12), using bovine serum albumin (BSA) as a standard. The yellow precipitate caused by Triton X-100 in the samples was pelleted before the absorbence at 750 nm was determined.

III. RESULTS

A. Specificity of ^{125}I-Toxin Binding to Electric Organ Membrane

The cobra α-neurotoxin used in this study was purified from the lyophilized venom of the India cobra *Naja naja* (17). Both native toxin and ^{125}I-toxin were homogeneous by the criteria of gel filtration on Sephadex G-75 and electrophoresis on acrylamide gels containing SDS.

In order to study binding of ^{125}I-toxin to receptor containing membrane fragments, a fraction containing membrane fragments in the form of vesicles was made from the main electric organ of *Electrophorus electricus* by a modification of the method of Kasai and Changeux (10). When ^{125}I-toxin was incubated with a suspension of the vesicle fraction, ^{125}I-toxin was observed to bind to the vesicles (Fig. 1). At low ^{125}I-toxin concentrations, 90% or more of the toxin binding was eliminated by adding acetylcholine receptor ligands such as acetylcholine [using vesicles depleted of esterase by extraction with 1 M NaCl (22) and in the presence of esterase inhibitors],

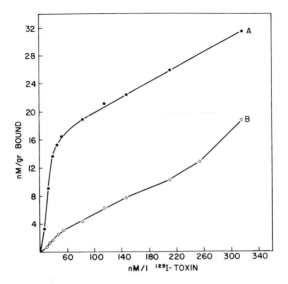

FIG. 1. Binding of ^{125}I-toxin to vesicles. Binding was performed as described in Methods, allowing 50-min incubation at 24°C. *A* = Total binding to vesicle-containing fraction. *B* = Binding in the presence of 10^{-3} M decamethonium.

decamethonium, carbamylcholine, or benzoquinonium to the suspension before adding ^{125}I-toxin. This result suggested that all these agents prevented binding of ^{125}I-toxin by competing for occupany of the acetylcholine binding site of the receptor. The number of sites which were protected from binding ^{125}I-toxin saturated at low toxin concentrations, but binding to sites which were not protected increased with increased ^{125}I-toxin concentration. Native toxin added at even 100-fold molar excess over ^{125}I-toxin gave no more protection than did receptor ligands or native toxin plus receptor ligands. This suggested that the only binding site native and ^{125}I-toxin had in common was the acetylcholine binding site of the receptor, and that although iodinated toxin molecules retained the ability to bind to receptors, they also acquired the capacity to bind to other sites.

In order to determine if the sites protected from binding to ^{125}I-toxin by agonists and antagonists corresponded to physiologically significant receptor sites, the activity of the receptors in the vesicles was studied *in vitro*, using the $^{22}Na^+$ efflux assay devised by Kasai and Changeux (10). This method involved diluting vesicles formed from receptor-containing membranes which had been equilibrated with $^{22}Na^+$ into nonradioactive media and measuring the efflux of $^{22}Na^+$. The efflux of $^{22}Na^+$ from the vesicles was more rapid than that observed by Kasai and Changeux and only approximately one-fourth of the bound $^{22}Na^+$ was affected by agonists (Fig. 2); these differences probably resulted from the differences in our methods of preparing vesicles. Nonetheless, agonists caused a marked increase in the

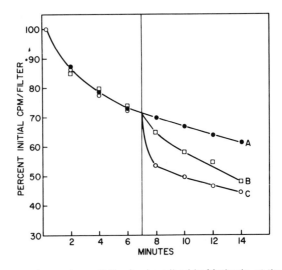

FIG. 2. *In vitro* assay of receptor activity. As described in Methods, at time zero, vesicles "loaded" with $^{22}Na^+$ were diluted into nonradioactive Ringer's solution in an ice bath. At the times indicated, vesicles contained in aliquots of this suspension were collected on Millipore filters and the $^{22}Na^+$ still retained was measured. *A:* Illustrates the efflux of $^{22}Na^+$. *B:* Illustrates the increased efflux of $^{22}Na^+$ due to 1.2×10^{-4} M carbamylcholine added at 7 min. *C:* Illustrates the maximum response obtained with 1×10^{-3} M carbamylcholine.

efflux of $^{22}Na^+$ from the vesicles, as would be expected from their action at acetylcholine receptors to increase cation permeability. The enhanced efflux of $^{22}Na^+$ caused by carbamylcholine (at 10^{-3} M) was completely antagonized by benzoquinonium (at 10^{-6} M) or native toxin (at 6×10^{-8} M); but unaffected by ouabain or tetrodotoxin, which would not be expected to affect the receptor. By arbitrarily defining the response to carbamylcholine as the difference between the efflux curves with and without carbamylcholine 3 min after addition of carbamylcholine, dose/response curves were constructed which indicated a carbamylcholine concentration giving a half maximal response of $8.9 \pm 2.2 \times 10^{-5}$ M (n = 4), which was similar to the value of 1.0×10^{-4} M obtained by Kasai and Changeux (10) (Fig. 3). This value was only slightly affected (decreased 13%) by defining the response at 7 min after the addition of carbamylcholine.

When the curve for decamethonium protectable binding of ^{125}I-toxin to vesicles was compared with the curve for blockage of *in vitro* receptor activity by ^{125}I-toxin in the same fractions, it was evident that both functions saturated over the same narrow range of ^{125}I-toxin concentrations (Fig. 4). This provided strong support for the interpretation that the sites protected from binding ^{125}I-toxin by decamethonium were the physiologically significant receptors. Data presented later showing that the decamethonium

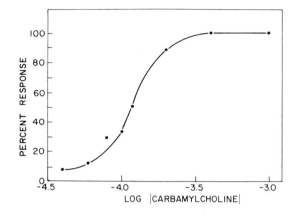

FIG. 3. Dose/response curve for *in vitro* receptor activity. Curves of $^{22}Na^+$ efflux from vesicles like those in Fig. 2 were prepared using several concentrations of carbamylcholine. The difference between the $^{22}Na^+$ bound at 10 min with no carbamylcholine added and that bound at 10 min using a particular concentration was defined as the response and expressed as a percent of the response to 1.0×10^{-3} M carbamylcholine.

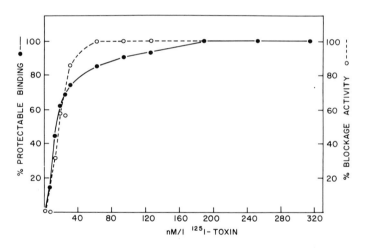

FIG. 4. Dose/response curves for decamethonium protectable binding of ^{125}I-toxin to vesicles and blockage of *in vitro* receptor activity. Protectable binding of ^{125}I-toxin is the difference between curves A and B of Fig. 1. The *in vitro* receptor response to 1×10^{-3} M carbamylcholine of each fraction used in Fig. 1A was determined and compared with that of an aliquot of vesicles not exposed to ^{125}I-toxin but pelleted and resuspended in parallel with the fractions in A.

protectable sites were homogeneous in their binding affinity for ^{125}I-toxin argued even more strongly that the protectable sites for ^{125}I-toxin binding were all receptor sites.

B. Mechanism of ^{125}I-Toxin Binding to Membrane

The binding properties of the ^{125}I-toxin binding sites were studied in greater detail by plotting the binding curve data in the form of Scatchard plots (21). A Scatchard plot of total ^{125}I-toxin bound to the vesicles fit two lines of different slopes, indicating the presence of two distinct populations of sites, one exhibiting very high affinity, corresponding to the specific receptor site; and another exhibiting much lower affinity, corresponding to a nonspecific site (Fig. 5A). Scatchard plots for binding to each site were constructed by plotting separately the nonspecific binding which occurred in the presence of decamethonium (Fig. 5B) and the specific receptor binding which was prevented by decamethonium (Fig. 5C). The plots indicated that this preparation contained 16 nM receptor sites/g protein to which ^{125}I-toxin bound with a $K_D = 2.2 \times 10^{-9}$ M and also 18 nM nonspecific sites/g protein to which ^{125}I-toxin bound with a $K_D = 2.1 \times 10^{-7}$ M. With three preparations, the concentration of receptor sites varied from 6 to 16 nM/g protein and the K_D varied from 0.97 to 2.3 $\times 10^{-9}$ M.

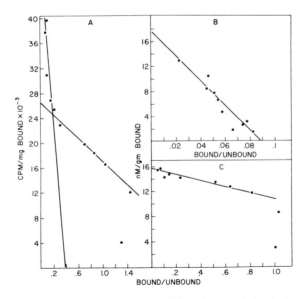

FIG. 5. Scatchard plots of A = total binding of ^{125}I-toxin to vesicles (using data from Fig. 1A); B = binding to a nonspecific site (using data from Fig. 1B); C = binding to the receptor site (using data from the difference of Figs. 1A and 1B). Failure of the two points obtained with the lowest ^{125}I-toxin concentrations to fit the line may have resulted from allowing only 50 min for binding.

If ^{125}I-toxin were bound to receptors reversibly with high affinity as indicated by the Scatchard plots, it should have been possible to demonstrate that ^{125}I-toxin spontaneously dissociated from receptors. When vesicles were labeled with ^{125}I-toxin (so that 60% of the labeling was specific), pelleted, and resuspended in the same volume of Ringer's solution (at 37°C to speed dissociation) and then pelleted again at intervals to determine the ^{125}I-toxin still bound, the amount bound decreased very slowly; but if the labeled vesicles were diluted 10-fold and rapidly stirred, the amount of ^{125}I-toxin bound rapidly decreased (Fig. 6). Rapid dissociation was also obtained if decamethonium or native toxin were added; however, addition of very high concentrations of choline (which has extremely low affinity for the receptor) did not increase the apparent rate of dissociation of ^{125}I-toxin. The simplest explanation for these observations was that ^{125}I-toxin spontaneously dissociated from the receptor, but since receptor and ^{125}I-toxin were at concentrations in excess of their K_D for binding, the ^{125}I-toxin was quickly rebound unless there was a competitor for the receptor site present which occupied the site after ^{125}I-toxin dissociated (Fig. 7). The site at which competitors acted showed the specificity expected of the acetylcholine binding site—choline was without effect and native toxin was effective at much lower concentrations than was decamethonium.

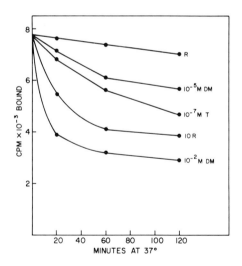

FIG. 6. Reversibility of ^{125}I-toxin binding. Vesicles (1 mg/ml giving a receptor concentration of 8.0×10^{-9} M) were labeled with ^{125}I-toxin (1.6×10^{-7} M) so that 60% of the binding was to sites protectable by 10^{-4} M decamethonium. The vesicles were pelleted, unbound ^{125}I-toxin was discarded with the supernatant, and then the pellet was resuspended at 37°C in an equal volume of Ringer's solution (R), 10^{-5} decamethonium (10^{-5} M DM), 10^{-7} M native toxin (10^{-7} M T), 10^{-2} M decamethonium (10^{-2} M DM), or in 10 volumes of Ringer's solution (10 R). At the times indicated aliquots of these suspensions were pelleted and the remaining bound ^{125}I-toxin measured.

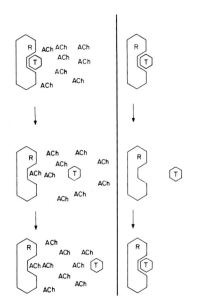

FIG. 7. Mechanism by which unlabeled ligands displace ^{125}I-toxin from the receptor site. The spontaneous dissociation of ^{125}I-toxin from receptor is depicted in the presence *(left)* or absence *(right)* of an excess of acetylcholine showing that acetylcholine could occupy the receptor after dissociation of ^{125}I-toxin and then protect the site from rebinding ^{125}I-toxin.

Another feature expected of reversible binding was that the receptor should be unaltered by binding and dissociation of toxin. Therefore an experiment was designed to test whether receptors from which ^{125}I-toxin had dissociated could again bind ^{125}I-toxin. Table 1 shows that labeled vesicles incubated with decamethonium at 37°C for 2 hr and then extensively washed free of decamethonium by pelleting and resuspension lost virtually all their bound ^{125}I-toxin, and yet that most of the receptor sites were intact and could again be labeled with ^{125}I-toxin. The slight loss of receptor sites observed could have resulted from the four cycles of pelleting and resuspension before relabeling. Table 1 also shows that labeled vesicles incubated without decamethonium and then washed extensively also lost some of the ^{125}I-toxin initially bound due to spontaneous dissociation.

In order to measure the first order rate constant, k_d, for dissociation of the ^{125}I-toxin-receptor complex $[(TR) \xrightarrow{k_d} T + R]$, the apparent dissociation rate was determined in the presence of high concentrations of decamethonium to prevent any rebinding of dissociated ^{125}I-toxin to receptor (Fig. 8). Rate constants at the various temperatures were determined from log plots of these data (Table 2).

The second-order reaction rate constant, k_a, for formation of the ^{125}I-toxin-

TABLE 1. *Dissociation and reassociation of* ^{125}*I-toxin-receptor complexes on vesicles*

Sample	% ^{125}I-toxin initially bound
(1) Vesicles labeled with ^{125}I-toxin (1.6×10^{-8} M)	100
(2) Vesicles labeled with ^{125}I-toxin then incubated 2 hr at 37°C, washed	45
(3) Vesicles labeled with ^{125}I-toxin then incubated 2 hr at 37°C with 10^{-2} M decamethonium, washed	9.5
(4) Vesicles labeled with ^{125}I-toxin then incubated 2 hr at 37°C with 10^{-2} M decamethonium, washed, then relabeled with ^{125}I-toxin	72

Suspensions of vesicles (0.5 ml at 1 mg protein/ml containing receptor at a concentration of 7.5×10^{-9} M) were incubated 1 hr at 24°C with ^{125}I-toxin (1.6×10^{-8} M). All suspensions were pelleted and the radioactivity bound to the vesicles determined (1). Pellets identical to (1) were then resuspended in 0.5 ml of either Ringer's solution (2) or 10^{-2} M decamethonium in Ringer's solution (3, 4) and incubated at 37°C for 2 hr. The samples were then pelleted and resuspended in 5 ml of 4°C Ringer's solution three times and left overnight at 4°C in 0.5 ml of Ringer's solution. The suspensions were then incubated at 24°C for 1 hr while those designated (4) were relabeled with ^{125}I-toxin at 1.6×10^{-8} M . All suspensions were then pelleted and the amount of ^{125}I-toxin bound determined. The values shown are the average of two experiments performed in duplicate.

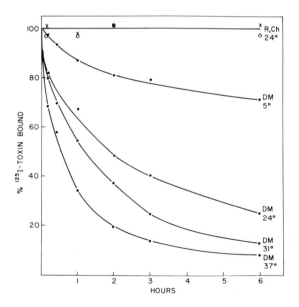

FIG. 8. Rate of dissociation of ^{125}I-toxin from vesicles. Aliquots of vesicles (1 ml at 3×10^{-8} M in receptor) were labeled with ^{125}I-toxin (2×10^{-8} M) resulting in 93% specific labeling. The aliquots were pelleted and resuspended at the indicated temperature in an equal volume of either Ringer's solution (R), 10^{-2} M choline in Ringer's solution (Ch), or 10^{-2} M decamethonium in Ringer's solution (DM). At the times indicated the vesicles were again pelleted and the remaining bound ^{125}I-toxin determined.

TABLE 2. *Kinetic parameters of toxin binding*

Temperature (C)	k_a ($M^{-1}\,s^{-1}$)	k_d (s^{-1})	$K_D = k_d/k_a$ (M)	$K_A = K_D^{-1}$ (M^{-1})
5°	2.8×10^4	8.8×10^{-6}	3.1×10^{-10}	3.2×10^9
24°	5.2×10^4	6.9×10^{-5}	1.3×10^{-9}	7.6×10^8
31°	5.6×10^4	1.3×10^{-4}	2.3×10^{-9}	4.4×10^8
37°	7.1×10^4	2.7×10^{-4}	3.9×10^{-9}	2.6×10^8

Values for k_d were derived from data shown in Fig. 8 and the values for k_a from the data shown in Fig. 9. The K_D determined by Scatchard plot of decamethonium protectable binding to this batch of vesicles at 24°C was 1.6×10^{-9} M and there were 9.5 nmole receptor sites/g protein.

receptor complex on vesicles $[T + R \xrightarrow{\;k_a\;} (TR)]$ was calculated from the initial reaction rate estimated from curves of the type shown in Fig. 9. Determining ^{125}I-toxin binding by collecting a "crude vesicle fraction" on Millipore filters as shown in Fig. 10 gave a value for k_a (3.6×10^4 $M^{-1}s^{-1}$ at 24°C) similar to that obtained by the centrifugation method used in Fig. 9 (5.2×10^4 $M^{-1}s^{-1}$ at 24°C). The filtration method was not applicable to the "vesicle containing fraction" because it passed through the filters used. The values for the rate constant determined in these cases were similar to the

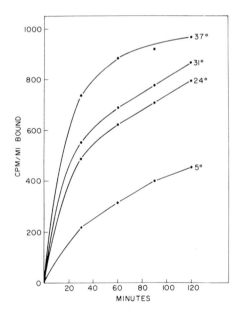

FIG. 9. Rate of association of ^{125}I-toxin with vesicles. In order to slow the reaction rate sufficiently to allow determination of the binding rate by pelleting, vesicles were diluted at the indicated temperatures to give a receptor concentration of 1.6×10^{-9} M and then ^{125}I-toxin was added at 7.4×10^{-10} M. At the times indicated, vesicles were pelleted and the amount of bound ^{125}I-toxin determined.

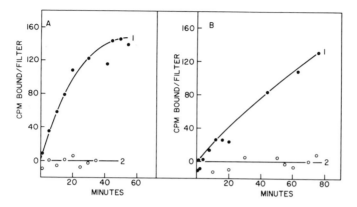

FIG. 10. Rate of association of ^{125}I-toxin with crude vesicle fraction. Suspensions containing receptor at 8.6×10^{-11} M were stirred with ^{125}I-toxin at 5.8×10^{-9} M and at intervals 1-ml aliquots were filtered through 0.22 μm EGWP Celotate filters. The filters were washed three times with 5 ml of Ringer's solution, dried, and the bound ^{125}I-toxin determined. In *A* the suspensions were at 24°C; in *B* at 0°C. In both cases (1) contained only ^{125}I-toxin and membrane fragments and (2) had 10^{-4} M decamethonium added before ^{125}I-toxin. The cpm bound shown include a background subtraction for ^{125}I-toxin bound to filters in the absence of membrane fragments.

value obtained for binding of the same preparation of ^{125}I-toxin to a cultured muscle cell line [9×10^4 $M^{-1}s^{-1}$ (17)] or to the value obtained for binding of tritiated *Naja nigricollis* toxin to vesicles of electric organ [1×10^5 $M^{-1}s^{-1}$ (14)]. All the estimates of the association rate constant indicated a value much slower than expected of a diffusion limited reaction (6).

The equilibrium dissociation constant for the ^{125}I-toxin-receptor complex was estimated on one preparation of vesicles by both the equilibrium method employing Scatchard plots and independent measurement of association and dissociation rate constants (Table 2). A Scatchard plot indicated $K_D = 1.6 \times 10^{-9}$ M which was quite close to the value of $K_D = 1.3 \times 10^{-9}$ M computed from k_d/k_a. This further supported the hypothesis that binding of ^{125}I-toxin to receptors could be described by a mechanism involving high affinity, reversible binding: $R + T \xrightleftharpoons{K_D} (RT)$. By determining rate constants at several temperatures, estimates were made of the thermodynamic constants describing this reaction (Fig. 11). At 24°C $\Delta G = -12$ Cal/mole, $\Delta H = -15$ Cal/mole, and $-T\Delta S = +2.4$ Cal/mole.

C. Binding of ^{125}I-Toxin to Receptors Solubilized from the Membrane

Several groups have demonstrated that complexes of toxin and receptor can be solubilized from membranes by mild detergent treatment or that receptors can be solubilized and then labeled with toxin (2, 3, 14–16, 18). Extraction of ^{125}I-toxin-labeled vesicles with the nonionic detergent Triton

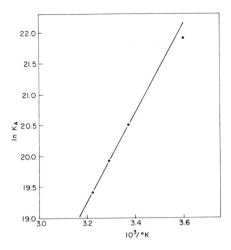

FIG. 11. Temperature dependence of the equilibrium constant for binding of ^{125}I-toxin to the receptor. Data is from Table 2.

X-100 resulted in the solubilization of a complex between ^{125}I-toxin and a high molecular weight component which could be separated from free ^{125}I-toxin by sedimentation on sucrose or glycerol gradients in the ultracentrifuge. In order to determine if the component to which ^{125}I-toxin was bound was the acetylcholine receptor, specific dissociation of the complex and protection of the binding component by acetylcholine receptor ligands were studied. It was found that the complex with ^{125}I-toxin could be dissociated by incubation in the presence of acetylcholine or other specific receptor ligands, but not by choline (Fig. 12, Table 3). This indicated that the binding component reversibly bound ^{125}I-toxin with the specificity expected of the receptor. That this specificity depended on the native structure of the receptor was further indicated by the observations that addition of the denaturing detergent SDS (20) to a concentration of 1% eliminated the complex observed by sedimentation on gradients, and did not result in a complex detectable by electrophoresis on acrylamide gels containing SDS. The use of specific receptor ligands to protect the solubilized component from binding ^{125}I-toxin further suggested that the receptor could be solubilized in a form which allowed it to specifically bind ^{125}I-toxin (Fig. 13). Experiments to be described later demonstrated that solubilized receptor eluted from toxin conjugated to agarose was still capable of binding ^{125}I-toxin, further indicating the reversibility of the labeling reaction.

In agreement with the results of others (2, 14) the toxin receptor complex obtained from either the vesicle-containing fraction or the bulk membrane fraction sedimented with an apparent sedimentation constant of 9.5 S (Fig. 14). Meunier, Olsen, and Changeux (13) have shown that for the complex of toxin and receptor $S_{20,w} = 12.5$. The discrepancy between the apparent

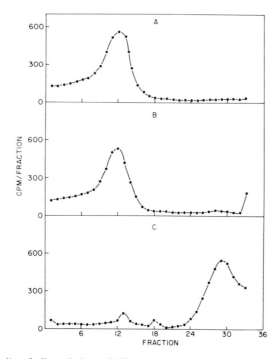

FIG. 12. Specificity of dissociation of ^{125}I-toxin from solubilized receptor. ^{125}I-toxin receptor complexes essentially without free ^{125}I-toxin were prepared by labeling vesicles with a low concentration of toxin and then pelleting and washing to remove unbound ^{125}I-toxin before solubilizing the vesicles with Triton X-100. The complex of ^{125}I-toxin with receptor in the Triton X-100 extract was resolved from free ^{125}I-toxin by centrifugation for 18 hr at 39,000 rpm in the SW39 rotor on glycerol gradients as described in Methods, except that the gradient also contained the ligand present in the incubation medium. In *A* the complex was incubated at 24°C for 4 hr with 10^{-5} M neostigmine (to inhibit acetylcholinesterase) before being centrifuged. In *B* the complex was incubated with 10^{-2} M choline plus neostigmine, and in *C* the complex was incubated with 10^{-2} M acetylcholine plus neostigmine.

sedimentation constant and the $S_{20,w}$ was shown to result from the low density of the complex due to large amounts of bound detergent, and they estimated the molecular weight of the actual receptor protein to be of the order of 3.6×10^5 daltons. In agreement with the results of others (15), we observed that the continued presence of Triton X-100 in the gradients was necessary to prevent aggregation of the solubilized receptor.

D. Purification of the Solubilized Receptor by Affinity Chromatography

Demonstration that receptor solubilized by Triton X-100 retained its native ability to reversibly bind toxin immediately suggested that the receptor could be eluted from an affinity adsorbent of toxin by means of receptor ligands, offering a method for achieving a large degree of purifica-

TABLE 3. *Dissociation of solubilized ^{125}I-toxin-receptor complexes*

Protector	Concentration	Dissociation (in 4 hr at 24°C)
Acetylcholine ($K_D = 1 \times 10^{-6}$ M) (10)	10^{-2} M (10^{-5} M neostigmine + esterase depleted vesicles)	69%
Decamethonium ($K_D = 1 \times 10^{-6}$ M) (10)	10^{-2} M	68%
	10^{-3} M	37 to 38%
Curare ($K_D = 2 \times 10^{-7}$ M) (10)	10^{-4} M	13%
Benzoquinonium ($K_D = 1 \times 10^{-8}$ M) (24)	10^{-4} M	67%
Unlabeled toxin ($K_D = 2 \times 10^{-9}$ M)	6×10^{-7} M	20%
Atropine	10^{-2} M	30%
Choline	10^{-2} M	2%

As described in Fig. 12, ^{125}I-toxin-receptor complexes were incubated 4 hr at room temperature with the indicated ligand and then the fractions sedimenting as complex and free ^{125}I-toxin were determined. Samples incubated without ligand contained 9% free toxin, so 9% was subtracted from the percent of ^{125}I-toxin migrating as free toxin to compute the percent dissociation due to the ligand.

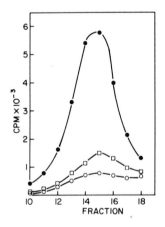

FIG. 13. Protection of solubilized receptor against binding of ^{125}I-toxin. Solubilized receptor at a concentration of 1.0×10^{-7} M was made 4.2×10^{-7} M in ^{125}I-toxin for several hours at 4°C and the ^{125}I-toxin-receptor complex formed resolved from free ^{125}I-toxin by sedimentation 10 hr at 45,000 rpm in the SW50. 1 rotor on 5 to 20% sucrose gradients as described in Methods (●——●); or the solubilized receptor was made 10^{-5} M (□——□) or 10^{-4} M (○——○) in benzoquinonium before ^{125}I-toxin was added and then the sample was sedimented on a gradient containing the same concentration of the appropriate ligand. Only the fractions of the resulting gradients containing the ^{125}I-toxin-receptor complex are shown.

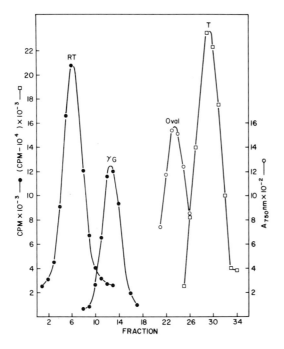

FIG. 14. Sedimentation of solubilized ^{125}I-toxin-receptor complexes. Sucrose gradients as described in Methods were centrifuged 10 hr at 45,000 rpm in the SW50.1 rotor. One gradient contained ^{125}I-toxin-receptor complexes (RT) and free ^{125}I-toxin (T). Another contained a sample of 1 mg/ml ovalbumin (Oval) and the third [^{14}C] gamma globulin (γG) produced by cultured mouse plasmacytoma cells.

tion in one step. So an affinity adsorbent was synthesized by conjugating native toxin to CNBr-activated agarose.

When Triton X-100 extracts of bulk membrane were applied to small columns of these toxin-agarose conjugates, it was found that these extracts were depleted of receptor as assayed by the formation of a specific complex with ^{125}I-toxin on sucrose gradients (Fig. 15). Since unsubstituted agarose did not bind receptor, this indicated that toxin conjugated to agarose retained its native ability to bind to the receptor. The maximum binding capacity of the adsorbents used was determined by applying sufficient Triton X-100 extract to columns so that substantial amounts of receptor were observed in the extract which passed through the column. Conjugates made with 5 mg/ml toxin appeared to have a maximum binding capacity for receptor of approximately 10^{-5} moles of receptor sites/liter of gel. Even though the slow rate of association of toxin with receptor could limit the apparent capacity of such columns, it seemed probable that much of the toxin conjugated under these conditions was inactive or inaccessible to receptor. Conjugates of 0.17 mg toxin/ml gel exhibited a binding capacity approximately 2×10^{-6} moles of receptor sites/liter of gel.

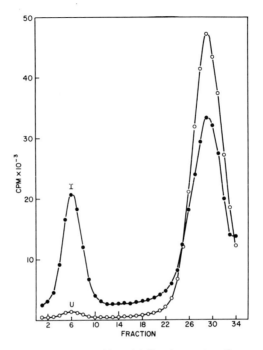

FIG. 15. Loading of affinity column with solubilized receptor. Over a period of 9 hr at 4°C 25 ml of Triton X-100 extract was passed through a column containing 0.7 ml of 5 mg toxin/ml substituted agarose gel. An aliquot of the extract applied to the column and of the extract after passage through the column was made 5.0×10^{-7} M in ^{125}I-toxin and left several hours at 4°C before being sedimented on sucrose gradients for 10 hr at 45,000 rpm in the SW50.1 rotor. The initial extract (I) was found to contain receptor at 3.1×10^{-7} M, but virtually all the receptor was depleted in the material passed through the column (U) which contained only 1.7×10^{-8} M receptor.

Receptor could be eluted from toxin-agarose conjugates by decamethonium, benzoquinonium, or ^{125}I-toxin, but not by choline (Fig. 16). The results with these eluents, like the results with ligands which produced dissociation of ^{125}I-toxin from vesicles or solubilized receptor, were those expected if the mechanism of elution was competition for the acetylcholine binding site of the receptor between the eluent and the conjugated toxin. In this series of experiments 25 ml of Triton X-100 extract was applied to 1-ml columns of toxin-agarose over a 6 to 8-hr period at 4°C. In each experiment the amount of receptor bound to the column was determined by the difference between the amount of receptor in the initial extract and the amount of receptor in the extract passed through the column. After extensive washing of the column with Triton buffer, the column was incubated with 1 volume of the eluent in Triton buffer for a period of time that the previous dissociation experiments indicated should allow dissociation of most of the toxin-receptor complexes before the eluate was collected. When the eluent

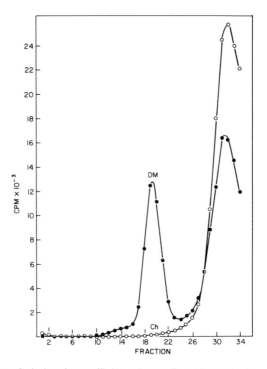

FIG. 16. Specificity of elution from affinity column. For this particular experiment toxin-agarose (5 mg/ml) was agitated overnight at 4°C with a Triton X-100 extract containing solubilized receptor, and then the gel was washed several times by centrifugation before being divided into two equal fractions. One fraction was agitated 4 hr at room temperature with 3 volumes of 10^{-2} M decamethonium in 0.5% Triton X-100, 0.1 M NaCl, 10^{-3} M Tris pH 7.4 while the other was similarly treated with 10^{-2} M choline. The gel was then pelleted and the supernatants extensively dialyzed against 0.5% Triton X-100 buffer to remove decamethonium and choline. Then aliquots of the decamethonium eluate (DM) and the choline eluate (Ch) were labeled with ^{125}I-toxin and sedimented on glycerol gradients for 5.5 hr at 45,000 rpm in the SW50.1 rotor. Decamethonium eluted a significant amount of receptor whereas choline did not elute any.

was ^{125}I-toxin, receptor was eluted in the form of ^{125}I-toxin-receptor complexes which could be measured directly by sedimenting the eluate on sucrose gradients. When the eluent was a nonradioactive ligand, the eluate was first dialyzed to remove the ligand, and then an aliquot was incubated with ^{125}I-toxin and sedimented on a gradient so that the amount of receptor eluted could be determined. As expected of the highest affinity eluent used, ^{125}I-toxin eluted significant amounts of the receptor bound to the columns at lower concentrations than did the other eluents. For example, ^{125}I-toxin at 5×10^{-5} M incubated on the column 4 hr at room temperature eluted 30% of the bound receptor from a column which exhibited a binding capacity of 1×10^{-5} M. Elution was routinely performed at room temperature in order to speed the dissociation of receptor from the toxin conjugate, although the receptor was less stable than at 4°C. In another experiment the column was incubated with ^{125}I-toxin for 90 hr at 4°C which resulted in the elution of 67% of the bound receptor. However, elution with ^{125}I-toxin was not extensively used because it presented the problem of removing the excess ^{125}I-toxin. Under the same conditions described for elution of 67% of the bound receptor by ^{125}I-toxin at 5×10^{-5} M, decamethonium at 10^{-2} M eluted only 3% of the receptor. Decamethonium at 10^{-2} M eluted up to 8% of the bound receptor from 5-mg toxin/ml columns in 4 hr at room temperature. Higher concentrations of decamethonium could not be used because the ionic strength of such solutions was found to be sufficient to irreversibly denature the receptor, thus preventing relabeling with ^{125}I-toxin. The alternative approach was taken of lowering the degree of substitution of the gel to 0.17-mg toxin/ml gel. It was found that incubation with 10^{-2} M decamethonium for 1 hr at room temperature eluted 25% of the bound receptor from the column. The higher affinity ligand benzoquinonium at 10^{-3} M was observed to elute 40 to 50% of the bound receptor under these conditions. Many nonspecific methods were tried for eluting receptor using treatments which were observed to disrupt the ^{125}I-toxin-receptor complex on gradients such as low pH, high salt, urea, and chaotropic reagents, but none eluted receptor in a form which could bind ^{125}I-toxin, indicating that all the treatments probably irreversibly denatured the receptor.

In order to purify large amounts of receptor for further study, a 20-ml packed volume of 0.17 mg toxin/ml gel was used in a 1 × 11 cm column. A typical experiment is shown in Table 4. A Triton X-100 extract of the bulk membrane fraction was applied to this column at approximately 20 ml/hr at 4°C to allow for the slow rate of the binding reaction. Then the column was extensively washed at 4°C, and for 1 hr at room temperature, before 1 column volume of 10^{-3} benzoquinonium was applied and allowed to incubate for 1 hr. Then 1.5 column volume was eluted (which contained ap-

TABLE 4. *Purification of solubilized acetylcholine receptor by affinity chromatography*

Sample	Volume (ml)	Receptor sites		Protein		Specific activity (nmoles/g)
		(moles/liter)	(nmoles total)	(mg/ml)	(mg total)	
Homogenate	9.4×10^2	8.3×10^{-8}	78	14.	1.3×10^4	5.9
Triton extract	3.3×10^2	1.9×10^{-7}	37	4.6	1.5×10^3	25.
Unbound to column	1.6×10^3	0	0	0.94	1.5×10^3	0
Benzoquinonium eluate (concentrated)	4.5	3.2×10^{-6}	15	0.79	3.6	4.1×10^3

The concentration of receptor in each fraction was determined by labeling with ^{125}I-toxin plus or minus 10^{-4} M benzoquinonium. The experiment described in the table used a preparation derived from 470 g main electric organ from a single eel.

proximately 70% of the eluted receptor) and 2 hr later another 1.5 column volume was collected and pooled with the first. The pooled eluates were concentrated by ultrafiltration, using an Amicon PM10 membrane which is designed to retain proteins larger than 10^4 daltons. This filter also retained much of the Triton X-100, hence the Triton concentration of the eluate rose to several percent. The concentrated eluate was then extensively dialyzed to remove benzoquinonium before being assayed for binding activity with ^{125}I-toxin. Meanwhile, the column was eluted with several volumes of 8 M urea to remove the 3 or 4 mg of protein not specifically eluted by benzoquinonium. The typical experiment shown in Table 4 achieved 170-fold purification of the receptor from the Triton extract and a final purification of 690-fold over the crude homogenate.

The eluate from the affinity column was substantially purified. When sedimented on sucrose gradients the eluate exhibited one major protein component which corresponded to the ^{125}I-toxin binding component of that fraction or of the initial extract (Fig. 17). In order to further purify the receptor, eluted material was sedimented on a sucrose gradient and the peak fractions pooled. In this way the eluate from the experiment described in Table 4 was further purified to a specific activity of 7.5×10^3 nmoles ^{125}I-toxin binding sites/g BSA equivalent protein, which corresponded to 1 mole of sites/133,000 g protein (and a total purification of 1.3×10^3-fold).

The polypeptide chains contained in the eluate were studied by electro-

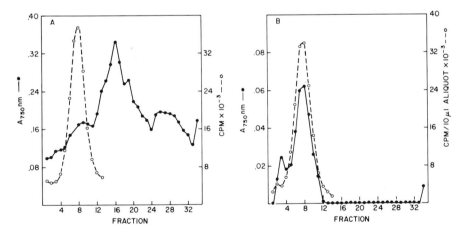

FIG. 17. Distribution of ^{125}I-toxin binding activity and protein of the initial Triton X-100 extract *(A)* and of purified acetylcholine receptor *(B)*. Aliquots labeled with ^{125}I-toxin were sedimented on sucrose gradients for 10 hr at 45,000 rpm in the SW50.1 rotor. Fractions from one gradient of the initial extract were collected for determination of radioactivity and from a second for protein assay. Ten-μl aliquots of the fractions from the gradient of purified receptor were assayed for radioactivity, while the remainder of each fraction was used for assay of protein.

phoresis on acrylamide gels containing SDS (Fig. 18). The eluate was always diluted at least 10-fold into the SDS sample buffer and heated briefly at 100°C to avoid problems which might arise from the presence of Triton X-100. Removal of Triton by extraction with ether or by precipitation with TCA followed by extraction with acetone did not alter the results, but allowed the use of higher concentrations of sample without altering the migration of the tracking dye, which occurred when large amounts of Triton X-100 were present in the sample. The eluates contained two principal components and small, variable amounts of higher molecular weight components which were probably contaminants. Most of the faint bands of high molecular weight could be removed by sedimenting the eluate on a sucrose gradient and pooling the peak fractions for analysis on SDS acrylamide gels. The eluate was clearly different and greatly reduced in heterogeneity with respect to the Triton X-100 extract, as expected from the large

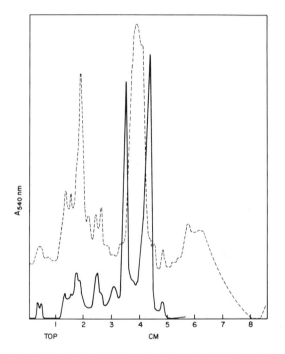

FIG. 18. SDS acrylamide gel electrophoresis of the initial Triton X-100 extract (---) and purified acetylcholine receptor eluted from an affinity column (——). Electrophoresis of a 114-μg sample of the initial extract and of a 33-μg sample of purified receptor from the experiment described in Table 4 was conducted as described in Methods. The Coomasie blue stained gels were scanned at 540 nm using the same settings for both gels. The scans shown begin immediately below the tops of the gels and extend to the dye marker in the case of the initial sample or to beyond the last protein band in the case of the purified receptor after which the scan was deleted because it contained a destaining artifact.

purification achieved (Fig. 18). The two principal bands observed in the eluate migrated with apparent molecular weights of 4.2 and 5.4 × 10⁴ daltons.

IV. DISCUSSION

The experiments described are consistent with the interpretation that the α-neurotoxin of *Naja naja* venom binds to acetylcholine receptors reversibly, but with very great affinity. The binding affinity of ^{125}I-toxin for receptor is so large that when a preparation contains one or both species at concentrations in large excess over their equilibrium binding constant (as is frequently the case), equilibrium strongly favors formation of the ^{125}I-toxin-receptor complex. Under these conditions, binding of ^{125}I-toxin appears irreversible unless a specific receptor ligand is present at concentrations which can prevent ^{125}I-toxin from rebinding to the receptor after it spontaneously dissociates.

Advantage was taken of the reversibility of toxin binding to achieve substantial purification of the receptor by affinity chromatography. Receptor solubilized from electric organ membrane by Triton X-100 in a form capable of specifically binding ^{125}I-toxin was adsorbed to an affinity adsorbent consisting of toxin conjugated to agarose. Receptor was eluted from the adsorbent with specific ligands which competed with the toxin-agarose conjugate for binding to the receptor. Although the method as described offers an easy method for achieving a several hundred-fold total purification of the receptor, it is not yet perfected in that elution of only 40 to 50% of the receptor bound to the adsorbent is achieved and the eluate is not completely homogeneous. Purification to homogeneity should be possible through conventional procedures, or by developing procedures for exhaustively removing traces of protein nonspecifically bound to the affinity adsorbent. One possible explanation for the limited elution of receptor from the column may be multiple toxin binding sites on the receptor molecule. For example, if a receptor were bound to the affinity adsorbent through two sites instead of one, its equilibrium dissociation constant might be of the order of 10^{-18} M instead of 10^{-9} M, making it virtually irreversibly bound. The large size of the receptor solubilized by Triton X-100 (approximately $3.6 × 10^5$ daltons) (13) makes it likely that it contains more than one acetylcholine binding site.

Electrophoresis of the β-mercaptoethanol-treated eluate on acrylamide gels containing SDS showed that it contained two main polypeptide chains with apparent molecular weights of 5.4 and 4.2 × 10⁴ daltons. Affinity labeling (23) is the method of choice for identifying the specific polypeptide chain and amino acid residues composing the active site of a protein. Reiter, Cowburn, Prives, and Karlin (19) have used an affinity labeling reagent which reacts with sulfhydryl groups to specifically label receptor on the surface of intact electroplax. This labeling reagent is covalently bound to a polypeptide chain of molecular weight 4.2×10^4 daltons. This suggests that the 4.2×10^4 molecular weight component may be the same as that labeled by Reiter et al. (19) and may contain some or all of the amino acid residues composing the acetylcholine binding site of the receptor. It seems likely that the 5.4×10^4 molecular weight component of the eluate is also a subunit of the receptor, and, although it may also contribute amino acid residues to the acetylcholine binding site of the receptor, it is also possible that it is the "ionophore" subunit of the receptor proposed by Changeux, Podleski, and Meunier (4). At present it is unknown if the solubilized receptor even retains an ionophore activity. Regardless of the role hypothesized for each polypeptide chain in the receptor, if it were supposed that both polypeptide chains were present, the receptor would have a molecular weight of 0.96×10^5 daltons/^{125}I-toxin binding site. The highest specific activity preparations obtained thus far contain 1.3×10^5 g protein/mole binding sites, which is reasonably close to the value of 0.96×10^5 daltons. If the figure of 0.96×10^5 g/mole toxin binding sites and the figure of 3.6×10^5 daltons (13) for the receptor as solubilized from the membrane were both accurate, there would be four toxin binding sites per aggregate.

Affinity chromatography of the type described here appears to offer a method for efficiently achieving substantial purification of the acetylcholine receptor, which should allow detailed biochemical study of this macro-molecule.

V. SUMMARY

Acetylcholine receptors on membrane fragments derived from the electric organ of *Electrophorus electricus* were studied using an α-neurotoxin purified from the venom of *Naja naja*. Toxin labeled with ^{125}I was found to bind to the acetylcholine binding site of these receptors with great specificity by a mechanism involving high affinity, reversible binding. Study of the specificity of binding by protection experiments and assay of receptor activity *in vitro* showed that at low concentrations ^{125}I-toxin bound almost exclusively to receptors, but (unlike native toxin) also bound to a non-specific site with much lower affinity. Estimates were made of the equilibrium dissociation constant for the formation of the ^{125}I-toxin-receptor complex, of the rate constants for its association and dissociation, and of the thermodynamic parameters of the reaction. Receptor was solubilized from the membranes in a form which retained the ability to specifically and reversibly bind toxin. Solubilized receptor was substantially purified by means of affinity chromatography using an adsorbent of toxin conjugated to agarose from which receptor was eluted by acetylcholine binding site ligands. Receptor was eluted from the adsorbent with a specific activity for binding of ^{125}I-toxin several hundred-fold greater than that of the crude homogenate of electric organ. Purified receptor consisted of one major protein component by sedimentation on sucrose gradients and was resolved into two major polypeptide chains by electrophoresis on SDS-acrylamide gels.

ACKNOWLEDGMENT

This work was supported by National Institutes of Health grant No. AI 06544 to E. S. Lennox.

REFERENCES

1. Barnard, E. A., Wieckowski, J., and Chiu, T. H. (1971): Cholinergic receptor molecules and cholinesterase molecules at mouse skeletal muscle junctions. *Nature*, 234:207–209.
2. Berg, D. K., Kelly, R. B., Sargent, P. B., Williamson, P., and Hall, Z. (1972): Binding of α-bungarotoxin to acetylcholine receptors in mammalian muscle. *Proc. Nat. Acad. Sci.*, 69:147–151.
3. Bosmann, H. B. (1972): Identification and biochemical characteristics of a cholinergic receptor of guinea pig cerebral cortex. *J. Biol. Chem.*, 247:130–145.
4. Changeux, J. P., Podleski, T., and Meunier, J. C. (1969): On some structural analogies between acetylcholinesterase and the macromolecular receptor of acetylcholine. *J. Gen. Physiol.*, 54–225s–244s.
5. Cuatrecasas, P. (1970): Protein purification by affinity chromatography. *J. Biol. Chem.*, 245:3059–3065.
6. Eigen, N., and Hammes, G. G. (1963): Elementary steps in enzyme reactions. *Adv. in Enzymol.*, 25:1–38.
7. Eldefrawi, M. E., Eldefrawi, A. T., Seifert, D., and Obrien, R. D. (1972): Properties of lubrol-solubilized acetylcholine receptor from torpedo electroplax. *Arch. Biochem. Biophys.*, 150:210–218.
8. Fambrough, D. M., and Hartzell, H. C. (1972): Acetylcholine receptors: Number and distribution at neuromuscular junctions in rat diaphragm. *Science*, 176:189–191.
9. Karlsson, E., Eaker, D., and Porath, J. (1966): Purification of a neurotoxin from the venom of *Naja nigricollis*. *Biochim. Biophys. Acta*, 127:505–520.
10. Kasai, M., and Changeux, J. P. (1971): *In vitro* excitation of purified membrane fragments by cholinergic agonists. *J. Membrane Biol.*, 6:1–88.
11. Laemmli, U. K. (1970): Cleavage of structural proteins during the assembly of the head of bacteriophage T4. *Nature*, 227:680–685.
12. Lowry, O. H., Rosebrough, N. J., Farr, A. L., and Randall, R. J. (1951): Protein measurement with the folin phenol reagent. *J. Biol. Chem.*, 193:265–275.
13. Meunier, J. C., Olsen, R. W., and Changeux, J. P. (1972): Effect of detergents on some hydrodynamic properties of the receptor protein in solution. *F.E.B.S. Letters*, 24:63–68.
14. Meunier, J. C., Olsen, R. W., Menez, A., Fromageot, P., Boquet, P., and Changeux, J. P. (1972): Some physical properties of the cholinergic receptor protein from *Electrophorus electricus* revealed by a tritiated α-toxin from *Naja nigricollis* venom. *Biochemistry*, 11:1200–1210.
15. Miledi, R., Molinoff, P., and Potter, L. T. (1971): Isolation of the cholinergic receptor protein of torpedo electric tissue. *Nature*, 229:554–557.
16. Miledi, R., and Potter, L. T. (1971): Acetylcholine receptors in muscle fibres. *Nature*, 233:599–603.
17. Patrick, J., Heinemann, S. F., Lindstrom, J., Schubert, D., and Steinbach, J. H. (1973): Appearance of acetylcholine receptors during differentiation of a myogenic cell line. *Proc. Nat. Acad. Sci. (in press)*.
18. Raftery, M. A., Schmidt, J., Clark, D. G., and Wolcott, R. G. (1971): Demonstration of a

specific α-bungarotoxin binding component in *Electrophorus electricus* electroplax membranes. *Biochem. Biophys. Res. Comm.*, 45:1622–1629.

19. Reiter, M. J., Cowburn, D. A., Prives, J. A., and Karlin, A. (1972): Affinity labeling of the acetylcholine receptor in the electroplax: Electrophoretic separation in sodium dodecyl sulfate. *Proc. Nat. Acad. Sci.*, 69:1168–1172.

20. Reynolds, J., and Tanford, C. (1970): Binding of dodecyl sulfate to proteins at high binding ratios. Possible implications for the state of proteins in biological membranes. *Proc. Nat. Acad. Sci.*, 66:1002–1007.

21. Scatchard, G. (1949): The attractions of proteins for small molecules and ions. *Ann. N.Y. Acad. Sci.*, 51:660–672.

22. Silman, H. J., and Karlin, A. (1967): Effect of local pH changes caused by substrate hydrolysis on the activity of membrane-bound acetylcholinesterase. *Proc. Nat. Acad. Sci.*, 58:1664–1668.

23. Singer, S. J. (1970): Affinity labeling of protein active sites. In: Ciba Foundation Symposium on *Molecular Properties of Drug Receptors*, edited by R. Porter and M. O'Connor, pp. 229–242. J. A. Churchill, London.

24. Webb, G. (1964): Affinity of benzoquinonium and ambenonium derivatives for the acetylcholine receptor, tested on the electroplax and for acetylcholinesterase in solution. *Biochim. Biophys. Acta*, 102:172–184.

Synaptic Transmission and Neuronal Interaction
Raven Press, New York 1974

Biochemical Studies on Cholinergic Synaptic Vesicles

V. P. Whittaker and H. Zimmermann

Department of Biochemistry, University of Cambridge, Cambridge CB2 1QW, England*

I. INTRODUCTION

Highly homogeneous preparations of synaptic vesicles can be obtained from mammalian nervous tissue (Whittaker, Michaelson, and Kirkland, 1964), but such preparations suffer from two main disadvantages: the vesicles are derived from many types of nerve endings differing in the chemical transmitters which they utilize and the yield is low—a few micrograms of vesicle protein per gram of brain cortex.

More recently milligram quantities of pure cholinergic synaptic vesicles have been successfully prepared in single zonal runs from the electric organ of *Torpedo* spp. (Whittaker, Essman, and Dowe, 1972*b*). We now present a combined morphological, electrophysiological and biochemical study which shows (1) that acetylcholine is packaged in such vesicles in association with ATP; (2) that the vesicles contain, in addition to acetylcholine and ATP, four main protein constituents, three of which are membrane constituents and the fourth a core protein; and (3) that on stimulating the organ at 5 stimuli/sec, vesicles are depleted in number and become smaller in size and that this is accompanied by a fall in vesicle proteins and a much greater fall in acetylcholine and ATP.

Finally, we will draw some tentative conclusions about what is going on.

Torpedos are elasmobranch fish related to skates and rays and, more distantly, to dogfish and sharks. Their body fluids are approximately 800 milliosmolar, which poses special problems in subcellular fractionation, since 0.8 M sucrose is a very dense and viscous medium for such purposes. Following some improvements made to the original fractionation procedure of Sheridan, Whittaker, and Israël (1966) by Israël, Gautron, and Lesbats (1970), we have been using 0.2 M sucrose made isoosmotic with elasmobranch plasma by the addition of 0.3 M sodium chloride for our initial extractions, and 0.2 to 1.4 M sucrose, with the addition of varying amounts of sodium chloride, for the density gradient.

---

* Present address: Abteilung für Neurochemie, Max-Planck-Institut für Biophysikalische Chemie, 3400 Göttingen, West Germany.

II. ISOLATION OF SYNAPTIC VESICLES

A. Morphology of Tissue

Most of the work was done with *Torpedo marmorata*, (Fig. 1). The electric organs form two masses of tissue, one on each side of the head. The honeycomb pattern is formed by closely packed stacks of electroplaque

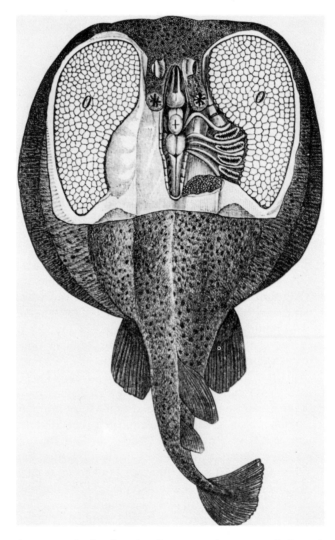

FIG. 1. *Torpedo marmorata* showing electric organ and nerve supply from electric lobe in the brainstem containing the cells of origin of the cholinergic tract. Note the honeycomb array of the stacks of electroplaques *(O)* each of which is profusely innervated on its ventral surface. Drawing taken from Fritsch (1890).

cells each of which is copiously innervated on the underside by branches of four cholinergic nerves; these pass through the gill arches from paired lobes in the brainstem. Vertical sections through the stacks (Fig. 2) (Sheridan, 1965) show that the nerve terminals are thickly applied to the underside (NT) and the highly invaginated noninnervated dorsal face (NI). Figure 2 *(right)* shows the nerve terminals with their synaptic vesicles at higher magnification.

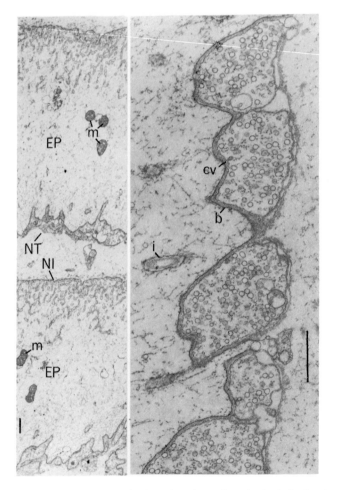

FIG. 2. Electron micrographs of vertical section through a stack of electroplaques. Left: two electroplaques *(EP)* are shown with nerve terminals *(NT)* applied to their ventral surfaces; the highly invaginated noninnervated *(NI)* surface is also seen. Note also mitochondria *(m)*. Right: enlargement of nerve terminals showing synaptic vesicles. To economize space the orientation of this micrograph is at right angles to its neighbor. Note basement membrane *(b)*, coated vesicle open to the synaptic cleft *(cv)*, and infolding of postsynaptic membrane *(i)*. Bars represent 1 μm.

B. Comminution of Tissue

Electric tissue is extremely difficult to homogenize using the conventional type of homogenizer. We have found (Whittaker et al., 1972b) that if the tissue is first frozen in liquid Freon 12, and, more recently, in liquid nitrogen, it becomes brittle and can be crushed to a coarse powder. Superficially, the fragments of tissue thus obtained (Fig. 3) look relatively undamaged at the ultrastructural level (Soifer and Whittaker, 1972). The invaginations of the innervated and noninnervated faces are readily recognized, and the nerve terminals can be applied to the innervated face. However, closer examination reveals, that over considerable areas, that part of the external presynaptic nerve membrane separate from the synaptic cleft has been damaged or torn away, and the nerve terminal is little more than a layer of frozen cytoplasm with vesicles embedded in it (Fig. 3, black arrow).

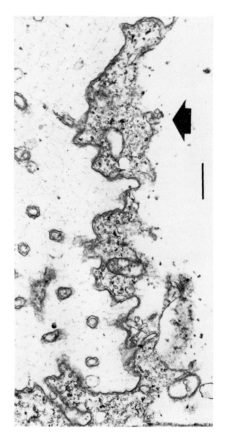

FIG. 3. Electron micrograph of fragment of frozen tissue showing damaged external presynaptic membrane *(arrow)* (Soifer and Whittaker, 1972). Bar represents 1 μm.

If these fragments of electroplaque are suspended in 0.2 M sucrose-0.3 M sodium chloride and the extracted fragments removed by relatively low-speed centrifugation (10,000 × g for 30 min), a supernatant is obtained which consists of terminal-soluble cytoplasmic protein and synaptic vesicles, diluted with the extraction medium and relatively uncontaminated with other membrane fragments.

C. Zonal Separation of Vesicles

This supernatant may now be placed on a density gradient in a zonal rotor and separated (Fig. 4) into three main fraction peaks: soluble proteins (SP), vesicles (VP), and larger membrane fragments (MP). Figure 4 shows the distribution down the gradient of protein, the enzymes lactate dehydrogenase, choline acetyltransferase, acetylcholinesterase, and acetylcholine. Lactate dehydrogenase is a soluble enzyme in most tissues so it is not

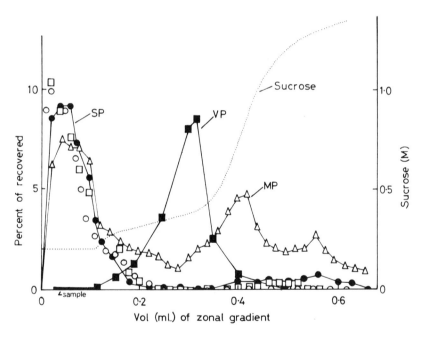

FIG. 4. Separation of synaptic vesicles from the electric organ (30 g) of the *Torpedo* by zonal centrifuging. The supernatant from a cytoplasmic extract of frozen, comminuted tissue after removal of coarse tissue fragments at 10,000 × g for 30 min is placed on a sucrose-NaCl density gradient in a Beckman Ti-14 zonal rotor and centrifuged at 48,000 rpm for 3 hr. Key to symbols and amounts recovered (enzyme units in μmole substrate transformed/min; percentages are of activity in supernatant sample): protein (●) 183 mg (91%); acetylcholine (■) 612 nmole (51%); lactate dehydrogenase (○) 8,360 units (69%); choline acetyltransferase (□) 177 units (110%); acetylcholinesterase (△) 1,530 units (56%). Data of Whittaker, Essman, and Dowe (1972*b*).

surprising that it is recovered, along with other soluble proteins, in the first peak (SP). Interestingly, choline acetyltransferase, the enzyme synthesizing acetylcholine, is also recovered entirely in the soluble protein peak. This confirms work with mammalian brain (Fonnum, 1967) and shows that the site of acetylcholine synthesis is the cytoplasm.

Acetylcholinesterase is, by contrast, bimodal in its distribution. Part of it is recovered in the soluble protein peak, but part is recovered in the peak of membrane fragments (MP), where it indicates the presence of fragments of postsynaptic membrane.

Acetylcholine has yet another distribution: it is recovered as a single peak (VP) with a density equivalent to 0.3 to 0.4 M sucrose. Electron microscopic investigation of this fraction shows it to be rich in particles of morphology identical to synaptic vesicles (Figs. 5 and 6). These are estimated to contain approximately 70,000 molecules of acetylcholine per vesicle (Whittaker et al., 1972b). The isolated vesicles are identical with those seen in the terminals and are somewhat larger than mammalian neuromuscular and CNS synaptic vesicles, approximately 84 nm in diameter.

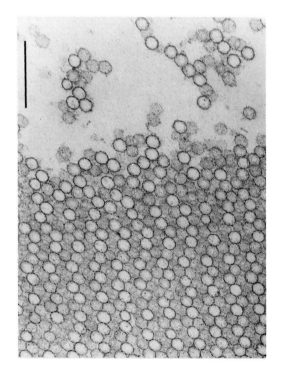

FIG. 5. Synaptic vesicles isolated from electric organ of *Torpedo,* using agar cup technique. Bar represents 0.5 μm.

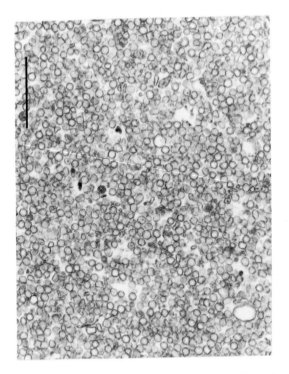

FIG. 6. Synaptic vesicles of VP fraction from electric organ of *Torpedo*, after pelleting. Note distortion of vesicles due to pelleting. Bar represents 1 μm.

The specific concentration of acetylcholine in this fraction is high, 600 to 1,300 nmole/mg of protein when allowance has been made for the small percentage of soluble protein that has diffused into VP from SP.

Two things need to be said about this acetylcholine. First it represents less than half of the acetylcholine originally present in the tissue. The rest disappeared during the initial comminution and extraction of the tissue with 0.2 M sucrose-0.3 M sodium chloride. This acetylcholine may have been cytoplasmic acetylcholine or acetylcholine belonging to a population of particularly fragile or easily discharged vesicles: we do not know, and this uncertainty is one of the limitations of the method.

The second point is that the acetylcholine that remains, and is recovered in VP, is acetylcholine that is stable in the presence of considerable amounts of acetylcholinesterase. Figure 4 shows that there are appreciable amounts of acetylcholinesterase activity even in the vesicle peak. If the acetylcholine is released from its bound state, for example, by detergents, it is immediately destroyed. So the acetylcholine in VP must be sequestered within the vesicle, not just adsorbed on its surface.

The association of acetylcholine with vesicles is further shown by gel filtration on columns of Agarose particles with an exclusion weight of five-million. Figure 7a shows the elution pattern of a sample of VP using a column pre-equilibrated with 0.4 M sucrose, 0.2 M sodium chloride. Acetylcholine comes out entirely in the void volume; protein mainly does also, but there is a small peak of lower molecular weight protein which evidently represents contamination by soluble proteins from SP. This is shown by the coincidence of this small peak with the main peak of SP proteins, which were run separately as a control and superimposed in this diagram.

III. COMPOSITION OF VESICLES

A. Protein

The vesicles are osmotically sensitive and can be lysed in water. A convenient way of doing this is to dialyze VP against water, freeze-dry the retentate, and then suspend the freeze-dried material in 0.2 M sodium chloride. If such material is gel filtered on Agarose 5 m, the effect of the treatment (Fig. 7b) is to release approximately 50% of the recovered vesicle protein as a low-molecular weight component (molecular weight approximately 10,000) (Whittaker, 1971, 1972). There are now two peaks, an initial peak of membrane protein coming through in the void volume and a second peak (of lower average molecular weight than the proteins of SP) in the nonexcluded volume of the gel.

Another similar experiment is shown in Fig. 8 where the dialyzed and freeze-dried vesicle peak from the zonal run has been filtered through Sephadex G-200. Note the void volume peak (1) of largely membrane protein; this fraction is rich in phosphorus, which is mainly lipid phosphorus. There then follows a small peak of soluble protein; this is SP contamination because this gel has good resolving power in the range 10,000 to 200,000 daltons. Finally (peak 2), we have the peak of the low-molecular weight vesicular protein: the core protein. We call this vesiculin (Whittaker, 1971, 1972).

The vesiculin peak also has phosphorus associated with it (Dowdall, M. J., *unpublished results*) but this is nonlipid phosphorus. From the absorption maximum at 260 to 265 nm which is shown by vesiculin (and which is seen in Fig. 8a) we think that this phosphorus is a nucleotide phosphorus. The amount of absorption at 260 to 265 nm/mole of phosphate would be consistent with a monophosphate, presumably AMP.

The results of disc gel electrophoresis of the material in the two main peaks is diagrammed in Fig. 8b. The membrane peak has two main, high-molecular weight components; the vesiculin peak has one main, low-molecular weight component and there is relatively little cross contamination.

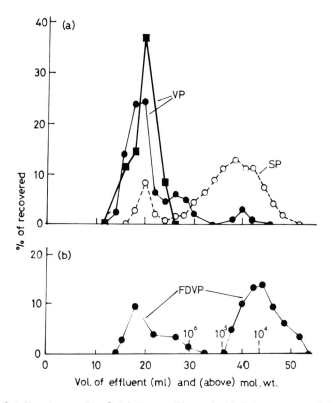

FIG. 7. (a) Gel filtration on Bio-Gel A-5m equilibrated with 0.4 M sucrose—0.2 M NaCl of samples of fractions VP and SP. Protein: VP (●); SP (○). Acetylcholine (■). Recovered: protein (VP) 191 μg (88%); (SP) 1.7 mg (62%); acetylcholine (VP), 43 nmole (71%). (b) Gel filtration under similar conditions of a dialyzed and freeze-dried sample of VP (FDVP). Protein (●). Recovered: 105 μg (80%). Results of Whittaker (1972).

The putative nucleotide that is associated with vesiculin isolated by gel filtration on Agarose and Sephadex G-200 columns can be separated out as shown in Fig. 9, which depicts the results of gel filtration through Sephadex G-50. The resolving power in the range 20,000 to 500 daltons of G-50 is better than G-200. It will be seen from Fig. 9 that vesiculin dissociates under these conditions into two components: vesiculin A, a nucleotide-free dimer (note the disappearance of nucleotide absorption in the U.V. spectrum, insert, curve A) and vesiculin B, with enhanced nucleotide absorption (insert, curve B) and an apparent molecular weight of less than 1,000 daltons. We think this is the free nucleotide. The small peak in the middle is real and represents undissociated vesiculin.

Table 1 shows the amino acid composition of hydrolysates of vesiculin in 6 N HCl. On the basis of one tyrosine residue molecule, the molecular weight works out to be just under 10,000, which is in very good agreement

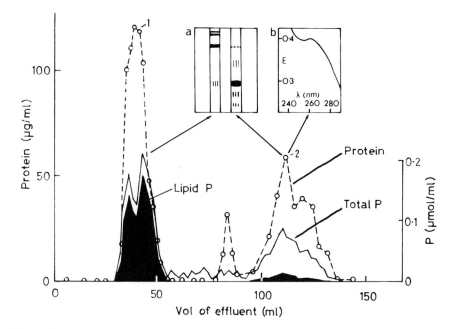

FIG. 8. Distribution of protein (○) and phosphorus (continuous lines) after gel filtration, through Sephadex G-200 of dialyzed and freeze-dried vesicles (FDVP) suspended in 0.2 M NaCl. The black profiles show the proportion of the total P in each peak that was chloroform-methanol soluble. Inserts: *(a)*, disc gel electrophoresis in sodium dodecyl sulfate of peaks 1 and 2; *(b)* U. V. absorption spectrum of peak 2. Recovered: protein, 2.23 mg (105%); phosphorus 4.57 μmole (51%). Results of M. J. Dowdall.

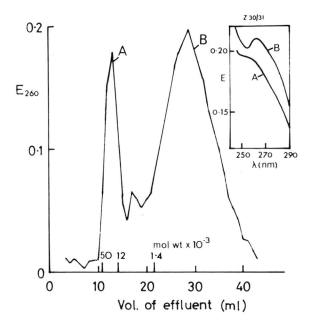

FIG. 9. Resolution of vesiculin (peak 2 of Fig. 8) into a protein *(A)* with reduced absorption (insert) at 260 to 265 nm and a putative nucleotide *(B)* with marked absorption in this region, using gel filtration through Sephadex G-50. Results of Whittaker (1971, 1972).

TABLE 1. *Amino acid content of hydrolysates of vesiculin*

Amino acid	Amino acid content		Assumed no. of vesicles/mole
	mole %	mole/mole of Tyr	
Ala	9.3 ± 0.24	7.7	8
Arg	2.4 ± 0.40	2.0	2
Asp	8.9 ± 0.54	7.4	7
Glu	18.8 ± 0.54	15.7	16
Gly	13.3 ± 1.50	11.1	11
His	2.0 ± 0.17	1.7	2
Ile	2.5 ± 0.02	2.1	2
Leu	4.5 ± 0.55	3.7	4
Lys	3.4 ± 0.66	2.8	3
Orn	2.8 ± 0.67	2.3	2
Phe	2.0 ± 0.32	1.7	2
Pro	4.8 ± 0.50	4.0	4
Ser	13.7 ± 1.69	11.4	11
Thr	5.2 ± 0.39	4.3	4
Tyr	1.2 ± 0.20	1.0	1
Val	4.1 ± 0.49	3.4	3
		Mol wt. (1 Tyr/mol)	9,891

Samples containing approximately 200 μg of Lowry-positive protein were hydrolyzed for 17 to 24 hr in 6 M HCl in an atmosphere of N_2. Values are means ± SEM of three determinations. The component here listed as Orn cochromatographed with authentic Orn.

with the gel estimate. Note the preponderance of acidic and hydroxy amino acids and the low content of basic amino acids. The acidic character of the protein was confirmed (Dowdall, M. J., *unpublished observations*) by its behavior on ion-exchange chromatography: it was strongly absorbed at neutral pH's and required buffers of pH 3.5 or less for elution. The excess of acidic over basic residues is 14, which would be sufficient to neutralize the positive charge on all of the vesicular acetylcholine.

B. Nucleotide

The association of a putative nucleotide, possibly AMP, with vesiculin suggested that nucleotides might be present in intact vesicles. Accordingly, the distribution of ATP in the zonal gradient was studied (Fig. 10) using the highly specific and sensitive luciferin-luciferase system (Whittaker, Dowdall, and Boyne, 1972a). It will be seen that there is a large peak of ATP in the soluble protein (SP) region of the gradient and a second peak in the vesicle (VP) region. When SP and VP are treated with an enzyme mixture (Fig. 11), which converts ATP into IMP (the mixture consists of potato apyrase, rabbit muscle myokinase, and calf intestine adenylate deaminase), the ATP in SP is rapidly hydrolyzed at the same rate as an equivalent amount of free ATP, whereas the vesicular ATP is quite stable. Thus,

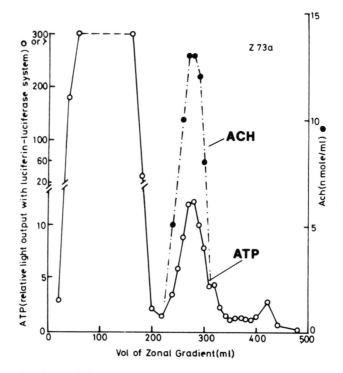

FIG. 10. Distribution of ATP in a zonal gradient. Materials and conditions are similar to those of Fig. 4. Results of Whittaker, Dowdall, and Boyne (1972*a*).

vesicular ATP, like vesicular acetylcholine, is protected against the action of hydrolytic enzymes.

This immunity of vesicular ATP to hydrolytic enzymes is again shown in Fig. 12. In this experiment the parent supernatant fraction was pre-incubated with the apyrase mixture until all free ATP was destroyed, at which point there is only one main peak of ATP, coinciding with the vesicle peak.

In this experiment the exchangeability of ATP with added ^{14}C-labeled ATP was also tested. All the added ^{14}C was recovered in the soluble protein peak and none was incorporated into the vesicles.

C. Stability of Vesicles

The release of vesicular acetylcholine and ATP as a result of various treatments is shown in Fig. 13. Both components are lost from vesicles on treatment with detergent *(c)*, exposure to hypo-osmotic shock *(d)*, and treatment with phospholipase at 26°C *(b)*. In each case, acetylcholine comes out first. Under milder conditions, for example, treatment with phospholi-

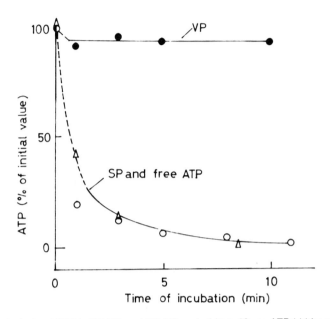

FIG. 11. Hydrolysis of ATP in VP (●) and SP (○) and of free, 20 μM, ATP (△) by an apyrase-myokinase-adenylate deaminase mixture. Results of Whittaker, Dowdall, and Boyne (1972*a*).

pase at 5°C *(a)*, acetylcholine may be induced to leak out with no loss of ATP. Morphological examination of the vesicles after phospholipase treatment by W. Edwards has shown that acetylcholine loss can occur with relatively little disturbance of vesicle morphology, but that loss of ATP is associated with considerable loss of structure in the vesicle membrane.

From preliminary studies with other methods of nucleotide analysis, we believe that ATP is the main, and probably the sole, nucleotide in the intact vesicle, and therefore is the nucleotide associated with the core protein vesiculin in the native state. The vesiculin-ATP complex may well serve as a macromolecular acidic counter-ion to acetylcholine. The cholinergic vesicle would thus appear to be constructed on similar lines to the chromaffin granule and the mast cell granule, both of which store small, molecular weight amines in combination with polyanions.

IV. EFFECT OF STIMULATION ON VESICLE YIELD AND COMPOSITION

The question may now be asked whether either of the two other components—ATP and vesiculin—is released along with acetylcholine. Preliminary results indicate that both acetylcholine and ATP are released when the organ is stimulated, whereas vesiculin is not released to the same extent.

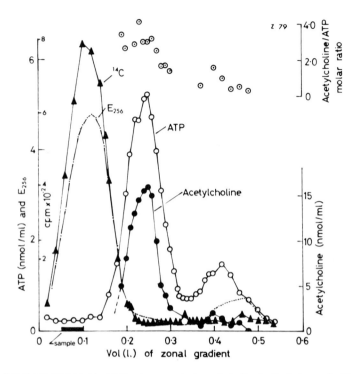

FIG. 12. Zonal separation of vesicles in an experiment similar to that shown in Figs. 4 and 10, except that the parent supernatant was pretreated with the ATP-hydrolyzing enzyme mixture described in the legend to Fig. 11 and [U-^{14}C]ATP was added to the tissue extract. Acetylcholine (●), ATP (○), molar ratio (☉), ^{14}C (▲), E256 (- . -). Results of Whittaker, Dowdall, and Boyne (1973).

A. Effect in Whole Organ

Figure 14 shows the arrangement for stimulating and recording the response of the organ. Stimulation is carried out under MS 222 anesthesia by applying a stimulating electrode through a hole in the skull to the electric lobe that contains the cells of origin of the cholinergic innervation of the organ. The effect of stimulation on the organ is controlled by denervating the organ on the other side at the beginning of the experiment and comparing the stimulated organ with the unstimulated control. Normally stimulation is continuous at 5 pulses/sec and this leads (Fig. 15) to a steady decline in the response of the organ as measured by an electrode applied to the surface of the skin covering it. Periodically, the ability of the response to recover is tested by stopping the repetitive stimulation and applying single shocks at 5, 10, 20, and 30 sec after stopping. After the recovery test is completed, the response of the organ is brought back to its pretest value by repetitive stimulation and this is continued to the next test point.

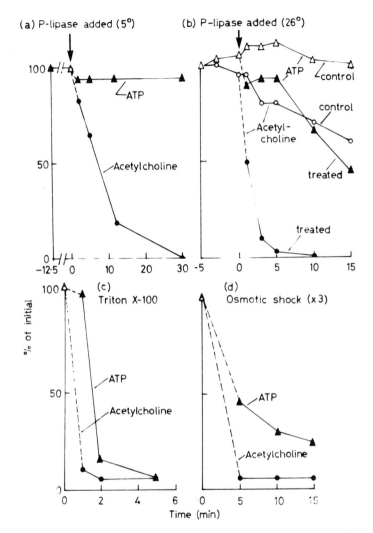

FIG. 13. Release of acetylcholine and ATP from VP by *(a)* phospholipase at 5°C and *(b)* at 26°, by *(c)* osmotic shock (2:1 dilution with water) and *(d)* by Triton X-100 (0.025%). Results of A. F. Boyne, M. J. Dowdall, and W. Edwards using a sample of phospholipase A₂ kindly provided by Dr. E. Heilbronn.

It was found (Fig. 15) that even an "exhausted" organ (i.e., one in which the response had been reduced to 1.0 V or less) has considerable powers of recovery, although never equal to more than half of the original response.

Electron microscopic examination of the organ at the end of the experiment showed a decline in the number of vesicles in the nerve terminals on the stimulated side to as low as 42% of that of the unstimulated control (Table 2); membrane blebs and what are interpreted as infoldings of the

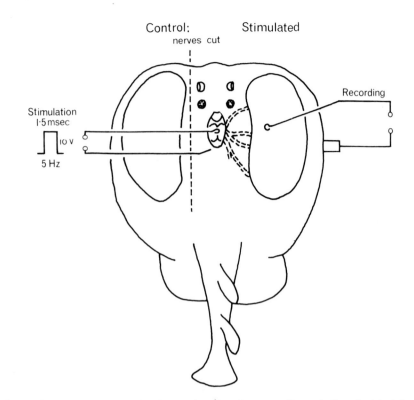

FIG. 14. Arrangements for stimulating the electric organ through the electric lobe. A nonstimulated control is provided by denervating the electric organ on the opposite side of the animal at the beginning of the experiment.

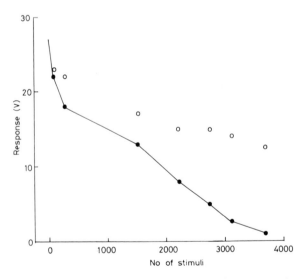

FIG. 15. Filled circles: response of organ (discharge in volts representing summed post-synaptic potentials of individual electroplaques) to repetitive stimuli (5 pulses/sec). At intervals represented by the circles, repetitive stimuli were stopped and the ability of the organ to recover was tested by single shocks at 5, 10, 20, and 30 sec. Recovery increased very little between 20 and 30 sec. The discharges at 30 sec are shown by the open circles. The discharge of the organ was brought back to its pretest value by repetitive stimulation, and this was then continued to the next point. The test procedure was then repeated. Note that even when the organ is virtually unable to respond further to repetitive stimuli (discharge ≤ 1 V), it still recovers rapidly.

TABLE 2. *Effects of stimulation on the electric organ*

Parameter	Stimulated tissue (as % of unstimulated)
Whole tissue	
Organ response[a] (V) after reduction of response to 1 V and 30-sec recovery	35 ± 8 (3)
No. of vesicle profiles/μm^2	49 ± 7 (2)
Fraction VP[b]	
Membrane protein[c]	45 ± 3 (2)
Vesiculin[c]	94 ± 14 (2)
ATP[d]	16 ± 3 (4)
Acetylcholine[d]	12 ± 3 (4)

Measurements relate to observations made with intact tissue or on fraction VP isolated at the end of the experiment. Values are means ± range (2) or SEM (more than two experiments; no. of experiments in parentheses) and are for tissue stimulated repetitively to exhaustion expressed (unless otherwise stated) as a percentage of the corresponding value for the unstimulated, denervated organ.

[a] Expressed as % of initial value.

[b] Isolated from tissue excised while stimulus was continued.

[c] Isolated on Sephadex G-200 after freeing fraction VP from traces of soluble protein by filtration through porous glass beads.

[d] Peak VP tubes.

external membrane also appeared (Fig. 16), as though extensive fusion of vesicle membranes with the external membrane had occurred. Similar results have recently been reported for the neuromuscular junction under the influence of repetitive stimulation (Korneliusson, 1972) or black widow spider venom (Clark, Hurlbut, and Mauro, 1972). In addition, a population of vesicles approximately 30% smaller in size than the vesicles of unstimulated terminals made their appearance (Fig. 17). Decreases in vesicle volume as a result of stimulation have also been reported for nerve terminals in muscle (Jones and Kwanbumbumpen, 1970).

B. Effect on the Vesicle Fraction

When fraction VP was prepared in two successive zonal runs from stimulated and unstimulated organs, the diminution of vesicle numbers noted in the intact tissue was reflected in an approximate 50% fall in vesicular membrane protein in the VP peak (Table 2, line 2). Vesiculin, oddly enough, did not fall appreciably as the result of stimulation (Table 2, line 3) although it might be expected to fall at least 50%. However, the estimate of the vesiculin content of the vesicles depends on separating it on a Sephadex G-200 column from membrane protein after dialysis and freeze-drying of the zonal vesicle peak; possibly vesiculin becomes more readily extractable after stimulation.

By contrast, the two small, molecular weight constituents of the vesicle

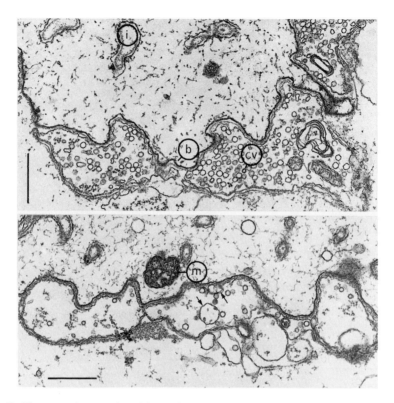

FIG. 16. Electron micrographs of *(upper)* unstimulated organ, and *(lower)* organ stimulated to "exhaustion" (discharge ≤ 1 V). Note blebs and infoldings *(arrows)* of external membrane and reduction in size and number of synaptic vesicles. Note coated vesicle *(cv)*, invagination of postsynaptic membrane *(i)*, basement membrane *(b)*, and mitochondria *(m)*. Bar represents 1 μm.

—ATP and acetylcholine—are greatly depleted by stimulation (Table 2, lines 5 and 6). Vesicular ATP and acetylcholine decline at the same rate as the response of the organ (Fig. 18) and acetylcholine tends to be more readily depleted than ATP. This is consistent with the observation in isolated vesicles that acetylcholine is lost more readily than ATP as the result of various treatments (Fig. 13). It is noteworthy that even after only 400 stimuli there is a significant fall in vesicular acetylcholine and ATP, which implicates the synaptic vesicles in transmission even during short periods of synaptic activity. Vesicles isolated from stimulated and non-stimulated tissue show size differences similar to, but less marked than, those observed in intact endings. The less marked character of the difference may be due to the greater vulnerability of the isolated vesicles to volume changes induced by isolation, fixation, and embedding. However, vesicle fractions isolated from stimulated organs also appear to contain more large

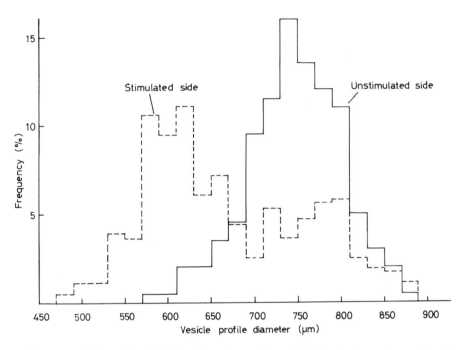

FIG. 17. Distribution of profile diameters of synaptic vesicles in electron micrographs of whole tissue preparations of stimulated and unstimulated electric organs. Note suggestion of bimodal distribution of vesicle size and increase in the proportion of the smaller vesicles on stimulation. Diameters are measurements of electron micrographs at a magnification of approximately 6,300.

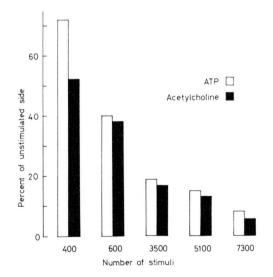

FIG. 18. Effect of stimulation on the acetylcholine and ATP content of isolated synaptic vesicles.

membrane contamination than vesicles derived from nonstimulated tissue (Fig. 19). This material preferentially sediments to the bottom of the tube when the vesicle fraction is centrifuged at high speed. It may be derived from the breakdown of the blebs and the infoldings noted above as characteristic of stimulated tissue. If these are created by vesicle fusion, then vesicular membrane fragments formed from them may have the same bouyant density as synaptic vesicles, and therefore be difficult to separate from the latter by density gradient centrifugation. Stimulation did not affect the levels of total protein, lactate dehydrogenase, and acetylcholinesterase in the cytoplasmic extracts put onto the density gradient; thus, zonal fractions other than VP could not have been affected.

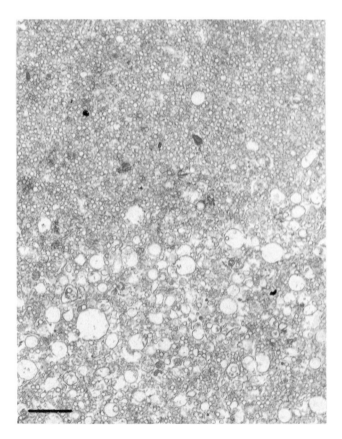

FIG. 19. Electron micrograph of the bottom portion of pellet of VP. Note the layer containing larger vesicles at the bottom of the pellet. Bar represents 1 μm.

V. DISCUSSION

Interpretation of the results is complicated by our ignorance of the extent to which the reduced response of the organ on repetitive stimulation is due to a failure in transmitter release or to a failure in the postsynaptic membrane to respond to normal transmitter release. Furthermore, comparisons of the properties of vesicle fractions isolated from stimulated and unstimulated tissue depend on the assumption that the yield of vesicles from stimulated and unstimulated tissue is identical. Evidence that the efficiency of extraction is not affected by stimulation comes from the constancy of composition of the parent cytoplasmic extract with respect to the soluble cytoplasmic markers already mentioned. However, the results seem to indicate that the cholinergic vesicle is built on somewhat similar lines to the chromaffin granule or the adrenergic vesicle in that in all three structures a biogenic amine is "packaged" with ATP and an acidic protein. On stimulation, vesicles are lost, and the remainder includes a considerable proportion of smaller vesicles which, on average, appear to store less ATP and acetylcholine, and to be less able to maintain transmission than the larger vesicles they have replaced. However, the remarkable, if partial, powers of recovery of the organ suggest that the surviving, depleted vesicles can be utilized through an unknown number of cycles of discharge and recharge before they too are discarded.

The role of ATP in the vesicles remains obscure. Is its only function to help neutralize the acetylcholine cation; or, could it be a trophic factor or auxiliary transmitter? Is it an intracellular energy source providing energy for vesicle translocation or fusion? Further work using a combination of biochemical, morphological, and electrophysiological techniques will be necessary for the solution of these problems.

ACKNOWLEDGMENTS

We are grateful to those colleagues, acknowledged in the text and legends to figures, who have allowed us to include their results: Mr. G. H. C. Dowe, Mr. C. Denston, Miss F. Henderson, Miss H. Potter, Mrs. G. Rowe, and Miss M. Talerman, for valuable technical and secretarial assistance, and Mr. P. Bystricky and Mr. B. Thurley, for help with the recording equipment. We are also most grateful to Professor C. Cazaux for arranging the supply of *Torpedos* and to Dr. E. Heilbronn for supplies of phospholipase A_2. The work was supported by a Programme Grant from the U.K. Medical Research Council (to V. P. Whittaker) and by a fellowship (to H. Zimmermann) from the Deutsche Forschungsgemeinschaft. Finally, we should like to thank Dr. D. Soifer for presenting the oral version of this manuscript to the 26th Annual Meeting of the American Society of General Physiologists.

REFERENCES

Clark, A. W., Hurlbut, W. P., and Mauro, A. (1972): Changes in the fine structure of the neuromuscular junction of the frog caused by black widow spider venom. *J. Cell Biol.*, 52:1–14.

Fonnum, F. (1967): The "compartmentation" of choline acetyltransferase within the synaptosome. *Biochem. J.*, 103:262–270.

Fritsch, G. (1890): *Die elektrischen Fische. Zweite Abteilung: Die Torpedineen.* von Weit and Co., Leipzig.

Israël, M., Gautron, J., and Lesbats, B. (1970): Fractionnement de L'Organe Electrique de La *Torpille:* Localisation Subcellulaire de L'Acetylcholine. *J. Neurochem.,* 17:1441–1450.

Jones, S. F., and Kwanbunbumpen, S. (1970): The effects of nerve stimulation and hemicholinium on synaptic vesicles at the mammalian neuromuscular junction. *J. Physiol.,* 207:31–50.

Korneliusson, H. (1972): Ultrastructure of normal and stimulated motor endplates. *Z. Zellforsch. Mikroskop. Anat.,* 130:28–57.

Sheridan, M. N. (1965): The fine structure of the electric organ of *Torpedo marmorata. J. Cell Biol.,* 24:129–141.

Sheridan, M. N., Whittaker, V. P., and Israël, M. (1966): The subcellular fractionation of the electric organ of *Torpedo. Z. Zellforsch. Mikroskop. Anat.,* 74:291–307.

Soifer, D., and Whittaker, V. P. (1972): Morphology of subcellular fractions derived from the electric organ of *Torpedo. Biochem. J.,* 128:845–846.

Whittaker, V. P. (1971): Origin and function of synaptic vesicles. *Ann. N.Y. Acad. Sci.,* 183:21–32.

Whittaker, V. P. (1972): La vesicule cholinergic. In: *La Système Cholinergique en Anesthésiologie et en Réanimation,* edited by G. G. Nahas, J. C. Salamagne, P. Viars, and G. Vourc'h, p. 45. Librairie Arnette, Paris.

Whittaker, V. P., Dowdall, M. J., and Boyne, A. F. (1972a): The storage and release of acetylcholine by cholinergic nerve terminals: Recent results with non-mammalian preparations. *Biochem. Soc. Symp.,* 36:49–68.

Whittaker, V. P., Essman, W. B., and Dowe, G. H. C. (1972b): The isolation of pure cholinergic synaptic vesicles from the electric organs of elasmobranch fish of the family torpedinidae. *Biochem. J.,* 128:833–845.

Whittaker, V. P., Michaelson, I. A., and Kirkland, R. J. A. (1964): The separation of synaptic vesicles from nerve ending particles ("Synaptosomes"). *Biochem. J.,* 90:293–303.

Synaptic Transmission and Neuronal Interaction
Raven Press, New York 1974

Synthesis, Axonal Transport, and Release of Acetylcholine by Identified Neurons of *Aplysia californica*

James H. Schwartz

Department of Microbiology, New York University Medical Center, and Neurobiology and Behavior, Public Health Research Institute of the City of New York, New York, New York 10016

I. INTRODUCTION

Much of our information about dynamic aspects of acetylcholine metabolism comes from studies with tissues composed predominantly of nerve terminals (Birks and MacIntosh, 1961; Whittaker, 1965; Collier, 1969; Marchbanks, 1969; Israel, Gautron, and Lesbats, 1970; and Potter, 1970). We know from these studies that acetylcholine turns over rapidly at cholinergic terminals, and that a major proportion of the transmitter substance released is made from choline taken up by the terminals from the synaptic cleft. Even though there has been some indication that cholinergic nerve cell bodies contain the synthetic enzyme choline acetyltransferase, the amount of the transmitter substance present in the cell body is relatively small compared with that in terminals. In cortex, for example, Whittaker (1965) found that approximately two-thirds of the total acetylcholine could be isolated in synaptosomes. Moreover, recent work of Heuser and Reese *(this volume)* suggests that formation of the vesicular apparatus for storage and release of acetylcholine can occur at the neuromuscular junction independently of the nerve cell body, at least for relatively short periods of time. It is therefore not surprising that the cell body and its proximal axon have been somewhat neglected in current views of the cholinergic mechanism; it is generally believed that somatic synthesis followed by axonal transport supplies at most an insignificant part of the acetylcholine needed for synaptic transmission.

We chose to work with the nervous system of *Aplysia* because it offers the chance of studying both identified cholinergic cell bodies and their terminals. During the past decade, neurons in the abdominal ganglion have been under intensive electrophysiological and pharmacological investigation in several laboratories; consequently much is known about their function. More than 30 neurons in the ganglion are large and can be reliably recognized from animal to animal (Frazier, Kandel, Kupfermann, Waziri, and Coggeshall, 1967); their size permits isolation of individual cell bodies for biochemical analysis (see Peterson, 1972, for review). Another important experimental advantage is that this invertebrate ganglion can be kept in simple organ culture for long periods of time (Strumwasser and Bahr, 1966).

All 30 of the identified cell bodies (Fig. 1, and see Frazier et al., 1967) were individually removed from the abdominal ganglion by free-hand

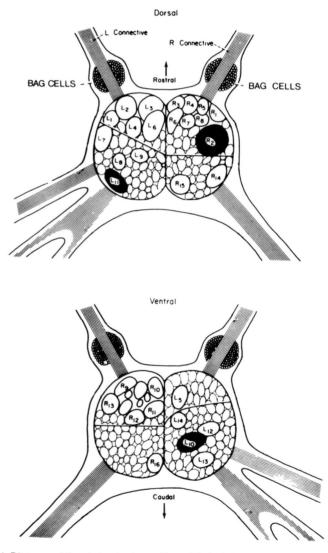

FIG. 1. Diagram of the abdominal ganglion of *Aplysia* (after Frazier et al., 1967).

dissection, and extracted and assayed for choline acetyltransferase using a sensitive radiochemical method (Giller and Schwartz, 1968, 1969, 1971). Extracts of three cells (R2, L10, and L11) had significant amounts of the enzyme; the others had less than 2% of that in any of the cholinergic neurons. These results were confirmed by McCaman and Dewhurst (1970). Electrophysiological and pharmacological studies of L10 have shown that it mediates cholinergic excitation to some cells, and inhibition to others (Kandel, Frazier, Waziri, and Coggeshall, 1967; Wachtel and Kandel, 1971). Unfortunately, similar neurophysiological information is not yet available for L11 and R2.

By measuring choline acetyltransferase in extracts of single neurons we identified some of the cholinergic cells in the ganglion. With *Aplysia,* however, we can inquire more deeply into the dynamic aspects of the cholinergic mechanism. Because the parts of neurons are anatomically rather easy to separate and isolate, we can see if synthesis of acetylcholine is confined to terminals, or if the transferase present in cell bodies actually functions under physiological conditions. We can determine what limits synthesis of the transmitter, and whether it is transported within the axon to be released at terminals. We have studied these questions using two experimental approaches: first, conventional uptake studies using radio-active choline, and second, direct pressure injection of ^{3}H-choline into cell bodies of individual identified neurons.

II. FORMATION OF ACETYLCHOLINE FROM EXOGENOUS CHOLINE

When the isolated abdominal ganglion is incubated for 1 hr in seawater supplemented with ^{3}H-choline, the cell bodies of R2, L10, and L11 synthesize radioactive acetylcholine (Table 1). We detected no synthesis in the cell bodies of identified neurons, which we previously have shown do not contain the transferase (Giller and Schwartz, 1971). Although these results provide additional evidence that R2, L10, and L11 are cholinergic neurons, the amount of transmitter synthesized in the three cell bodies was unexpectedly low. In *Aplysia* weighing 100 g nearly a quarter of the total transferase activity in the whole ganglion is contained in the cell bodies of R2, L10, and L11. But we found that they contained less than 1% of the total acetylcholine formed in the ganglion from exogenous choline. Thus the rate of synthesis is quite low in the cell body when compared to enzymatic capacity; the rate of synthesis in the rest of the ganglion (presumably neuropile) and connectives is considerably higher (Table 1). This suggests that synthesis of acetylcholine might be limited by the uptake of choline, and that an uptake mechanism is present in nerves and neuropile, but is deficient in the cell body.

TABLE 1. *Formation of acetylcholine from exogenous ³H-choline*

Neural component	Number of experiments	ACh (pmoles/hr)	Choline	Efficiency (% of enzymatic capacity)
Cells				
R2	7	0.21 ± .05	7.5 ± 1.4	0.023
L10	2	0.2, 0.29	4.8, 3.8	0.034
L11	4	0.21 ± .03	1.8 ± .32	0.036
Ganglia	7	49 ± 4.6	432 ± 47	0.6
Connectives (per cm length)	4	63 ± 19	327 ± 38	2.6

Isolated abdominal ganglia from *Aplysia* weighing 60 to 100 g were incubated at 15°C for 1 hr in the presence of 65 μM ³H-choline (Amersham-Searle, 16 C/mmole) in 50μl of artificial seawater containing 50 mM Tris-HCl buffer (pH 7.7), streptomycin (0.1 mg/ml), and penicillin G (200 units/ml) (Schwartz et al., 1971). Ganglia were washed with seawater; cell bodies were dissected from the ganglia, and frozen in 70% ethylene glycol (Giller and Schwartz, 1971). Cell bodies and nervous tissue were extracted with 1 M formic acid:acetone (15:85). Acetylcholine was separated from choline and other choline derivatives by high-voltage electrophoresis at pH 4.7 (Giller and Schwartz, 1971). Radioactivity in acetylcholine and choline was measured by scintillation directly on paper cut from electropherograms, and 853 cpm were equivalent to 1 pmole. Efficiency of acetylcholine synthesis is defined as *in vivo* rate of synthesis/*in vitro* activity of choline acetyltransferase at 15°C × 100. Values are presented ± SEM.

III. ENTRY OF CHOLINE INTO NERVOUS TISSUE

Measurements of biochemical parameters in identified neurons and in ganglia of *Aplysia* are quite variable (see, for example, Schwartz, Castellucci, and Kandel, 1971) and measurements of choline uptake were no exception. In order to obtain data suitable for kinetic analyses of the uptake mechanism, we needed an experimental design in which a single specimen of nervous tissue would provide its own normalization. A comparison of the rates of uptake by the same ganglion at two concentrations of external choline was found to yield data with little variation. An example of an experiment with this design is shown in Fig. 2. We covered each of three ganglia with a measured droplet of seawater containing one concentration of ¹⁴C-choline (here 20 μM). After 30 min, these droplets were removed and sampled. The difference between the amount of choline originally applied and the amount remaining after a 30-min interval was the amount taken up by the tissue. The ganglia were then covered with fresh droplets, and incubated for another 30-min period. The amount of choline taken up by each ganglion during 30-min intervals was constant in experiments lasting for 6 hr at concentrations of choline greater than 17 μM. (Shorter intervals must be used at concentrations below 17 μM.) After four intervals of 30 min at the one concentration, we increased the concentration of ¹⁴C-choline in the droplets to 209 μM, and continued the experiment in the same

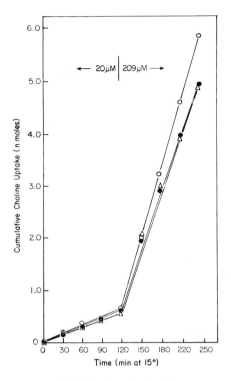

FIG. 2. Time course of uptake of ^{14}C-choline by *Apylsia* nervous tissue at two external concentrations of choline. See text.

way for another 2 hr. The ratio of the rates of uptake at various concentrations to that at the standard concentration of 209 μM was reproducible and reliable.

We found that at higher concentrations of choline the rate of uptake was proportional to the external concentration; no saturating concentration of choline was achieved. When data from a number of experiments using the protocol described above (Fig. 2) with concentrations of choline from 17 to 420 μM were analyzed kinetically, however, an important feature of the uptake mechanism emerged. We found that two apparently independent components of the uptake process operate at low and high concentrations of external choline. Below 25 μM, choline enters the tissue by a saturable mechanism with an affinity constant between 5 and 10 μM. This mechanism is completely dependent upon the presence of Na$^+$ and is inhibited by ouabain. At higher concentrations, choline enters by another mechanism with an apparent affinity constant of approximately 2,000 μM. This process also shows some dependence on Na$^+$, but is not affected by ouabain. Both uptake mechanisms are affected by the metabolic state of the tissue. They are both equally depressed at low temperatures, and in the presence of dinitrophenol and phenethylalcohol. Biphasic entry of choline has been noted previously in squid axon (Hodgkin and Martin, 1965) and in other nervous tissue (Marchbanks, 1968; Marchbanks and Israel, 1971). Uptake of choline in *Aplysia* in the range of low external concentrations, however, occurs with considerably greater affinity.

As might be expected, it is the uptake mechanism with the higher affinity which operates under physiological conditions. By bioassay using *Neurospora* 34486 CHOL-1, Eisenstadt, Cedar, and I *(in preparation)* have found that the choline concentration of *Aplysia* hemolymph is 11 μM ($n = 8$) with a range of 3.2 to 19.7 μM. These values are similar to those reported for human serum (5 to 50 μM, Bligh, 1952).

An indication that the high affinity uptake mechanism is important to the cholinergic process is our observation that little, if any, acetylcholine is synthesized from the excess choline which accumulates in nervous tissue at external concentrations greater than approximately 25 μM (Fig. 3). Synthesis of acetylcholine appears to be limited by a process with a Michaelis constant in the range of both the concentration of choline in the hemolymph and the affinity constant we have estimated for the saturable uptake mechanism. It seems likely therefore that entry of choline limits the synthesis of acetylcholine in *Aplysia*.

The fate of the choline taken up by the tissue also depends critically on the external choline concentration. At very low external concentrations, the fraction of the choline converted to acetylcholine approaches 60 to 70%. This fraction decreases as the external choline concentration is raised, and, between 20 and 100 μM, remains at a constant value of approximately 8 to 10%. This also indicates that the excess choline which enters by the low affinity mechanism is not readily available for synthesis of acetylcholine.

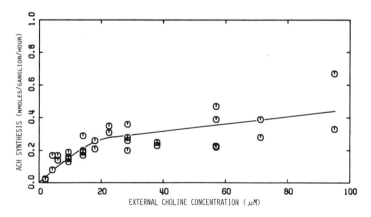

FIG. 3. Ganglia were incubated at 15°C for 45 min in the presence of various concentrations of ^{14}C-choline, and the acetylcholine formed was extracted and determined as described in the legend of Table 1.

If the notion that uptake of choline limits synthesis of acetylcholine is correct, choline cannot be formed at a significant rate endogenously. Studies with ^{3}H-methyl-labeled methionine supplied to isolated ganglia in the bath or to individual cell bodies by direct intracellular injection show that endogenous methylation of choline occurs at less than 0.5% of the rate at which choline enters nervous tissue when present in external concentrations normally found in the hemolymph (Schwartz, Eisenstadt, and Cedar, *in preparation*).

III. METABOLISM OF CHOLINE INJECTED INTO IDENTIFIED NEURONS

In order to investigate the metabolism of choline in the cell body, as well as for other studies, Koike, Eisenstadt, and I (1972a) developed a technique for injecting radioactive materials in relatively large amounts (Fig. 4). R2 is impaled with a double-barreled electrode with tip diameters broken to approximately 5 μ. One barrel, filled with 2 M potassium citrate, signals penetration, and is used to record resting membrane potentials and action potentials; the other is used to inject. About 1 nl of concentrated radioactive solution is drawn by suction into the tip of the injecting pipette. The progress of the injection can be monitored by watching the movement of the meniscus formed within the pipette at the interface between the radioactive solution and air. Usually all of the solution is injected within a few minutes by air pressure.

The fate of ^{3}H-choline injected into cholinergic neurons appears to be characteristic, and can be used to distinguish cholinergic from noncholiner-

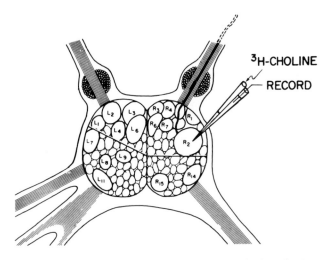

FIG. 4. Injection of cell R2 using double-barreled micropipettes.

gic neurons. R2 and L10, two cells which Giller and I found to contain choline acetyltransferase, convert between 75 and 85% of the injected radioactivity into acetylcholine within 1 hr. The remaining material is in the form of phosphorylcholine and betaine (together nearly 10%). Only a small fraction remains as unconverted choline (Koike et al., 1972a; Koike, Kandel, and Schwartz, 1972b). (During longer periods of time after the injection, an increasing proportion of the radioactivity is incorporated into lipid, although the proportion of the material in the form of acetylcholine usually remains above 50% for 24 hr.) In cells which do not contain choline acetyltransferase, the injected choline is largely converted to substances other than acetylcholine, with more than 85% in the form of phosphoryl-choline and betaine.*

Using the injection technique, Carew, Kandel, and I (1972) and Eisenstadt, Goldman, Kandel, Koester, Koike, and Schwartz (1973) have found additional cholinergic neurons in the ganglion. For one of these, LDG, a motor neuron to the gill, we were able to show that it contained the transferase, even though the cell is quite small and difficult to dissect out cleanly without damage. The other, LDHI, a motor inhibitor of the heart, was not tested by enzymatic assay. The injection technique is a general one: a wide variety of labeled precursors of transmitter substances might be injected. We are currently mapping serotonergic neurons in the ganglion by injecting ³H-tryptophan (Eisenstadt et al., 1973).

Besides being a simpler technique for mapping, injection also permits us to show directly that the synthesis of acetylcholine in cholinergic cell bodies is limited by the accessibility of exogenous substrate. Injected choline is converted to acetylcholine much more efficiently than is the choline taken up from the bath (Table 2). This is true even when similar amounts of choline are associated with the cell body. This again shows that the excess choline taken up from the bath is mainly unavailable for synthesis of transmitter substance. It is possible that this choline is not intraneural, but is situated either on the cell surface as a contaminant, or in glial cells which invest the large neurons of *Aplysia* (Bullock and Horridge, 1965; Giller and Schwartz, 1971). Alternatively it may be within the neuron, but located in a cellular compartment, for example, within membranes where it might be sequestered for the synthesis of lipids.

We have measured the rate of acetylcholine synthesis in more than 20 injections which gave an estimated intracellular concentration range from 0.01 to 74 mM. From that data, Eisenstadt and I *(in preparation)* have obtained the kinetic constants for choline acetyltransferase *in the living cell*. The maximal velocity is 33% of the expected enzymatic capacity and the apparent Michaelis constant is 5.9 mM, which checks well with

---

* Dewhurst (1972) recently reported that she found similar amounts of choline phospho-kinase in both cholinergic and noncholinergic neurons in the ganglion.

TABLE 2. *Efficiency of acetylcholine synthesis*

Source	Content of choline (pmoles/cell)	Estimated intracellular ^{3}H-choline concentration (mM)	ACh synthesis (pmoles/cell/hr)	Efficiency (% of enzymatic capacity)
Exogenous	7.6	0.11	0.25	0.023
Injection (small)	6.3	0.10	4.82	0.54
Injection (large)	2230	34	212	23
Calculated intracellular V_{max}	—	—	300	33

the value of 7.5 mM which Giller and I (1971) obtained for the extracted enzyme *in vitro*. The transferase has two substrates, choline and acetyl Coenzyme A(CoA). In order to find the Michaelis constant for choline in our *in vitro* studies (Giller and Schwartz, 1971) we saturated the enzyme with acetyl CoA. The constants obtained in the cell by injection are probably apparent, since we do not know the intracellular concentration of acetyl CoA but can assume that it is likely not to be saturating. We also do not know the concentration of choline normally present within the cell. Since the transferase in the cell was shown to be unsaturated over a wide range of ^{3}H-choline concentrations, we can argue that the endogenous, intracellular choline concentration available to the enzyme is normally below the Michaelis constant. Also consistent with the idea that the normal endogenous concentration of choline is limiting is our observation that synthesis of acetylcholine from ^{3}H-acetyl CoA injected into the cell body of R2 was stimulated by more than an order of magnitude when the co-substrate was injected with a saturating amount of unlabeled choline.

IV. AXONAL TRANSPORT OF ACETYLCHOLINE

The giant cell R2 is an ideal neuron for studying axonal transport, since it is thought to make few, if any, connections within the ganglion, and sends its major axon, which is 40 μ in diameter (Coggeshall, 1967; Frazier et al., 1967) into the right pleuroabdominal connective for up to 10 cm without arborizing or making synapses. After injecting ^{3}H-choline into the cell body of R2 and maintaining the nervous system for various periods of time in culture, we determined the chemical nature and the distribution of the injected radioactivity. Within 1 hr of the injection most of the ^{3}H-choline in R2 is converted to acetylcholine and the proportion of total radioactivity within the neuron (cell body and axon) in the form of acetylcholine usually remains above 50% for up to 24 hr (Fig. 5B). It is unlikely that the acetylcholine synthesized during the first hour after the injection is broken down and continuously resynthesized, since supplementation of the bathing solution with high concentrations of unlabeled choline did not appear to affect either the total amount or the proportion of radioactive acetylcholine in the neuron. Furthermore, studies with ^{3}H-acetyl CoA (labeled in the acetyl moiety) injected intrasomatically show directly that much of the acetylcholine synthesized initially is stable for long periods of time.

We found that radioactivity was localized only in those parts of the nervous system which contained the cell body of R2 and its axons. Immediately after the injection, almost all of the radioactivity was in the cell body. With time, an increasing proportion appeared in the right connective, reaching between 30 and 40% of the total in 24 hr after injection either of ^{3}H-choline (Fig. 5A) or of ^{3}H-acetyl CoA (data not shown). No significant radioactivity was present in the left connective.

This restriction to the right connective of the appearance of radioactivity with time suggested that the material moves from the cell body within the

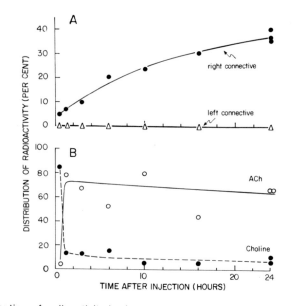

FIG. 5. Distribution of radioactivity in the nervous system after intracellular injection of ^{3}H-choline into R2. After various periods at 15°C following injection, the nervous system was subdivided and extracted. A. Appearance of radioactivity with time in the right (filled circles) and left *(open triangles)* connectives. The values are presented as percent total radioactivity recovered from the entire nervous system. B. The time course of conversion of injected ^{3}H-choline into acetylcholine *(open circles)* in the entire nervous system. Unconverted choline is shown with filled circles. Values are expressed as percent of total choline-containing compounds eluted from the electropherogram (from Koike, Eisenstadt, and Schwartz, 1972a).

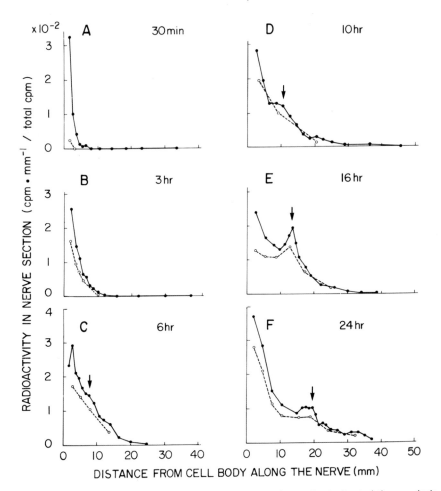

FIG. 6. Localization of radioactivity in the right connective at the indicated time periods after injection of ^{3}H-choline into R2. Following injection, the nervous system was cultured at 15°C for the indicated periods. The right connective was then stretched to the point where coiling was no longer observed. The nerve was rapidly frozen under powdered solid CO_2, and sectioned along its entire length by hand under a dissecting microscope. The cell body of R2 is at the origin in the figure, and the most proximal portion of the axon (approximately 1 mm in length) is within the ganglion itself. Nerve segments were extracted and prepared for scintillation counting. In some instances to obtain sufficient radioactivity for determining acetylcholine, extracts from several segments were combined and subjected to high-voltage electrophoresis. Values for acetylcholine *(open circles)* and for total radioactivity in the segments *(filled circles)* were normalized per millimeter length of nerve by dividing by the radioactivity in the entire nervous system, which was (in cpm): *A,* 184,747; *B,* 235,429; *C,* 124,900; *D,* 63,560; *E,* 135,903; *F,* 300,629. Arrows indicate the position of possible moving fronts (from Koike, Eisenstadt, and Schwartz, 1972a).

axon. After injecting the cell body of R2 with ^{3}H-choline, and keeping the nervous system in culture for various periods of time, we sectioned the right connective sequentially in order to determine both the amount and the chemical composition of the radioactivity in short segments of the nerve (Fig. 6). At 6 hr and thereafter, radioactivity clearly appears to move out along the connective as a wave (indicated by arrows, Fig. 6). This wave advances along the nerve at a constant rate of about 17 mm/day at 15°C.

Most of the labeled material in the nerve is acetylcholine at all times after the intrasomatic injection of either ^{3}H-choline (Fig. 6) or ^{3}H-acetyl CoA. With ^{3}H-choline, the proportion of radioactivity in the form of acetylcholine increased with the distance from the cell body, reaching a value of 95% in the most distal portion of the right connective from a nervous system kept for 24 hr after injection (Fig. 7). The greatest increase in the proportion of acetylcholine seems to occur in the region where the axon leaves the cell body. This suggests that acetylcholine is transported selectively in the axon, since phosphorylcholine and the other choline-containing substances migrate more slowly and tend to remain associated with the cell body.

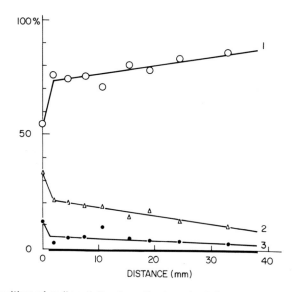

FIG. 7. Composition of radioactivity along the length of the right connective 24 hr after injection of ^{3}H-choline into the cell body of R2. The nerve was sectioned, and the individual segments were extracted and analyzed by high-voltage electrophoresis for their content of (1) acetylcholine, (2) phosphorylcholine and betaine, and (3) choline. Values for these compounds are presented as the percent of total radioactivity found in a segment.

V. SUBCELLULAR DISTRIBUTION OF ACETYLCHOLINE

Structures with the characteristic morphology of synaptic vesicles have been seen in electron micrographs of both the cell bodies and the axons of cholinergic neurons in *Aplysia* (Coggeshall, 1967; Elizabeth Thompson, *unpublished observations*). In support of the idea that a substantial amount of acetylcholine in the neuron is contained in synaptic vesicles, Koike et al. (1972*a*) found that up to 46% of the labeled acetylcholine in the right connective was sedimented during high-speed centrifugation (Table 3). Considerably less was sedimented in the cell body, suggesting the possibility that vesicles might be the vehicle for axonal transport. It is important to note that all of the radioactive material is derived primarily from the cell body and axon of a single cholinergic neuron and little if any from nerve terminals, since R2 is thought to make no synaptic contacts in the nervous tissue taken for homogenization.

Although high-speed pellets would be expected to contain synaptic vesicles, they also contain a large number of other structures. In order to study the subcellular distribution of acetylcholine further, Eisenstadt and I fractionated homogenates of nervous tissue which contained an R2 injected

TABLE 3. *Subcellular distribution of acetylcholine*

Time after injection (hr)	Neural component	Sedimentable radioactivity (% total)	
		Acetylcholine	Choline
1	Nerve	31	2.0
	Ganglion	4.7	2.8
18	Nerve	30	2.9
	Ganglion	11.6	10.7
24	Nerve	46.3	4.2
	Ganglion	15.5	9.0

Abdominal ganglia with nerves attached, cultured for the indicated periods after injection of ^{3}H-choline into R2, were incubated for an additional 10 min in artificial seawater containing 50 μM eserine sulfate. Seawater was then replaced with 0.2 M sucrose containing 0.3 M NaCl and eserine after washing three times. The right connective was cut from the ganglion, and eserinized *Aplysia* nervous tissue was added as carrier to both ganglion and nerve. The tissues were minced with an iris scissor at 0°C, and then homogenized in a glass tissue grinder with a loose-fitting Teflon pestle (0.25 to 0.3 mm clearance). The homogenates were centrifuged at 1,000 × *g* for 10 min, and the resulting pellets were rehomogenized. The combined 1,000 × *g* supernatants were centrifuged at 105,000 × *g* for 90 min. The resulting high-speed pellets and supernatants were analyzed for acetylcholine by high-voltage electrophoresis at pH 4.7 (Giller and Schwartz, 1971). (Data from Koike, Eisenstadt, and Schwartz, 1972*a*.)

with ³H-choline, using centrifugation in sucrose density gradients. After homogenization in the presence of 50 µM eserine, we concentrated particulate material by centrifugation at 300,000 × g for 30 min against a cushion of 2 M sucrose. The supernatant, containing the free acetylcholine, was saved for analysis. The concentrated particulate material was fractionated by flotation (Fig. 8). Substantial amounts of the total radioactivity appeared in fractions B and C which contain membranous structures, some with the morphological appearance of synaptic vesicles (Elizabeth Thompson, *unpublished observations*). These fractions are also enriched in their content of labeled acetylcholine (Table 4). Thus, although it is clear that in *Aplysia,* as in other animals, acetylcholine is present in homogenates in a free or unbound form, some of the transmitter also appears to be in vesicles.

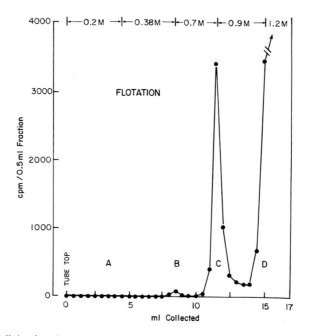

FIG. 8. Subcellular fractionation by flotation. A nervous system containing an R2 whose cell body was injected with ³H-choline was kept at 15°C for 4 hr and then homogenized. Particulate material was concentrated by centrifugation as described in the text. This material was placed at the bottom of a centrifuge tube and its density made equivalent to 1.2 M sucrose by addition of Ficoll® (Pharmacia) to a final concentration of 15%. Approximately 3.5 ml each of less dense solutions were layered above. The densities of these solutions were made equivalent to the sucrose concentrations indicated in the figure. Above 0.8 M sucrose, this was accomplished by adding Ficoll®. The osmolarity of all of the solutions was made 800 mOsmoles; below 0.8 M sucrose, this was accomplished by the addition of an appropriate amount of NaCl. Centrifugation was for 90 min at 2°C in a Spinco SW 27 rotor at 27,000 rpm. Fractions from the gradient, collected from the top of the tube by pumping, were immediately made pH 4.2 by adding 50 µl of 1 M ammonium acetate buffer. Radioactivity in the fractions was concentrated and analyzed as described in Table 4.

TABLE 4. *Composition of subcellular fractions*

Fraction	Distribution of soluble ^{3}H-choline derivatives (% of total Reinecke precipitable radioactivity)		
	ACh	Choline	Phosphorylcholine
High-speed supernatant	34.6	50.1	15.2
Gradient fractions			
B	60	40	0
C	80	20	0
D	58.3	32.9	8.8

The ^{3}H-choline derivatives were concentrated by precipitation with Reinecke salt from the centrifugal fractions described in the text and in Fig. 8. These were analyzed by high-voltage electrophoresis at pH 4.7.

VI. SYNAPTIC RELEASE OF RADIOACTIVITY FROM AN INJECTED CHOLINERGIC NEURON

We have seen that acetylcholine can be synthesized in the cell body of a cholinergic neuron, and can be transported down its axon. Some of the acetylcholine appears to be carried within synaptic vesicles. In order to determine whether the transmitter substance formed in the cell body and transported in the axon can be released at nerve terminals, we (Koike et al., 1972*b*) made use of another cholinergic neuron, L10, which is an interneuron in the abdominal ganglion. Unlike R2, which makes no known connections in the ganglion, L10 synapses with numerous follower cells close to its cell body (Kandel et al., 1967).

L10 normally fires spontaneously at a rate of 2 impulses/sec. A hint that, at its terminals, L10 might be releasing material which derived from the ^{3}H-choline injected into the cell body came from measurements of radioactivity in the perfusate collected after injection during 15-min periods (Fig. 9). Immediately after we had injected ^{3}H-choline, a relatively large amount of radioactivity appeared in the perfusate. We attributed this *immediate release* to leakage of choline from the site of the injection, since it occurred initially with all injections and was increased transiently whenever the electrode was withdrawn. During the next hour, radioactivity in the perfusate diminished rapidly. At approximately 70 min, the amount of radioactivity again increased, reaching a maximum at 100 min after the injection; it then gradually subsided. This pattern was seen in each of three similar experiments, and might be explained if the maximum represented the synaptic release of a wave of labeled acetylcholine that was transported from the cell body to the nerve terminals with an average delay of close to 70 min.

To examine this possibility we carried out experiments in which we

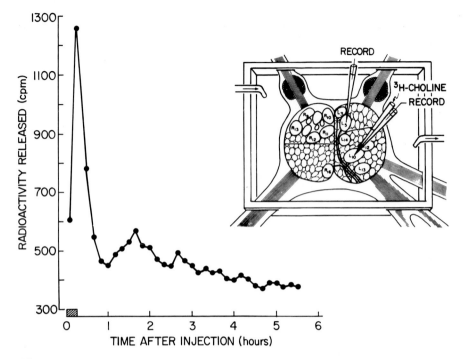

FIG. 9. Appearance of radioactivity after injection of ³H-choline into the cell body of L10 under conditions of *spontaneous* firing. Artificial seawater was delivered at a constant rate by a peristaltic pump to the inner chamber containing the ganglion with the injected cell body *(inset)*. Radioactivity in the perfusate collected during 15-min periods was counted by scintillation. The period during which the double-barreled electrode was kept in the cell is indicated in the figure by a crosshatched box on the abscissa.

controlled the rate of firing (Koike et al., 1972*b*). The electrodes were kept in the cell after the injection, and firing was suppressed by passing hyperpolarizing current. We alternated 15-min periods of silence with 15-min periods of spontaneous firing by applying and removing the hyperpolarizing current. The record of one of these experiments is shown in Fig. 10. In the first 2 hr after the injection, the amount of radioactivity was the same in the perfusates collected during periods of firing and during periods of rest. After this latency, firing the neuron increased the appearance of radioactivity. Typically, the amount of radioactivity which appeared during a 15-min period of firing *(firing release)* was nearly twice that appearing during periods which preceded or followed the suppression of action potentials *(resting release)*. We observed significant increases with stimulation in 14 successful injections of L10. Increased firing release occurred only after a latency of 99 ± 7 min (12 experiments).

As in other animals (del Castillo and Katz, 1954), release of transmitter in *Aplysia* is suppressed by elevated concentrations of Mg²⁺ and enhanced

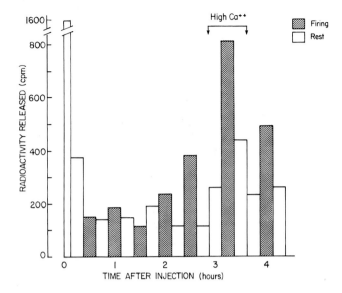

FIG. 10. Appearance of radioactivity after injection of ^{3}H-choline into the cell body of L10 under conditions of *controlled* firing. Each bar represents the radioactivity appearing in perfusate collected during 15-min periods of firing alternated with 15-min periods of rest (see text). At 3 hr, Ca^{2+} was increased sixfold from normal seawater to a concentration of 66 mM. Normal seawater was again delivered at 3.75 hr after the injection.

by elevated Ca^{2+}. Synaptic transmission and firing release in L10 was similarly affected. Ca^{2+} markedly and reversibly increased firing release (Fig. 10); in other experiments we found that Mg^{2+} decreased or abolished firing release. The concentrations of divalent ions had no significant effect on resting release. These results are consistent with the hypothesis that the increased appearance of radioactivity when L10 is firing is a consequence of synaptic activity, since firing release has characteristics expected of the release of a transmitter substance.

Firing release occurred in L10, a neuron which a) is cholinergic and b) makes synaptic connections within the ganglion. Both of these features of the cell are necessary. We also injected ^{3}H-choline into three noncholinergic neurons (L3, L5, and L12), and controlled firing of these neurons using the same protocol as for L10. We found that the appearance of radioactivity in the perfusate decreased exponentially with time after injection. Less radioactivity appeared in the perfusate, and it did not increase with firing. Thus leakage of radioactivity through noncholinergic cell membranes is small and is unaffected by the direction of the current or by changes in the membrane potential.

The fate of choline in noncholinergic cells is quite different from that in cholinergic neurons. Most of the radioactivity is converted to phosphoryl-choline, betaine, and lipid. Moreover, it might be argued that the cell membrane of cholinergic neurons could have a different permeability toward the radioactive material. We therefore injected ^{3}H-choline into the cell body of R2, which, although cholinergic, has no synapses in the ganglion, and collected the perfusate during firing and rest. Little radioactivity appeared in the perfusate; the rate was unaffected by hyperpolarizing current, spontaneous firing, or synaptic activation of the giant cell.

All attempts to isolate acetylcholine in the perfusate have so far failed even in the presence of the anticholinesterases eserine and diisopropyl flurophosphate (DFP), and high concentrations of unlabeled acetylcholine. We nevertheless still think it likely that the radioactivity is released in the form of acetylcholine and then broken down by residual cholinesterase activity in the ganglion. When we injected radioactive acetylcholine extracellularly into the neuropile region of the ganglion, we did not detect any acetylcholine in the perfusate even in the presence of 0.3 mM DFP, which irreversibly inhibits more than 95% of the cholinesterase as determined subsequently by assaying homogenates of a treated ganglion.

VII. SUMMARY AND CONCLUSIONS

We have shown that acetylcholine can be synthesized under physiological conditions throughout all parts of a cholinergic neuron. Synthesis is limited by the uptake of choline from hemolymph, and uptake mechanisms seem to be localized primarily in axons and in the neuropile, presumably at nerve terminals. Even though cell bodies are deficient in this uptake mechanism, transmitter made in the cell body can be transported down the axon to nerve terminals, some of it apparently in vesicles, and we have evidence that this material can be released synaptically by nerve impulse.

It is likely, however, that the amount of transmitter normally synthesized in the cell body is trivial compared to the amount formed at the terminals. What then is the significance of our observations of somatic synthesis and axonal transport? I believe that, by labeling somatic acetylcholine, we are able with great sensitivity to detect the axonal transport of the apparatus for release and storage of the transmitter, the synaptic vesicles, or their precursors. These organelles may or may not normally contain significant amounts of acetylcholine during their passage down the axon from the cell body. Our results suggest, however, that, at least over the long term, the macromolecular components of synaptic vesicles are replenished from the cell body.

REFERENCES

Birks, R., and MacIntosh, F. C. (1961): Acetylcholine metabolism of a sympathetic ganglion. *Can. J. Biochem. Physiol.,* 39:787.
Bligh, J. (1952): The level of free choline in plasma. *J. Physiol.* (London), 117:234–240.
Bullock, T. H., and Horridge, G. A. (1965): *Structure and Function in the Nervous System.* W. H. Freeman, San Francisco.

Carew, T., Schwartz, J. H., and Kandel, E. R. (1972): Innervation of *Aplysia* gill muscle fibers by two identified excitatory motor neurons using different chemical transmitters. *Physiologist* (Abstract), 15:100.

Coggeshall, R. E. (1967): A light and electron microscope study of the abdominal ganglion of *Aplysia californica. J. Neurophysiol.*, 30:1263.

Collier, B. (1969): The preferential release of newly synthesized transmitter by a sympathetic ganglion. *J. Physiol.*, 205:341.

del Castillo, J., and Katz, B. (1954): The effects of magnesium on the activity of motor nerve endings. *J. Physiol.*, 124:553.

Dewhurst, S. A. (1972): Choline phosphokinase activities in the ganglia and neurons of *Aplysia. J. Neurochem.*, 19:2217.

Eisenstadt, M., Goldman, J. E., Kandel, E. R., Koike, H., Koester, J., and Schwartz, J. H. (1973): Intrasomatic injection of radioactive precursors for studying transmitter synthesis in identified neurons of *Aplysia california. Proc. Natl. Acad. Sci.*, 70 (December).

Frazier, W. T., Kandel, E. R., Kupfermann, I., Waziri, I., and Coggeshall, R. E. (1967): Morphological and functional properties of identified neurons in the abdominal ganglion of *Aplysia californica. J. Neurophysiol.*, 30:1288.

Giller, E., Jr., and Schwartz, J. H. (1968): Choline acetyltransferase: Regional distribution in the abdominal ganglion of *Aplysia. Science*, 161:908.

Giller, E., Jr., and Schwartz, J. H. (1969): Distribution of choline acetyltransferase in single neurons of the abdominal ganglion *Aplysia. Fed. Proc.*, 28:734.

Giller, E., Jr., and Schwartz, J. H. (1971): Choline acetyltransferase in identified neurons of abdominal ganglion of *Aplysia californica. J. Neurophysiol.*, 34:93.

Hodgkin, A. L., and Martin, K. (1965): Choline uptake by giant axons of *Loligo. J. Physiol.*, 179:26–27.

Israel, M., Gautron, J., and Lesbats, B. (1970): Subcellular fractionation of the electric organ of *Torpedo marmorata. J. Neurochem.*, 17:1441.

Kandel, E. R., Frazier, W. T., Waziri, R., and Coggeshall, R. E. (1967): Direct and common connections among identified neurons in *Aplysia. J. Neurophysiol.*, 30:1352.

Koike, H., Eisenstadt, M., and Schwartz, J. H. (1972a): Axonal transport of newly synthesized acetylcholine in an identified neuron of *Aplysia. Brain Res.*, 37:152.

Koike, H., Kandel, E. R., and Schwartz, J. H. (1972b): Synaptic release of radioactive material after injection of ^{3}H-choline into single neurons in the isolated abdominal ganglion of *Aplysia. Fed. Proc.* (Abstract), 31:665.

Marchbanks, R. M. (1968): The uptake of (^{14}C) choline into synaptosomes *in vitro. Biochem. J.*, 110:533.

Marchbanks, R. M. (1969): Biochemical organization of cholinergic nerve terminals in the cerebral cortex. *Symposia of the Int. Soc. for Cell Biology*, 8:115.

Marchbanks, R. M., and Israel, M. (1971): Aspects of acetylcholine metabolism in the electric organ of *Torpedo marmorata. J. Neurochem.*, 18:439–448.

McCaman, R. E., and Dewhurst, S. A. (1970): Choline acetyltransferase in individual neurons of *Aplysia californica. J. Neurochem.*, 17:1421.

Peterson, H. P. (1972): Biochemical methods used to study single neurons of *Aplysia californica.* In: *Methods of Neurochemistry*, Vol. 2, edited by R. Fried, p. 73. Marcel Dekker, New York.

Potter, L. T. (1970): Synthesis, storage and release of (^{14}C) acetylcholine in isolated rat diaphragm muscles. *J. Physiol.*, 206:145.

Schwartz, J. H., Castellucci, V. F., and Kandel, E. R. (1971): The functioning of identified neurons and synapses in the abdominal ganglion of *Aplysia* in the absence of protein synthesis. *J. Neurophysiol.*, 34:939.

Strumwasser, F., and Bahr, R. (1966): Prolonged *in vitro* culture and autoradiographic studies of neurons in *Aplysia. Fed. Proc.* (Abstract), 25:512.

Wachtel, H., and Kandel, E. R. (1971): Conversion of synaptic excitation to inhibition at a dual chemical synapse. *J. Neurophysiol.*, 34:56.

Whittaker, V. P. (1965): The application of subcellular fractionation techniques to the study of brain function. *Prog. Biophys.*, 15:39.

Synaptic Transmission and Neuronal Interaction
Raven Press, New York 1974

Studies on the Development of Neuromuscular Junctions in Cell Culture

G. D. Fischbach,* M. P. Henkart, S. A. Cohen,* A. C. Breuer, J. Whysner, and F. M. Neal

Behavioral Biology Branch, National Institute of Child Health and Human Development, National Institutes of Health, Bethesda, Maryland 20014

I. INTRODUCTION

The past generation has seen great advances in the biophysics of membrane excitation and synaptic transmission on the one hand and morphologic analysis of neuron differentiation, migration, and, ultimately, synapse formation on the other. The two approaches have not as yet combined even though correlative studies are needed for analysis of specificity in synapse formation and of long-term changes in synaptic structure and function. A major roadblock has been the definition of a system appropriate for both intracellular microelectrode studies and direct observation of neuron growth.

Some of the problems encountered in studies of intact embryos have been overcome through the use of slices of embryonic neural tissue (explants) maintained *in vitro* (see reviews by Murray, 1965, and Crain, 1966). Synapses form within such explants and between spatially separated explants from different regions of the central nervous system. Functional neuromuscular junctions have been identified in combined muscle and spinal cord explant cultures (Crain, 1970; Robbins and Yonezawa, 1971; Kano and Shimada, 1971). However, even the smallest explants are highly complex in terms of cell density, number of cell types, and interneuronal connections, and little has been learned of the "minimum essential" requirements for synapse formation. With this in mind, we have begun a study of synapse formation in dissociated spinal cord and muscle cell cultures prepared by combined enzymatic and mechanical disruption of embryonic tissue.

In principle, the ability to visualize the entire extent of each pre- and postsynaptic cell including individual nerve terminals in sparse cell cultures, for periods as long as 2 months, should permit precise electrophysi-

* Present address: Department of Pharmacology, Harvard Medical School, Boston, Massachusetts 02115.

ologic description of initial stages of synapse formation and identification of structural correlates of each stage. We have focused on combined spinal cord–muscle cultures because the chemical mediating nerve–muscle transmission is known. The adult neuromuscular junction is the most completely analyzed chemical synapse and has provided a perfect model for synaptic excitation and inhibition, transmitter release, presynaptic inhibition, and trophic interactions at central synapses. It seems likely, therefore, that principles governing formation of functional nerve–muscle contacts and long-term interaction between neurons and muscle cells can also be generalized to central synapses.

An early impetus was provided by the demonstration by Shimada (1968) that dissociated spinal cord and muscle cells could be co-cultured if spinal cord cells are added at least 2 to 4 days after plating the myoblasts, and that some of the silver-impregnated nerve endings overlying muscle fibers resembled early embryonic or regenerating contacts (Tello, 1917; Gutmann and Young, 1944; Shimada, Fischman, and Moscona, 1969). Our strategy has been to simplify the cell cultures further by eliminating fibroblasts and other "supporting" cells and to adjust the plating density so that ideally, in older cultures, only one neuron and one or a few muscle fibers are present in each microscopic field. This strategy raises a basic issue. It might reasonably be thought that excitable cells separated from one another and from glia and satellite cells would not differentiate or, more precisely, would dedifferentiate in vitro and that chemical synapses, extremely differentiated entities from a neurobiologist's eye view, would not form. In that case, despite the advantages mentioned above, the cell cultures would be quite worthless as a model system. Our first studies, summarized in this chapter, were intended to document the occurrence of functional nerve–muscle contacts and to describe certain neuron and muscle membrane properties that might be relevant to synapse formation.

We chose the chick as a source of cells because the embryo has been precisely staged and is extremely convenient. Myoblasts were dissociated from the pectoral muscle of 10- to 11-day-old embryos and neurons from the brachial segments of 6- to 7-day-old spinal cords. Similar results were obtained in cultures of lower limb muscle and lumbar cord cells. The details of cell culture and electrophysiologic techniques have been published (Fischbach, 1972; Fischbach and Cohen, 1973).

II. THE CULTURES

Myogenesis in vitro has been extensively studied and reviewed (Konigs berg, 1963, 1970; Yaffe, 1969; Holtzer, 1970; Fischman, 1970). Mono nucleated muscle precursor cells divide several times after plating, migrate over the surface and, after 36 to 48 hr, fuse with one another to form thin multinucleated myotubes. Once incorporated into a myotube, muscle nuclei no longer synthesize DNA. Multinucleation results solely from repeated fusion.

Over the next few days, the multinucleated muscle cells increase in length (up to 2,000 μ) and diameter (up to 50 μ). Obvious cross striations and several hypolemmal nuclei are evident at this stage. Many of the mononucleated cells present in the initial suspension are fibroblasts. Konigsberg (1963) has shown by cloning single mononucleated cells that myogenic cells are usually spindle shaped and can be distinguished from flat, polygonal fibroblasts. Fibroblasts divide rapidly *in vitro,* form a confluent monolayer after about 5 to 7 days, and eventually embed the muscle fibers in a multilayered connective tissue mat which poses several problems. After addition of spinal cord cells, fine neurites can rarely be traced more than 200 μ with phase-contrast optics; it is difficult to penetrate deeply situated muscle fibers with microelectrodes and to position extracellular electrodes for focal stimulation or iontophoresis of drugs.

Fortunately, nearly all of the fibroblasts can be eliminated from the cultures by a simple protocol which includes treating young cultures with 10^{-5} M cytosine arabinoside (ara C), a drug that kills dividing cells (Graham and Whitmore, 1970). The drug is added, for 48 hr, 2 to 3 days after plating when most of the muscle nuclei are incorporated into myotubes and have withdrawn from the mitotic cycle but when fibroblasts are not yet confluent and are multiplying rapidly. Figure 1 shows typical fields in a 12-day-old untreated culture (A) and in a sister culture exposed to ara C on days 3 and 4 (B). Such "pure" muscle cultures approach the ideal assay system for presumptive motoneurons.

At 10^{-5} M, ara C does not alter protein or RNA synthesis in L-cells (Graham and Whitmore, 1970). It does not prevent differentiation of muscle cells. On the contrary, fibers exposed to the drug become obviously striated earlier than fibers in untreated cultures, and hypolemmal nuclei are more obvious. Purified cultures cannot be maintained as long as fibroblast-rich plates (1 vs. 2 months), and in older cultures the fibers are not, on the average, as large and they do not twitch as often. These differences are probably due to the fact that the dense mat of connective tissue prevents the most active cells from pulling up from the plate.

Ara C did not qualitatively alter the ultrastructure of the muscle fibers. As shown in Fig. 2, myofibrils are regularly aligned, and each sarcomere contains prominent A and I bands with Z lines, H zones, and often M-lines (Fig. 2). The sarcoplasmic reticulum (SR) is well developed and is especially prominent in the region of the I bands. A complex system of tubules and vesicles is prominent near the periphery of the cell. Ezerman and Ishikawa (1967) and Ishikawa (1968) first described this system in cultured chick muscle fibers and, on the basis of its appearance in different aged fibers and the fact that the tubules communicate with one another and the external medium, suggested that it represents a form of the transverse tubular system.

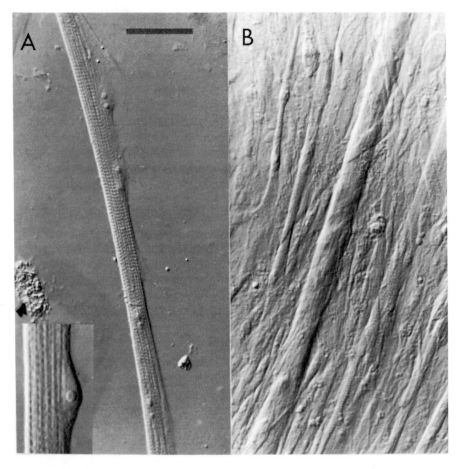

FIG. 1. Effect of cytosine arabinoside. Nomarski optics showing a "naked" muscle fiber in a 12-day-old culture that was treated with ara C (A) and fibers in an untreated culture plated at the same time (B). See text. Fibers in (B) appear to be covered in many areas by connective tissue. Inset in (A) shows a hypolemmal nucleus in another fiber. Bar = 50 μm (A) and (B), 20 μm inset (from Fischbach and Cohen, 1973).

Specialized contacts, diads and triads, can be identified between cisternae of the SR and both tubular and vesicular elements of the extensive T-system (see also Figs. 13 and 14). The peripheral nucleus shown in Fig. 2 is truly hypolemmal: it does not belong to a satellite cell. The most significant differences between fibers in ara C treated versus untreated cultures is that, several days after plating, the latter are covered by external lamina wheras the former are not (Fig. 2B,C). A few tufts of amorphous material have been found adjacent to the surface membrane of otherwise naked muscle cells.

Ara C does not significantly affect the electrical properties of the muscle

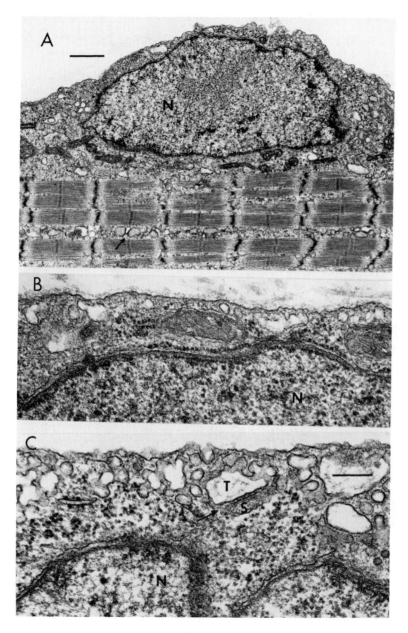

FIG. 2. Electron micrographs of muscle fibers from cultures without added neurons. The material was fixed in glutaraldehyde, post-fixed in OsO_4, and block-stained with uranyl acetate. The sections were stained with uranyl acetate and lead citrate. Symbols: N, nucleus; S, sarcoplasmic reticulum; T, portions of complex tubular system continuous with extracellular space. (A) shows a well-developed striation pattern typical of many vertebrate skeletal muscles. Overlying some of the I-bands in the center of the picture are networks of sarcoplasmic reticulum. The arrow indicates a triad: two cisternae of the sarcoplasmic reticulum forming junctions with a central "transverse" tubule. The bar indicates 1 μm. (B) is a portion of the surface of a muscle fiber from a culture not treated with ara C and, therefore, containing fibroblasts. The surface is covered by an external lamina (basement membrane). (C) is a portion of a fiber from an ara C treated muscle culture. The surface is virtually free of external lamina. (Because of fine irregularities in the contour of the surface membrane, small portions of the membrane are seen in tangential section. These views of the membrane account for most of the fuzzy-appearing patches.) The arrow indicates a junction between an expanded, vesicle-like portion of the tubular system and a cisterna of the sarcoplasmic reticulum which is distinguishable by its more opaque, granular content. The bar in (C) indicates 0.25 μm for (B) and (C).

membrane. In some regards, mature fibers in culture resemble denervated adult muscle (Fischbach, Nameroff, and Nelson, 1971; Powell and Fambrough, 1973): membrane potentials are relatively low (50 to 70 mV), membrane resistivity relatively high (ca. 2,500 Ω cm^2), spontaneous action potentials and twitches (fibrillation) are common, and all regions of the surface membrane are sensitive to iontophoretically applied acetylcholine (ACh). However, a comparison of each of these parameters in innervated and uninnervated fibers *in vitro* is necessary before the analogy can be taken seriously. It will be important in further studies of synapse formation to determine when characteristic membrane properties first appear. Some mononucleated cells are sensitive to ACh (Fambrough and Rash, 1973), and young myotubes can generate active responses (Fischbach et al., 1971).

Spinal cord cells dissociated from 7-day-old embryos do not segregate after addition to 3- to 5-day-old "purified" muscle cultures. Isolated cells settle either on the collagen coated surface or directly on the muscle fibers (Fig. 3A,B). Shortly after settling, the neuroblasts (a term used here rather loosely to describe small, round, freshly dissociated cells) extend processes that, depending on the initial location of perikaryon, contact nearby muscle fibers within 24 to 48 hr. In our cultures, the cells grow rapidly, and after 1 to 2 weeks, differences in perikaryon size and shape and in length and pattern of neurites indicate that, as expected, a variety of different neuron types are present. Large multiprocessed cells can unambiguously be identified as neurons because, when adequately stimulated through an intracellular microelectrode, they generate all-or-none action potentials. Variation in size and time course of spikes, in the sign and magnitude of after-potentials, and in degree of adaptation during sustained depolarization are consistent with our impression that different types of spinal cord neurons survive *in vitro* (Fischbach and Dichter, *in preparation*). Spinal cord neurons are not invested in satellite cells even in the oldest cultures, and neurites, perhaps because meninges were stripped from the cord prior to dissociation, are not invested in Schwann cells. Each of the spinal cord cell types is dramatically different both in morphology and action potential mechanism from dissociated dorsal root ganglion (DRG) cells grown under the same conditions. All of the spinal cord cell spikes are blocked by low concentrations (10^{-7} g/ml) of tetrodotoxin (TTX) whereas spikes evoked in DRG cell bodies are not. Other evidence suggests that the inward spike current in the sensory cells is carried by both Na$^+$ and Ca^{++} ions. Spikes conducted along DRG neurites are more, if not completely, dependent on Na$^+$ ions (Dichter and Fischbach, *in preparation*).

III. NEUROMUSCULAR JUNCTIONS

In older cultures, neuron–muscle pairs like that shown in Fig. 3C were tested by recording from the muscle fiber with an intracellular microelec-

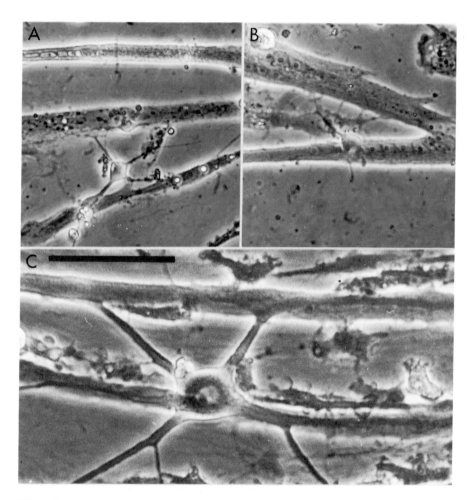

FIG. 3. Phase-contrast micrographs of nerve-muscle pairs. (A) and (B) one day after addition of dissociated spinal cord cells to 6-day-old muscle cultures. Spinal cord cells settle on the collagen-coated culture plate (A) or directly over a muscle fiber (B). (C) A typical "test" nerve-muscle pair in a 25-day-old culture. Bar = 50 μm applies to (A), (B), and (C).

trode and by stimulating the neuron through another intracellular electrode or through a fine-tipped extracellular electrode. As shown in Fig. 4A, some of the spinal cord cells are motoneurons—defined simply as a neuron that transmits signals to a muscle cell. The neuron spike evoked by a step of outward current is followed after 2 to 3 msec by a brief depolarization of the muscle fiber. In other cases similar responses were evoked by focal extracellular stimulation of fine neurites. Even though true endplates have not yet been identified in cell cultures, we will, for convenience, refer to these synaptic responses as endplate potentials (epps). Epps in different muscle

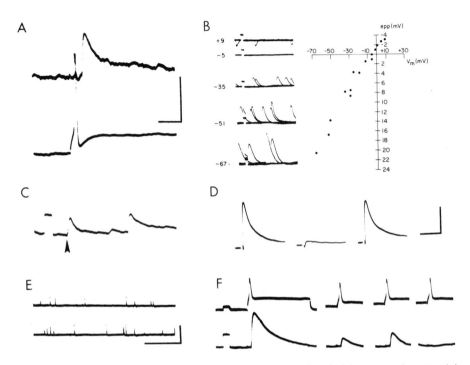

FIG. 4. Synaptic physiology. (A) A functional contact: a depolarizing synaptic potential (upper trace) follows an action potential in a nearby neuron evoked by intracellular stimulation (current pulse not shown). Bars = 3.5 and 50 mV for muscle and neuron records, respectively, and 10 msec for both. (B) Superimposed traces show the change in epp amplitude as the muscle membrane potential (V_m) was altered to the values shown at the left of each record by steady currents injected through a second intracellular microelectrode. Calibration pulse = 5 mV, 5 msec. Each point in the graph represents the mean amplitude of 5 to 10 epps. (C) An ACh response (arrow) evoked by a 1-msec pulse of ACh precisely mimics a spontaneous synaptic potential recorded on the same trace. Calibration = 5 mV, 10 msec. (D) Reversible reduction in epp size by d-tubocurare (10^{-7} g/ml). Third record obtained 30 min after removal of the drug. Bars = 15 mV, 15 msec. (E) Mepps recorded on contiguous segments of moving film. Bars = 5 mV, 2 sec. (F) Variation in amplitude (and one failure) of successive epps in a series evoked at a rate of 1/sec despite a constant stimulus (action potential) in the innervating neuron (upper traces). Calibration pulse = 5 mV, 5 msec. (A), (B), (D), and (F) from Fischbach (1972); (C) from Fischbach and Cohen (1973).

fibers range widely in amplitude between approximately 1 and 30 mV. Some but not all of the largest responses trigger muscle action potentials. It is not yet clear whether failure in impulse initiation is a sign of real differences between muscle fibers or is simply due to membrane damage caused by the microelectrode.

The basic principles of synaptic transmission at contacts that form in cell culture are identical to those of the adult neuromuscular junction (see Katz, 1966). (1) Synaptic potentials are caused by a change in conductance of the postsynaptic membrane — the hallmark of chemical transmission. Epps invariably increased in size when the muscle membrane was hyperpolarized, decreased when the membrane was depolarized, and, in several cases in which the inside of the cell was made sufficiently positive, inverted in polarity near 0 mV (Fig. 4B). We have not determined the reversal potential precisely. This will require precise localization of the site of transmitter release. (2) The transmitter is probably ACh. Synaptic potentials can be mimicked by iontophoretically applied ACh (Fig. 4C), and they can be blocked by 10^{-7} g/ml d-tubocurare (Fig. 4D) or 2×10^{-8} M α-bungarotoxin, a component of snake venom that combines with nicotinic ACh receptors at the adult neuromuscular junction (Chang and Lee, 1963; Changeux, Kasai, and Lee, 1970; Miledi, Molinoff, and Potter, 1971). (3) Transmitter release is quantal. Miniature epps (mepps) — small, TTX-resistant, curare-sensitive potentials that recur in an apparently random manner are detected at many functional contacts (Fig. 4E). The amplitudes of successive epps in series evoked at approximately 1/sec fluctuate (Fig. 4F), and amplitude histograms are often clearly multimodal. Both mean mepp frequency (ca. 1 to 10/min) and estimates of mean quantum content of evoked epps based on the Poisson probability law (ca. 1 to 30) are low compared to values recorded at adult neuromuscular junctions (1 to 5/sec and 200 to 400, respectively).

This low level of transmitter output is consistent with the idea that the simple terminal boutons seen in silver-stained preparations are, in fact, the sites of transmitter release. This correlation is facile, however, and perhaps misleading. Terminal swellings may simply represent a stereotyped change which occurs in a growth cone as it palpates a foreign object or another cell. In any case, the existence of a terminal enlargement does not preclude the possibility that transmitter is released at other sites along the fine neurite. In the same vein, it will be difficult to define the minimum ultrastructural correlates of a newly formed synapse. Certainly the existence of small vesicles in a neurite that is apposed to a muscle fiber is not, in itself, sufficient. The low quantal output may be associated with only a few release sites so that membrane specializations associated with the release of 50- to 55-nm vesicles may be contained within one or two thin sections. Thus, it is clear that any statement about the morphology of early synapses must be based on analysis of sets of serial sections through nerve-muscle contacts demonstrated physiologically to contain functional synapses. It might be possible to localize sites of transmitter release to within a few microns by extracellular recording of synaptic currents.

The occurrence of mepps is not a good assay for synapse formation in these cultures. In several innervated fibers, they appeared only after one or a few epps were evoked, and in a few cases they could not be detected at all. Further experiments are required to control for electrotonic decrement and postsynaptic input resistance, but it is possible that although both stimulus-evoked and spontaneous leakage of transmitter depend on Ca^{++}, other factors, which are unique to one or both forms of transmitter release, develop at different times. The opposite sequence has been observed at regenerating frog neuromuscular junctions (Miledi, 1960): mepps due to nerve terminal quanta (distinguished from mepps of Schwann cell origin) reappear and increase in frequency before stimulus-evoked transmission is reestablished. This sequence may be explained, as suggested by Miledi, by failure of action potentials to invade regenerating terminals.

One significant difference from adult cholinergic neuromuscular junctions is that the enzyme acetylcholinesterase is apparently absent or nonfunctional. Epps are relatively slow (rise time ca. 2.9 msec) and prolonged (half fall ca. 11 msec), and their time course is not altered following addition of inhibitors of the enzyme to the bath (Fig. 5A). The fibers contain true

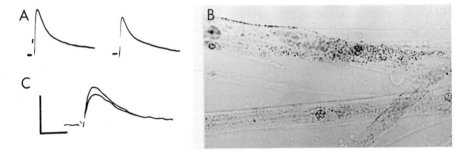

FIG. 5. Failure of anticholinesterase drugs to increase the size of or prolong an evoked epp (A) or an ACh potential (C). The second record in (A) was obtained 30 min after addition of physostigmine (10^{-6} g/ml) to the bath. Compare to control (first record). Superimposed tracings of two ACh potentials evoked at the same point on an uninnervated fiber are shown in (C). The smaller response was preceded by a 1-sec "conditioning" pulse of edrophonium delivered from another, adjacent microelectrode. (B) "True" acetylcholinesterase demonstrated by the method of Karnovsky and Roots (1964) in the presence of iso-OMPA, an inhibitor of pseudo cholinesterase. Note the diffuse and uneven distribution of reaction product and the variation between fibers. Calibration bars = 15 mV, 15 msec in (A) and 5.8 mV, 22.5 msec in (C); from Fischbach (1972).

acetylcholinesterase as determined by the limited criteria accepted in light-microscopic histochemical techniques, but specks or patches of reaction product appear to be diffusely distributed throughout the cytoplasm (Fig. 5B). We have not observed focal accumulations in the region of nerve terminals and electrophysiologic data indicate that catalytic sites are not present anywhere on the surface membrane (Fig. 5C). Interestingly, cholinesterase could not be demonstrated at embryonic junctions (Diamond and Miledi, 1962) or at early contacts that formed in culture between muscle fibers and neurons in spinal cord explants (Robbins and Yonezawa, 1971; Kano and Shimada, 1971). Cholinesterase activity, apparently, is not involved in the initial stages of synapse formation.

Direct electrical coupling has been detected in five nerve–muscle pairs in which both neuron and muscle fiber were penetrated with microelectrodes. Figure 6 shows electrotonic potentials in a muscle fiber during injection of prolonged current pulses into a nearby neuron. Coupling ratios which ranged between 0.03 and 0.25 in different pairs did not depend on the direction of current flow. Muscle fibers in ara C treated cultures are not covered by a basal lamina (see Fig. 2C), so close contact between nerve and muscle membranes and, perhaps, formation of gap junctions are possible. Embryonic muscle fibers at the time of invasion by motor neurites are apparently not enclosed in a basal lamina and "close" contacts (Kelly and Zacks, 1969), and striking interdigitations between neurites and muscle cells (James and Tresman, 1969) have been described by electron microscopy. The fact that typical chemical synaptic potentials were recorded in four of the five coupled pairs suggests the possibility that electrical coupling is a stage in formation of a chemical synapse. Clearly, other interpretations are possible if not likely: electrotonic transmission has been demonstrated in embryos and between a variety of cell types in culture (see

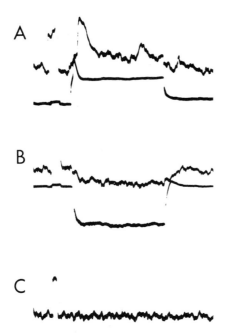

FIG. 6. Electrical coupling between a muscle fiber and a nearby neuron. Outward and inward current pulses (not shown) injected into the neuron depolarized and hyperpolarized the muscle membrane (upper traces in (A) and (B), respectively. The voltage response of the neuron is shown in the lower trace in each pair. Note that the nerve cell action potential in (A) is followed by a synaptic potential in the muscle cell. Two mepps appear on the same trace. (C) Absence of a potential change to identical current pulses after the muscle electrode was withdrawn to a position just outside of the fiber. Calibration pulse = 2 mV, 5 msec. From Fischbach (1972).

Fischbach, 1972, for references). Further experiments are required to locate the site of coupling and to demonstrate a sufficient and necessary relation.

Not every large neuron formed a functional contact on a muscle cell, and, conversely, many fibers were enmeshed in a network of neurites but were not innervated. As a limiting statement, therefore, it seems clear that muscle fibers do not "create" cholinergic motoneurons and neurons do not induce appropriate receptive sites on muscle fibers. Dissociated sensory ganglion cells contact but do not synapse on muscle fibers. It is likely that the low incidence of synapses is simply due to the fact that relatively few cholinergic neurons (anterior horn or lateral column) were present in the initial suspension.

IV. ACh SENSITIVITY

The motor neuron is important in regulating the distribution of ACh sensitivity over the muscle membrane: adult innervated fibers are sensitive to ACh only in the immediate vicinity of nerve terminals whereas denervated muscle and embryonic muscle prior to innervation are sensitive over their entire length (Axelsson and Thesleff, 1959; Miledi, 1960; Diamond and Miledi, 1962). As this interaction was one of the motivating factors in beginning our studies on synapse formation *in vitro*, we asked the question: Is innervation sufficient for reduction in extrajunctional chemosensitivity? The answer was clearly no (Fischbach and Cohen, 1973). The background extrajunctional sensitivity of innervated fibers is comparable to that of uninnervated fibers. Histograms of all values of sensitivity (measured as mV depolarization/nanocoulomb of ACh ejected) recorded in 18 innervated and 36 uninnervated (in cultures to which no spinal cord cells were added) fibers are shown in Fig. 7.

Despite the wide range in both groups—due to variation between fibers and between different sites along the same fiber—the shape of the two histograms and the modal values are nearly identical. Although the mean input resistance and membrane potential of innervated and uninnervated fibers were comparable, small differences in sensitivity might be overlooked after pooling values. But, we were not looking for small differences: the extrajunctional region of adult innervated fibers is 10^3- to 10^4-fold less sensitive than the endplate zone (Miledi, 1960).

Although disappointing at first glance because it might imply that dissociated motoneurons *in vitro* are not sufficiently differentiated to exert a trophic influence on the muscle membrane, this negative result is, in fact, quite consistent with the recently resurrected suggestion that the amount of activity generated by the motoneuron is an important determinant of extrajunctional sensitivity (references in Lømø and Rosenthal, 1972). Partial disuse of the intact rat soleus neuromuscular junction produced by limb immobilization results in a small increase in extrajunctional sensitivity

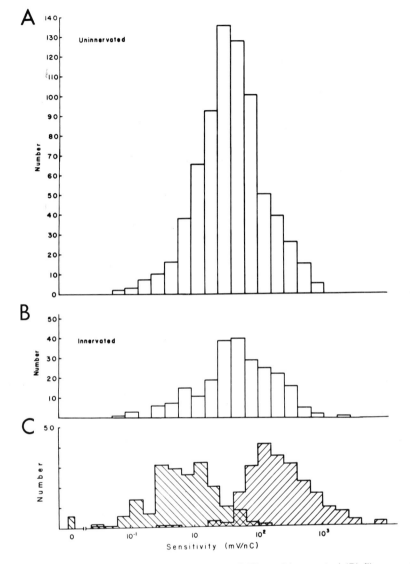

FIG. 7. ACh sensitivity histograms of uninnervated (A), and innervated (B) fibers and of active and inactive fibers (C). The modal values and range of uninnervated and innervated fibers are similar. Active fibers (stimulated intermittently for 2 to 3 days at 10/sec) are less sensitive and inactive fibers (grown for the same period in 2×10^{-7} g/ml TTX) are more sensitive than controls. All of the cells represented in (C) were uninnervated. (A) and (B) from Fischbach and Cohen (1973); (C) from Cohen and Fischbach (1973).

(Fischbach and Robbins, 1972), whereas complete disuse of the same junction effected by application of an anesthetic cuff around the sciatic nerve results in a spread of sensitivity as great as that which follows denervation (Lømø and Rosenthal, 1972). The essential factor may be inactivity (impulse and/or mechanical) of the muscle itself because chronic, direct stimulation of denervated muscle prevents the increase in extrajunctional sensitivity (Lømø and Rosenthal, 1972; Drachman and Witze, 1972). We have found that activity is an important determinant of sensitivity of uninnervated muscle cells in culture: inactive fibers grown in the presence of TTX were about 50 times as sensitive as active fibers—stimulated through large electrodes fixed in the culture dish (Fig. 7, lower histograms; geometric means ca. 450 mV/nC vs. 9 mV/nC; Cohen and Fischbach, 1973). Therefore, muscle activity is sufficient to reduce ACh sensitivity *in vitro*, and this finding may explain why innervated but relatively inactive fibers remain extremely sensitive.

It might be possible, in these cell cultures, to uncouple excitation from contraction and to maintain the fibers for longer periods than have been possible in adult muscle and then further analyze the complex phenomenon of muscle activity.

On detailed mapping of innervated fibers, it became apparent that although the entire exposed surface was quite responsive to ACh, the distribution of sensitivity was not uniform. In most cases, one or more relative peaks of sensitivity or "hot spots" (2 to 10 times background levels) were detected in the immediate vicinity of fine nerve fibers (Fig. 8A). With the phase

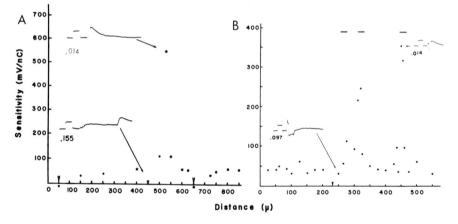

FIG. 8. Peaks of ACh sensitivity along an innervated (A) and an uninnervated (B) muscle fiber. Ordinate: mV/nC. Abscissa: distance along the fiber; origin arbitrary. Arrowheads on abscissa indicate recording electrode positions. Different symbols refer to different recording sites (arrowheads). Representative traces are shown as insets. Numbers refer to estimated nC of ACh ejected. Notice the spontaneous synaptic potential in the lower inset of (A). Calibration for insets: 5 mV and 10 msec. Horizontal bars above (B) plot indicate positions and lengths of hypolemmal muscle nuclei. Modified from Fischbach and Cohen (1973).

optics employed in these experiments, we could not determine the precise position of the nerve terminals — especially when the neurites lay over striated, refractile muscle fibers. The peaks identified with brief (1 to 2 msec) ACh pulses were extremely sharp. The sensitivity usually returned to base-line levels within 5 to 10 μ. Harris, Heinemann, Schubert, and Tarakis (1971) found similar relative peaks of sensitivity in co-cultures of muscle fibers that formed from a transformed line of myoblasts and neuroblastoma cells. The identified peaks were located in the immediate vicinity of neuro-blastoma nerve terminals. They proposed that the peaks were caused by the nerve terminals and that this interaction represented an early stage in synapse formation.

No evidence concerning the second part of this hypothesis is available. Synaptic potentials could not be evoked by stimulation of the neuroblastoma cells. It is possible that the firmly attached neurites "caused" hot spots by local irritation of the muscle membrane (see Katz and Miledi, 1964). The causal relation, although a plausible and interesting hypothesis, cannot be accepted without further evidence because, in the chick primary culture system, striking peaks have been found over uninnervated cells in cultures to which no neurons have been added (Figs. 8B and 9). Thus, it is not clear whether nerve terminals (or fine neurites) correspond to hot spots because they create them or because they seek them out. The suggestion that motor nerve terminals search for hot spots does not necessarily imply that receptor molecules are involved in nerve–muscle recognition. The membrane at these sites may be specialized in other ways.

We have noted that hot spots in mature fibers are often associated with bulging, hypolemmal nuclei. The bars above the three peaks shown in Fig. 8B represent the position and length of three hypolemmal nuclei. Two

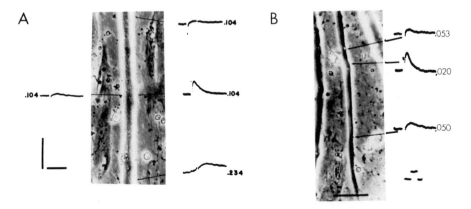

FIG. 9. Variation in ACh response at different points on a relatively thick (A) and thin (B) myotube. Note the larger, faster responses at a point between the two muscle nuclei in (A) and over the bulging nucleus in (B). Numbers refer to the estimated nC of ACh ejected. Vertical bar 24.6 mV and 50 μm; horizontal bar 70 msec in (A). Calibration: 5 mV and 10 msec; horizontal bar 50 μm in (B). Modified from Fischbach and Cohen (1973).

examples of hot spots located in the immediate vicinity of obvious nuclei in a thick striated fiber and in a thin myotube are shown in Fig. 9A and B, respectively. The perinuclear sensitivity was about three times greater than that over a nearby comparable area on the same fiber in 37 of 48 paired comparisons. Autoradiography of cultures exposed to blocking concentrations of $^{125}I-\alpha$-bungarotoxin is consistent with this electrophysiologic result. Grains are rarely distributed uniformly over the fibers. Dense patches of grains are common, and they are usually located over or immediately adjacent to obvious muscle nuclei (Fig. 10). This apparent correlation is extremely interesting in light of the possibility that nerve terminals seek out rather than induce membrane patches that are relatively sensitive to ACh. Several studies conclude that embryonic or regenerating motor neurites terminate near clusters of muscle nuclei (Tello, 1917; Gutmann and Young, 1944; Couteaux, 1955). Also, it is well known that the mound

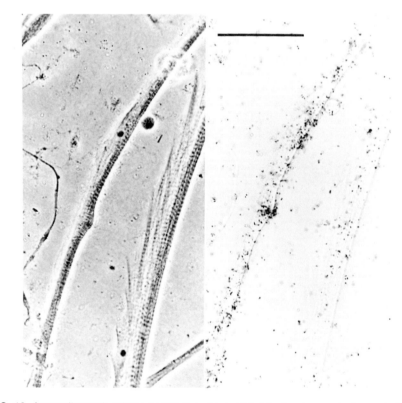

FIG. 10. Autoradiograph (phase contrast and bright field) of uninnervated muscle fibers exposed to 2×10^{-8} M $^{125}I-\alpha$ bungarotoxin (sp. ac. $\approx$ 50,000 C/mole) for 30 min. Toxin was added in Earle's salt solution + 1% horse serum, and the plate was washed eight times before fixation. Exposure time was 7 days at 4°C. Note the nonuniform distribution of grains along individual fibers and the correlation between patches of grains and muscle nuclei. Also note the variation in average grain density between adjacent fibers. The bar indicates 50 μm. From Fischbach and Cohen (1973).

of sarcoplasm that marks mammalian and avian endplates contains several "sole plate nuclei." Nuclear accumulations are less obvious at amphibian junctions.

It should be emphasized that the correspondence between iontophoretically defined hot spots or ^{125}I-toxin grains and muscle nuclei is not invariant. Not every bulging nucleus is hot, and hot spots have, on a few occasions, been identified in regions where nuclei were not distinguishable with the optics employed. Most muscle fibers contain many centrally located nuclei; we have only systematically tested peripherally located nuclei. Thus, although extremely suggestive, a definite relationship will be hard to "prove."

Some of the discrepancies may be explained by the fact that some nuclei migrate within the muscle fiber (see Capers, 1960; Nakai, 1969). We have observed by time-lapse cinematography that nuclei migrate several hundred microns at rates as fast as 40 μ/hr. In the example shown in Fig. 11, several nuclei move along both arms of a branched myotube and accumulate at the branch point. Other nuclei rotate about the long axis of the fiber or oscillate over a few microns along the long axis but show no net migration

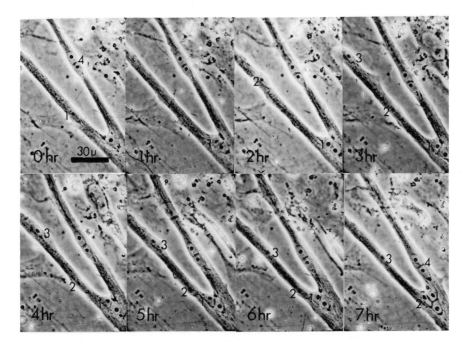

FIG. 11. Nuclear migration in a 6-day-old myotube. Frames at 1-hr intervals selected from a 16-mm, phase-contrast, time-lapse film (six frames/min) demonstrate net movement of several nuclei to form a cluster at the lower right. Nuclei numbered in each frame could be unambiguously followed. Different nuclei migrate at different mean rates; the rate of a given nucleus varied at different times.

over a 5- to 10-hr period. It is our initial impression that nuclei in thick, striated fibers are less mobile than those in thin, less obviously striated cells.

A more exact description of the relation between hot spots, muscle nuclei, and ingrowing motor nerve fibers might result from monitoring these phenomena over long periods of time (24 to 48 hr) with both electrophysiologic and time-lapse cinematography techniques. It will be necessary to describe the relation between nerve terminals and hot spots (and ^{125}I-toxin grains) more precisely and to determine the fate of hot spots that are not contacted by neurites. These studies would be facilitated if we could identify motoneurons and their growing axons prior to initial muscle contact or junction formation. It might be possible to isolate motoneurons from the initial dissociated cell suspension on the basis of size (cells at this stage range from 10 to 40 μ in diameter), density (motoneurons, at some stage, become tetraploid), or surface specificities (they might bind to specific agonists or antibodies immobilized on sepharose beads).

The relation between hot spots and early neuromuscular junctions might be clarified if we could discover the "reason" for hot spots. Either a focal increase in number of receptors[1] per unit area of membrane or surface specializations that increase the number of receptors exposed to a test pulse of ACh could account for peaks of sensitivity. Even though we have no conclusions regarding these alternatives, we will describe some preliminary results because they are intriguing and because the techniques involved point out some advantages of the cell culture system.

Scanning electron microscopy of "naked" fibers in ara C treated cultures has shown that the muscle surface is indeed complex. The micrograph in Fig. 12 illustrates coarse folds of membrane near a nucleus, longitudinally oriented furrows, and patches of microvilli. These features vary somewhat depending on the conditions of fixation, so it is not clear that they are equally as prominent in living cells. Structures which are probably microvilli have been identified on unfixed cells with Nomarski optics, but a rigorous correlative study of living, fixed, and dried material is needed.

The extensive network of communicating tubules and vesicles (T-system) is continuous with the extracellular space and could account for hot spots if the bounding membranes contain ACh receptors. The networks are prominent near nuclei (perhaps because there is more cytoplasm unoccupied by myofilaments) and are sometimes interposed between the nuclear and surface membranes. Openings of tubules at the surface membrane are often seen (Fig. 13), but their number and distribution are difficult to evaluate in thin sections; they are small (ca. 50 nm) and difficult to resolve by scanning electron microscopy. Indirect evidence for this explanation

---

[1] The term "receptor" is used loosely here to describe both the ACh binding site and the associated ionic channel.

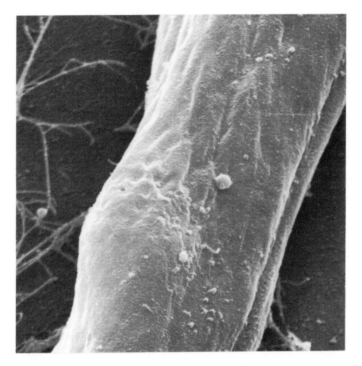

FIG. 12. A scanning electron micrograph of a muscle fiber fixed in glutaraldehyde, de-hydrated in ethanol, and critical-point dried from amyl acetate. The prominent bulge in the lower half of the fiber is a hypolemmal nucleus. Coarse membrane folds and patches of microvilli occur, in this preparation, in the vicinity of the nucleus. The fibrous material in the background is the prepared collagen coating of the coverslip on which the muscle was grown. The negative was kindly provided by Bruce Wetzel.

would be obtained if hot spots disappear following procedures which disrupt the communication between the T-system and the extracellular space (e.g., Howell and Jenden, 1967; Eisenberg and Eisenberg, 1968).

Foci of increased receptor density might occur in several ways. For ex-ample, they may correspond to sites of insertion into the surface membrane of newly synthesized receptors. As in other cells, Golgi complexes in the cultured muscle fibers are often located in the immediate vicinity of nuclei (Fig. 14). In addition to its role in packaging proteins destined for secretion, this structure has been implicated in the synthesis of glycoproteins and other molecules (see Beams and Kessel, 1968, for review) which, according to a scheme proposed by Palade (1959), might then be incorporated into the surface membrane by fusion of Golgi vesicles with the preexisting membrane. ACh receptors may follow the same route. It is possible that some vesicles in continuity with the elaborate T-system represent new, receptor-rich membrane coming from the Golgi rather than invaginations of the surface membrane.

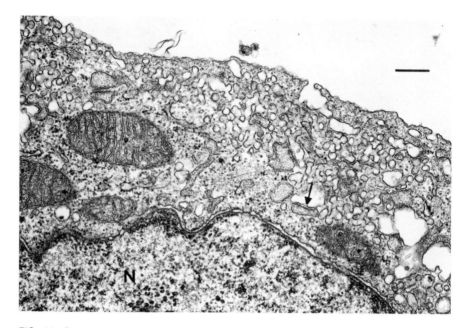

FIG. 13. Openings of the tubular system at the surface membrane in the vicinity of a nucleus (N). The complex network of the tubular system forms junctions with cisternae of the sarcoplasmic reticulum at arrow. This fiber was from a culture treated with ara C. The bar indicates 0.25 μm.

Obviously, studies designed to explore these possible explanations for hot spots will require a high resolution and specific tag for individual receptors. With the help of Vincent Marchesi we have begun experiments with α-bungarotoxin covalently linked to ferritin, a large protein that contains a dense iron core which can be visualized by electron microscopy using both thin-section and freeze-etch techniques. Immunologists have employed ferritin–antibody conjugates for several years to localize the sites of surface antigens (see review by Morgan, 1972). Purified toxin–ferritin conjugates, prepared by mixing the two proteins in the presence of glutaraldehyde (Avrameus, 1969), block ACh responses and epps but have only about $^1/_{10}$ the potency of unconjugated toxin. Figure 15A shows a replica obtained by the freeze-etch technique. Following incubation with toxin-ferritin conjugate, the cells were fixed (0.05% glutaraldehyde) scraped from the dish, pelleted, frozen, and fractured. Some of the surrounding ice was then sublimed (etched), exposing the outer surface of the membrane. (See Pinto de Silva and Branton, 1970, for discussion of interpretation of freeze-etch images.) Clusters of ferritin molecules are distributed over the exposed outer membrane surface. No clusters were detected on cells preincubated in 10^{-4} g/ml d-tubocurare. Since these experiments were performed on ara C treated cultures, the great majority, if not all, of the mem-

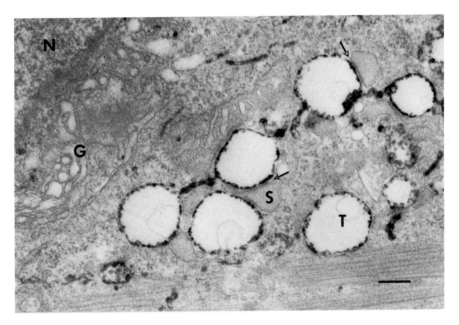

FIG. 14. An unstained section from a muscle culture incubated with horseradish per-oxidase (HRP) before fixation. HRP reaction product outlines or fills areas continuous with the extracellular space. Below the nucleus (N) is a Golgi complex (G) not filled with tracer. The tracer-filled vesicles may be identified as part of the T-system (T) and distinguished from pinocytotic vesicles by their continuity with tracer-filled tubules and by the fact that they form extensive junctions with cisternae of the sarcoplasmic reticulum. The arrows indicate examples of such junctions. The bar indicates 0.25 μm.

branes examined belonged to muscle cells. Clusters of ferritin associated with the surface membrane have also been demonstrated in thin sections (Fig. 15B). The clusters are unevenly distributed over the surface of the muscle fiber and occasionally are found in vesicles and tubules of the T-system. They have also been found in a few of the frequently encountered coated vesicles in the periphery of the muscle fibers. The preliminary nature of these results should, perhaps, be reemphasized. We must de-termine the efficiency of the coupling procedure and the stability and purity of the resulting conjugates.

Nevertheless, several questions are rather obvious. Are receptors lo-calized in clusters in the membrane? Is it possible that receptors clump after binding the complex ligand or that toxin–ferritin conjugates them-selves aggregate during the coupling procedure? If a cluster corresponds to more than one receptor, what is the relation between these aggregates and hot spots? The resolution of iontophoretic (and autoradiographic) techniques employed to date is not less than 2 to 5 μ, so a brief ACh pulse probably tests an area that is larger than the entire field shown in Fig. 15A. Significant variation in numbers of ferritin clusters has been found on

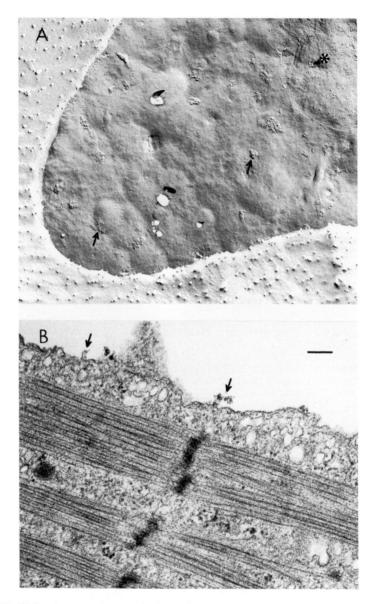

FIG. 15. (A) An electron micrograph of a replica prepared by the freeze-etch technique as described in the text. Clumps of ferritin-toxin conjugate (arrows) are distributed over the outer surface of the muscle membrane which has been exposed by etching. The upper and right area (asterisk) represents the outer aspect of the inner membrane leaflet (see Pinto de Silva and Branton, 1970). The negative was kindly provided by Vincent Marchesi. (B) An electron micrograph of a thin section of muscle treated with ferritin–α-bungarotoxin conjugate. Clumps of ferritin in association with the surface membrane are indicated by arrows. The bar indicates 0.25 μm and applies to both (A) and (B).

different etched surfaces, and it seems more likely that this scale corresponds to the electrophysiologic measurements.

Although the size of the ferritin molecule (ca. 100 Å diameter) sets a limit to its usefulness in counting receptors — which in an adult postsynaptic membrane may be as closely packed as $10^5/\mu^2$ (centers separated by ca. 40 Å; Miledi and Potter, 1972) — the conjugates should be useful for a qualitative description of relative receptor density in different regions of the membrane and for precise localization of new surface receptors. It might also be possible to identify intracellular sites of receptor assembly (if they exist) by adding the conjugates to protein-embedded or frozen sections of muscle fibers (McLean and Singer, 1970; Kraehenbuhl and Jamison, 1972) or to the outside of cells made leaky by various treatments, or after direct intracellular injection of the conjugates.

Hot spots may be due to foci of qualitatively different receptors rather than to increased numbers of the same receptor present elsewhere on the fiber. There is some evidence that extrajunctional receptors may be different from junctional receptors in adult denervated muscle fibers. Extrajunctional receptors are less sensitive to d-tubocurare and more sensitive to succinyl choline (Beranek and Vyskocil, 1967); they desensitize more rapidly (Miledi, 1960); and Feltz and Mallart (1971) reported that ACh potentials elicited at extrajunctional sites reverse in polarity at a more negative muscle membrane potential (-40 vs. -10 mV). We have no data, as yet, relating to these phenomena in cultured fibers.

V. SUMMARY

Chemical cholinergic neuromuscular junctions form in sparse cell cultures, and this relatively simple system should allow more precise study of the initial events during synapse formation. Two observations — direct electrical coupling between nerve and muscle cells and postsynaptic membrane specializations which to date have been simply identified as patches of increased ACh sensitivity — provide interesting leads. In addition, since there is no obvious limit to the degree of differentiation of dissociated neurons and muscle cells, it might be possible to study the specificity of connections and various long-term interactions between synaptically connected cells.

REFERENCES

Avrameus, S. (1969): Coupling of enzymes to proteins with glutaraldehyde. *Immunochem.*, 6:43–52.

Axelsson, J., and Thesleff, S. (1959): A study of supersensitivity in denervated mammalian skeletal muscle. *J. Physiol.*, 147:178–193.

Beams, H. W., and Kessel, R. G. (1968): The golgi apparatus: Structure and function. *Int. Rev. Cytol.*, 23:209–276.

Beranek, R., and Vyskocil, F. (1967): The action of tubocurarine and atropine on the normal and denervated rat diaphragm. *J. Physiol.*, 188:53–66.

Capers, C. R. (1960). Multinucleation of skeletal muscle *in vitro*. *J. Biophys. Biochem. Cytol.*, 7:559–566.

Chang, C. C., and Lee, C. Y. (1963). Isolation of neurotoxins from the venom of *Bungarus multicinctus* and their modes of neuromuscular blocking action. *Arch. Int. Pharmacodyn.*, 144:241–257.

Changeux, J.-P., Kasai, M., and Lee, C. Y. (1970). Use of a snake venom toxin to characterize the cholinergic receptor protein. *Proc. Nat. Acad. Sci.*, 67:1241–1247.

Cohen, S. A., and Fischbach, G. D. (1973): Regulation of muscle acetylcholine sensitivity by muscle activity in cell culture. *Science* 181:76–78.

Couteaux, R. (1955): Localization of cholinesterases at neuromuscular junctions. *Int. Rev. Cytol.*, 4:335–375.

Crain, S. (1966): Development of "organotypic" bioelectric activities in central tissues during maturation in culture. *Int. Rev. Neurobiol.*, 9:1–45.

Crain, S. (1970): Bioelectric interactions between cultured fetal rodent spinal cord and skeletal muscle after innervation *in vitro*. *J. Exp. Zool.*, 173:353–370.

Diamond, J., and Miledi, R. (1962): A study of fetal and newborn rat muscle fibers. *J. Physiol.*, 162:393–408.

Drachman, D., and Witzke, F. (1972): Trophic regulation of acetylcholine sensitivity of muscle: Effect of electrical stimulation. *Science*, 176:514–516.

Eisenberg, B., and Eisenberg, R. S. (1968): Selective disruption of the sarcotubular system in frog sartorius muscle. A quantitative study with exogenous peroxidase as marker. *J. Cell Biol.*, 39:451–467.

Ezerman, E. B., and Ishikawa, H. (1967): Differentiation of the sarcoplasmic reticulum and T system in developing chick skeletal muscle *in vitro*. *J. Cell Biol.*, 35:405–420.

Fambrough, D., and Rash, J. E. (1973): Development of acetylcholine sensitivity during myogenesis. *Devel. Biol.*, 26:55–68.

Feltz, A., and Mallart, A. (1971): Ionic permeability changes induced by some cholinergic agonists on normal and denervated frog muscles. *J. Physiol.*, 218:85–100.

Fischbach, G. D. (1972): Synapse formation between dissociated nerve and muscle cells in low density cell cultures. *Devel. Biol.*, 28:407–429.

Fischbach, G. D., and Cohen, S. A. (1973): The distribution of acetylcholine sensitivity over uninnervated and innervated muscle fibers grown in cell culture. *Devel. Biol.*, 31:147–162.

Fischbach, G. D., and Robbins, N. (1971): Effect of chronic disuse of rat soleus neuromuscular junctions on post-synaptic membrane. *J. Neurophysiol.*, 34:562–569.

Fischbach, G. D., Nameroff, M., and Nelson, P. G. (1971): Electrical properties of chick skeletal muscle fibers developing in cell culture. *J. Cell. Physiol.*, 78:289–300.

Fischman, D. A. (1970): The synthesis and assembly of myofibrils in embryonic muscle. *Cur. Top. Devel. Biol.*, 5:235–280.

Graham, F. L., and Whitmore, G. F. (1970): The effect of 1-β-D-arabino-furanosylcytosine on growth, viability and DNA synthesis of mouse L-cells. *Cancer Res.*, 30:2627–2634.

Gutmann, E., and Young, J. Z. (1944): The re-innervation of muscle after various periods of atrophy. *J. Anat.*, 78:15–43.

Harris, A. J., Heinemann, S., Schubert, D., and Tarakis, H. (1971): Trophic interaction between cloned tissue culture lines of nerve and muscle. *Nature*, 231:296–301.

Holtzer, H. (1970): Myogenesis. In: *Cell Differentiation*, edited by O. Scheide and J. de Vellis, pp. 476–503. Van Nostrand Reinhold, Princeton, N.J.

Howell, J. W., and Jenden, D. J. (1967): T-tubules of skeletal muscle: morphological alterations which interrupt excitation–contraction coupling. *Fed. Proc.*, 26:553.

Ishikawa, H. (1968): Formation of elaborate networks of T-system tubules in cultured skeletal muscle with special reference to T-system formation. *J. Cell Biol.*, 38:51–66.

James, D. W., and Tresman, R. L. (1969): An electron-microscopic study of the *de novo* formation of neuromuscular junctions in tissue culture. *Z. Zellforsch. Mikrosk. Anat.*, 100:126–140.

Kano, M., and Shimada, Y. (1971): Innervation of skeletal muscle cells differentiated *in vitro* from chick embryo. *Brain Res.*, 27:402–405.

Karnovsky, M., and Roots, L. (1964): A "direct-coloring" thiocholine method for cholinesterases. *J. Histochem. Cytochem.*, 12:219–221.

Katz, B. (1966): *Nerve, Muscle and Synapse*. McGraw Hill, New York.

Katz, B., and Miledi, R. (1964): The development of acetylcholine sensitivity in nerve-free segments of skeletal muscle. *J. Physiol.*, 170:389–396.

Kelly, A. M., and Zacks, S. J. (1969): The fine structure of motor endplate morphogenesis. *J. Cell Biol.*, 42:154–169.

Konigsberg, I. (1963): Clonal analysis of myogenesis. *Science*, 140:1273–1284.

Konigsberg, I. (1970): The relationship of collagen to the clonal development of embryonic skeletal muscle. In: *Chemistry and Molecular Biology of the Intercellular Matrix*, edited by E. A. Balazs, pp. 1779–1810. Academic Press, New York.

Kraehenbuhl, J. P., and Jamieson, J. D. (1972): Solid-phase conjugation of ferritin to Fab-fragments of immunoglobulin G for use in antigen localization on thin sections. *Proc. Nat. Acad. Sci.*, 69:1771–1775.

Lømø, T., and Rosenthal, J. (1972): Control of ACh sensitivity by muscle activity in the rat. *J. Physiol.*, 221:493–514.

McLean, J. D., and Singer, S. J. (1970): A general method for the specific staining of intracellular antigens with ferritin-antibody conjugates. *Proc. Nat. Acad. Sci.*, 65:122–128.

Miledi, R. (1960): The acetylcholine sensitivity of frog muscle fibers after complete or partial denervation. *J. Physiol.*, 151:1–23.

Miledi, R. (1960): Properties of regenerating neuromuscular synapses in the frog. *J. Physiol.*, 154:190–205.

Miledi, R., Molinoff, P., and Potter, L. (1971). Isolation of the cholinergic receptor protein of torpedo electric tissue. *Nature*, 229:554–557.

Miledi, R., and Potter, L. (1972): Acetylcholine receptors in muscle fibers. *Nature*, 233:599–603.

Morgan, C. (1972): The use of ferritin-conjugated antibodies in electron microscopy. *Int. Rev. Cytol.*, 32:291–326.

Murray, M. (1965): Nervous tissues *in vitro*. In: *Cells and Tissues in Culture*, Vol. 2, edited by E. N. Willmer, p. 373. Academic Press, New York.

Nakai, J. (1969): The development of neuromuscular junctions in cultures of chick embryo tissues. *J. Exp. Zool.*, 170:85–106.

Palade, G. (1959): In: *Subcellular Particles*, edited by T. Hayashi. Ronald Press Co., New York.

Pinto de Silva, P., and Branton, D. (1970): Membrane splitting in freeze-etching. *J. Cell Biol.*, 45:598–605.

Powell, J., and Fambrough, D. (1973). Electrical properties of normal and dysgenic mouse muscle in culture. *J. Cell. Physiol. (in press)*.

Robbins, N., and Yonezawa, T. (1971): Physiological studies during formation and development of rat neuromuscular junctions in tissue culture. *J. Gen. Physiol.*, 58:467–481.

Shimada, Y. (1968): Suppression of myogenesis by heterotypic and heterospecific cells in monolayer culture. *Exp. Brain Res.*, 51:564–578.

Shimada, Y., Fischman, D. A., and Moscona, A. A. (1969): Formation of neuromuscular junctions in embryonic cell cultures. *Proc. Nat. Acad. Sci.*, 62:715–721.

Tello, J. F. (1917): Genesis de las terminaciones nervidsas moterices y. sensitivas. I. En la sistema locomotor de los vergebrados speriores. Histogenesis muscular. Trabajos del Laboratorio de Investigaciones Biologicas de la Universidad de Madrid, 15, 101–199.

Yaffe, D. (1969): Cellular aspects of muscle differentiation *in vitro*. *Curr. Top. Devel. Biol.*, 4:37–77.

Synaptic Transmission and Neuronal Interaction
Raven Press, New York 1974

On the Differentiation and Organization of the Surface Membrane of a Postsynaptic Cell—the Skeletal Muscle Fiber

Douglas M. Fambrough, H. Criss Hartzell, Jeanne A. Powell,*
John E. Rash,** and Nancy Joseph

*Department of Embryology, The Carnegie Institution of Washington, Baltimore, Maryland
21210*

I. INTRODUCTION

The vertebrate neuromuscular junction has long served as a model for chemical synapses in general. The mechanisms of transmitter release and the transduction of a chemical to an electrical signal which take place at the neuromuscular junction are represented by apparently quite similar mechanisms at other chemical synapses. It seems reasonable to suppose that the close resemblance between the neuromuscular junction and other chemical synapses extends past the level of physiological function to the more subtle aspects of synaptology: the biochemical processes and regulatory mechanisms involved in synaptogenesis and maintenance of functional connections.

One might argue that the neuromuscular junction and all other chemical synapses represent only especially interesting manifestations of the cellular control mechanisms and activities operative generally in cell differentiation and cell-cell interactions. If this is so, then it is likely that much of the research which is presently building the foundations for an understanding of synapse formation may be oriented toward membrane chemistry and biosynthesis, the physical properties of real and artificial membranes, the control mechanisms involved in the topological organization of the cell surface, and the relationship between cell surface and genetic regulation. All of these subjects can be pursued in "simpler" systems, using cells which,

---

* Present Address: Division of Biological Sciences, Smith College, Northampton, Massachusetts 01060.
** Present Address: Department of Molecular, Cellular Developmental Biology, University of Colorado, Boulder, Colorado 80302.

at least up to now, neurobiologists have generally considered both unexcitable and unexciting. A happier point of view for neurobiologists is that although the chemical synapse may be a particular manifestation of basic cellular activities, it is such a striking one that it constitutes a very attractive context in which to study such basic cellular phenomena as membrane biosynthesis and organization and the control mechanisms which govern them.

II. THE ADULT NEUROMUSCULAR JUNCTION

Before considering developmental changes, let us look for a moment at the end point of the developmental sequence – the adult neuromuscular junction. Figures 1, 2, and 3 represent three experimental views of the neuromuscular junction. In Fig. 1, we see part of a whole-mount of a rat diaphragm. This preparation has been stained to reveal the location of cholinesterases (Crevier and Bélanger, 1955; Koelle and Horn, 1968), particularly the acetylcholinesterase which is mainly located at neuromuscular junctions. The neuromuscular junctions appear as irregular

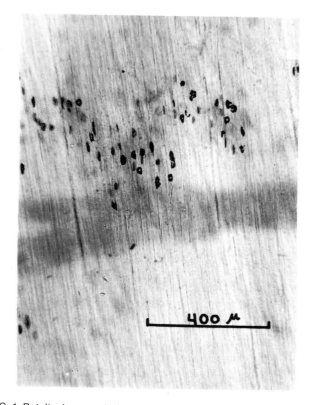

FIG. 1. Rat diaphragm whole-mount stained for acetylcholinesterase.

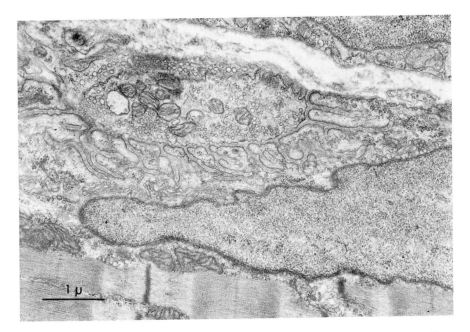

FIG. 2. Electron micrograph of rat diaphragm neuromuscular junction, red fiber. Note the nucleus, Golgi apparatus, granular endoplasmic reticulum, and free ribosomes in the subsynaptic area. Also note extensive folding of postsynaptic surface membrane and its association with extracellular amorphous layer. Courtesy of Dr. Geraldine Gauthier (cf. Padykula and Gauthier, 1970).

"cartwheel" figures approximately 25 μm in diameter. Each muscle fiber bears one such figure. One impression obtained from this view of the neuromuscular junction is that the surface area of the muscle fiber involved in synaptic transmission represents a very small fraction of the total fiber surface membrane. The concentration of acetylcholinesterase at the neuromuscular junction is remarkably high. Rogers, Darzynkiewicz, Salpeter, Ostrowski, and Barnard (1969) have measured the number of active sites of acetylcholinesterase in the rat neuromuscular junction as 11,000,000 per junction. Acetylcholinesterase would seem to be an ideal marker for probing the nature and development of the neuromuscular junction, but despite much research over the past two decades, several fundamental questions remain unanswered. The biochemical characterization of acetylcholinesterase remains confusingly complex (Leuzinger, Goldberg, and Cauvin, 1969; Massoulie and Rieger, 1969; Hall, 1972; Rieger, Bon, and Massoulie, 1972); the location of acetylcholinesterase, which is often thought to be in the postsynaptic membrane, remains in doubt (Albuquerque, Sokoll, Sonesson, and Thesleff, 1968; Betz and Sakmann, 1971; Hall and Kelly, 1971); and it is not known whether acetylcholinesterase is

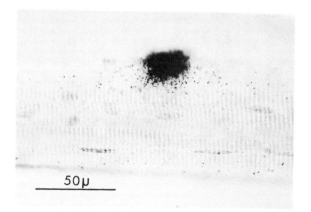

FIG. 3. Autoradiograph of the end plate region of a single skeletal muscle fiber after incubation with $^{125}I\text{-}\alpha$-bungarotoxin and staining for the enzyme acetylcholinesterase.

synthesized by muscle fiber, motoneuron, Schwann cells, or some combination of these.

Figure 2 is an electron micrograph of a section through a neuromuscular junction, again from the rat diaphragm. The impression one takes from this view is of concentrated specialization in both pre- and postsynaptic elements of the synapse. The nerve terminal is packed with components essential for synaptic transmission whereas the postsynaptic membrane, the end plate, is highly and rather regularly infolded, increasing the chemoreceptive surface five- to 10-fold. The subsynaptic cytoplasm shows signs of synthetic activity (nuclei, polysomes, Golgi), but the extracellular sheath extending over the end plate and deep into all the junctional folds suggests that the end plate may be a rigid and fairly static structure. This latter impression is strengthened by data on the long-term survival of the end plate structure after denervation (Birks, Katz, and Miledi, 1960; Bauer, Blumberg, and Zacks, 1962; Miledi and Slater, 1968; Nickel and Waser, 1968).

Figure 3 shows a very recent view of the neuromuscular junction. In this case a muscle biopsy specimen was incubated in a medium containing α-bungarotoxin (α-BGT) which had been labeled with ^{125}iodine (Hunter and Greenwood, 1962) to a high specific activity. The radioactive toxin molecules formed complexes with acetylcholine (ACh) receptors (Chang and Lee, 1963; Lee, Tseng, and Chiu, 1967; Changeux, Kasai, and Lee, 1970; Miledi, Molinoff, and Potter, 1971); the unbound toxin was washed away, and a single muscle fiber was dissected free, mounted on a microscope slide, and coated with photographic emulsion. After several days the emulsion was developed so that silver grains remained near the sites of radioactive decay. Over the neuromuscular junction the grains are clustered so tightly that they form a solid mass, whereas there are few grains over the fiber surface a short distance away. This distribution of silver grains bespeaks a tight clustering of ACh receptors in the end plate. In fact, since the resolution in [125]iodine autoradiography is only moderate (Ada, Humphrey, Askonas, McDevitt, and Nossal, 1966), the clustering of ACh receptors is even tighter than the autoradiograph (Fig. 3) suggests.

Using different radioisotope-labeled α-BGT derivatives and different experimental designs, Barnard, Wieckowski, and Chiu (1971) and Fambrough and Hartzell (1972) have derived estimates of the packing density of ACh receptors in the postsynaptic membrane. The values for mouse and rat are very similar: 1.2×10^4 and 1.3×10^4 sites per μm^2 of membrane. In Table 1 some of the properties of ACh receptors are compared with proper-

TABLE 1. *Comparison of rhodopsin[a] and ACh receptor properties*

	Rhodopsin	ACh receptor
Molecular weight	40,000	$\geqslant 96,000$
Molecular size	50 Å diameter	$\sim$ 50 to 100 Å diameter[b]
Molecules per μm^2 membrane	20,000	12,000 to 13,000[c]
Average center to center spacing in membrane	70 Å	$\sim$ 100 Å

[a] Data on rhodopsin taken from Blasie and Worthington (1969) and references therein and from Heitzmann (1972).
[b] Assuming a molecular shape similar to rhodopsin.
[c] Miledi and Potter (1971) have estimated a packing density of 100,000/μm^2 and a center-to-center spacing of 30 Å for ACh receptors in frog end plates.

ties of the vertebrate photoreceptor rhodopsin. Rhodopsin is a protein which constitutes 80 to 90% of the membrane protein in rod outer segment membranes (Heitzmann, 1972). In these membranes the packing density of rhodopsin is approximately 2.0×10^4 molecules per μm^2 of membrane, thus similar in packing density to ACh receptors in the end plate. The size of the ACh receptor is still unsettled as is the stoichiometry of α-BGT binding. By all estimates, however, the size of the ACh receptor per toxin-binding site appears to be larger than rhodopsin (see discussions by Klett, Fulpius, Cooper, and Reich, and Lindstrom, *this volume*). Thus it appears likely that the ACh receptor constitutes the major protein species in the postsynaptic membrane at neuromuscular junctions.

As a focal point in studies of neuromuscular synaptogenesis, the ACh receptor appears to be the molecule of choice. It is a major functional component of the postsynaptic cell; it is definitely located in the postsynaptic membrane, where it is a major structural component as well; and it is readily identified both by iontophoresis and intracellular recording and by interaction with radioisotope-labeled α-BGT.

III. DENERVATION SUPERSENSITIVITY TO ACETYLCHOLINE

The ACh receptor also plays a central role in a curious phenomenon known as "denervation supersensitivity" (Fig. 4). Sensitivity to ACh in vertebrate skeletal muscle fibers is confined almost exclusively to the immediate vicinity of the neuromuscular junction (del Castillo and Katz, 1955), but, following denervation, the entire muscle fiber surface becomes sensitive to ACh (Axelsson and Thesleff, 1959; Miledi, 1960a), and this sensitivity increases with time until it approximates that typically measured at the end plate. The rise in sensitivity occurs approximately synchronously along the fiber (Albuquerque and McIsaac, 1970; Fambrough, 1970) and is not accompanied by a significant diminution in end plate sensitivity. The noninnervated portions of transected muscle fibers also quickly become ACh sensitive (Katz and Miledi, 1964). In Fig. 5 the ACh sensitivity of extrajunctional surface membrane of denervated rat diaphragm fibers is plotted as a function of time following denervation (data from Hartzell and Fambrough, 1972). After a lag of approximately 2 days, ACh sensitivity begins to increase rapidly. During the lag period, inhibitors of protein and of RNA synthesis will block the subsequent development of sensitivity (Fambrough, 1970; Grampp, Harris, and Thesleff, 1972).

Studies employing radioisotope-labeled α-BGT have extended the

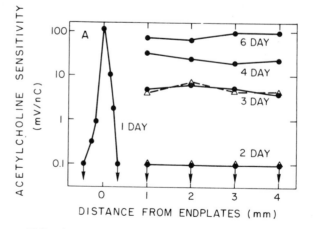

FIG. 4. ACh sensitivity along rat diaphragm muscle fibers following denervation. ACh sensitivity was measured by intracellular recording and iontophoretic application of ACh (from Fambrough, 1970).

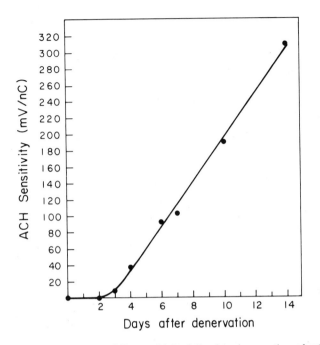

FIG. 5. Time course of increase in ACh sensitivity following denervation of rat diaphragm.

electrophysiological analysis (Miledi and Potter, 1971; Berg, Kelly, Sargent, Williamson, and Hall, 1972; Hartzell and Fambrough, 1972). Denervation supersensitivity is accompanied by an approximately 20-fold increase in ACh receptor sites (α-BGT-binding sites) on rat diaphragm fibers. These new sites are distributed rather evenly over the muscle fiber surface (Fig. 6), and, as shown in Fig. 7, the ACh receptor density in extrajunctional surface membrane rises from less than five ACh receptors per μm^2 to nearly $1,700/\mu m^2$ (data from Hartzell and Fambrough, 1972). Thus the ACh receptor density finally reaches a value approximately eightfold less than the end plate density. Even at this lower density, ACh receptors surely constitute several percent of the surface membrane protein, conceivably as much as 10%.

IV. DEVELOPMENT OF ACETYLCHOLINE SENSITIVITY DURING MYOGENESIS

Denervation supersensitivity has been thought of over the years as an expression of the return of skeletal muscle to its intrinsic state of differentiation, following removal of an overriding, modifying influence from the motoneuron. The similarities between denervated and embryonic muscle may offer some clues to control mechanisms operating in synaptogenesis.

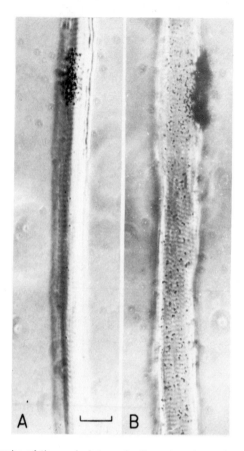

FIG. 6. Autoradiographs of the end plate and adjacent regions of rat diaphragm muscle fibers after incubation with ^{125}I-α-bungarotoxin. A. Control fiber. B. 10-day denervated fiber. Note change in extrajunctional receptor density and maintenance of high receptor density at end plate (from Hartzell and Fambrough, 1972).

At this point let us go back to the beginning of the developmental sequence — to the fusing myoblasts — and trace some early differentiative trends. After that, we will consider some parallels between embryonic and denervated muscle and finally discuss some hypothetical mechanisms for controlling receptor distribution and some ways in which we are attempting to test them.

ACh receptors begin to appear during myogenesis at about the same time that myoblasts begin to fuse and to synthesize contractile proteins and to construct specialized internal membranes (Fig. 8) (Fambrough and Rash, 1971). In general, mononucleate myoblasts are dividing, undifferentiated cells that will become muscle. These cells are not depolarized in response to ACh and do not bind α-BGT. Once committed to differentiate, they do not divide, but they readily fuse with myotubes and other myoblasts to form

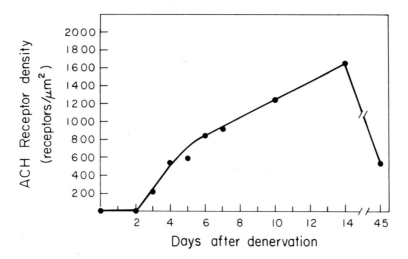

FIG. 7. Time course of increase in ACh receptor density in extrajunctional membranes following denervation of rat diaphragm muscle fibers.

multinucleate cells (for reviews see Yaffe, 1969; Holtzer, 1970; Fischman, 1970). All multinucleate cells and some differentiating mononucleate ones are sensitive to ACh and bind α-BGT. We have suggested (Fambrough and Rash, 1971) that the commitment to differentiate may entail activation of the set of genes that code all of the special proteins characteristic of the differentiated state. Thus ACh receptor synthesis begins at the same time as myosin synthesis even though ACh receptors have no apparent function in the morphogenesis of skeletal muscle fibers. The expression of chemosensitivity coincident with cytological and morphological differentiation may be a general phenomenon for postsynaptic cells. Woodward, Hoffer, Siggins, and Bloom (1971) have reported that as the cerebellar Purkinje cells begin to differentiate morphologically they begin to respond to applied glutamate, norepinephrine, and gamma-aminobutyric acid even though the processes which will terminate presynaptically on Purkinje dendrites and cell body have not yet arrived. Apparently postsynaptic cells anticipate the nature of the chemical transmitters they will later respond to and, as they begin to differentiate, they display appropriate chemoreceptor molecules in their surface membranes. This behavior is consistent with the general observation that neuronal circuitry is to a large extent predetermined (cf. Jacobson, 1970).

Binding selectively to ACh receptors, α-BGT binds to myotubes but not to fibroblasts and dividing myoblasts (Fig. 9). The kinetics of binding to myogenic cell cultures are illustrated in Fig. 10. There are two components to the binding curve. The faster binding component represents the saturation of surface ACh receptors by α-BGT. After a 20-min exposure to

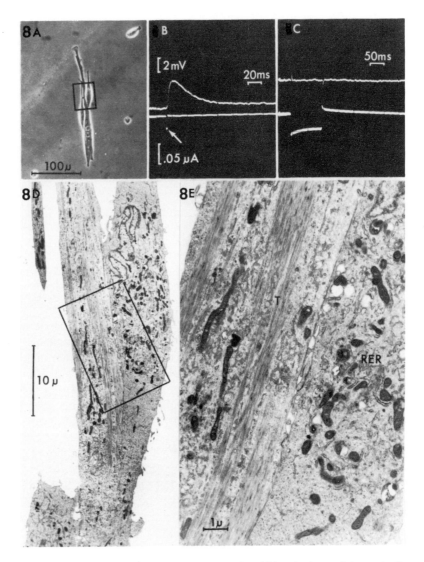

FIG. 8. *A, D,* and *E:* Light and electron micrographs of binucleate myotube and adjacent myoblasts. Note bundles of oriented myofilaments and anastomosing tubules (T) in myotube, general absence of these structures in myoblasts which contain many small polysomes, and occasional rough endoplasmic reticulum (RER). *B* and *C:* Electrophysiological records from binucleate myotube *(B)* and myoblast *(C)*. Upper trace, intracellular record; lower trace, ACh iontophoretic current (from Fambrough and Rash, 1971).

α-BGT, the myotubes are no longer sensitive to iontophoretically applied ACh. The second, slower binding component represents the continued addition of new receptors to the myotube surface (Hartzell and Fambrough, 1973). In support of this interpretation are the observations that bound toxin does not wash off even after long-term extensive washing and that the

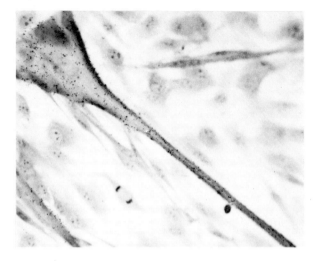

FIG. 9. Autoradiograph of rat myotube in tissue culture after incubation with ^{125}I-α-bungarotoxin. Note rather even distribution of α-bungarotoxin-binding sites (grains) over myotube and lack of binding sites on mononucleate cells. Autoradiograph has been counter-stained with Ehrlich's hematoxylin.

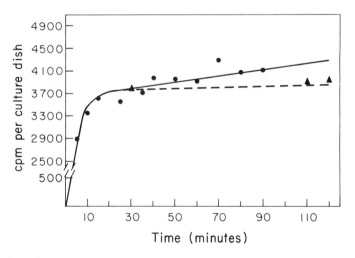

FIG. 10. ●——● Kinetics of ^{125}I-α-bungarotoxin binding to cultured chick muscle. Each of 11 sets of cultures (between four and 12 dishes/set) was incubated in medium containing 0.2 μg/ml ^{125}I-α-BGT for the length of time shown on abscissa. ▲——▲ Retention of bound ^{125}I-α-BGT during washout after 30-min incubation in toxin (from Hartzell and Fambrough, 1973).

toxin-binding sites appearing after a saturating α-BGT exposure have the same kinetics of binding as the original set of surface receptors (Fig. 11). The slower binding component represents the binding of α-BGT to myotubes at a rate limited by the rate of appearance of new receptors in the surface membrane.

α-BGT-receptor complexes are not internalized and α-BGT does not affect the rate of appearance of new receptors. In the experiment illustrated in Fig. 12, the rate of appearance of new binding sites in myogenic cell cultures was the same for cells exposed to a saturating dose of α-BGT as for cells grown without α-BGT block. These myotubes are rapidly growing in size. There is evidence for a small amount of turnover of surface membrane glycoproteins in other growing cells in culture (Warren and Glick, 1968).

The incorporation of new receptors into surface membranes can be inhibited (Fig. 13) by treatment of myotubes with cycloheximide, by low temperature, by combinations of dinitrophenol and iodoacetate or dicoumerol and fluoride, but not by actinomycin D. The inhibition by cycloheximide is particularly interesting. It takes several hours for this inhibition to develop even though inhibition of protein synthesis is maximally effective within a minute. In Fig. 14 the ability of myotubes to recover ACh sensitivity during 1 hr following α-BGT treatment is plotted as a function of total time in cycloheximide. From this plot it appears that myotubes must be treated with cycloheximide for 2 to 3 hr before receptor incorporation into membranes is maximally depressed. There is a low-level return of sensitivity even after long-term cycloheximide treatment.

The slow inhibition of receptor appearance by cycloheximide suggests

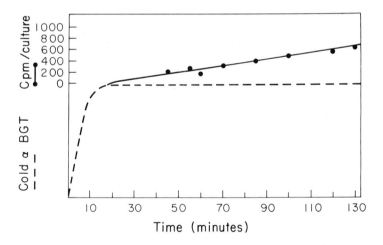

FIG. 11. Appearance of new α-BGT-binding sites after α-BGT block. At zero time, eight groups of eight culture dishes were given a 20-min saturating exposure to unlabeled α-BGT to block surface sites. This is indicated by the dashed line. The unbound toxin was washed out and the cultures incubated in toxin-free medium. The number of new binding sites appearing during various toxin-free incubation periods was then determined by exposing groups of cultures to ^{125}I-α-BGT *for 20 min*. The slope of the line generated in this experiment is not different from the slow component of α-BGT binding shown in Fig. 10 (from Hartzell and Fambrough, 1973).

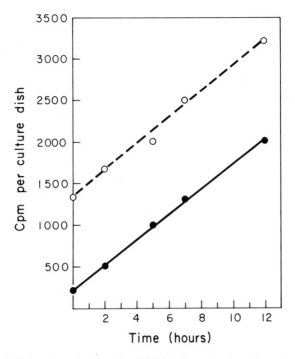

FIG. 12. ○----○ Rate of production of α-BGT-binding sites in cultured muscle. At each time indicated on abscissa, six cultures were incubated in saturating ^{125}I-α-BGT to determine relative number of binding sites. ●----● Rate of appearance of new α-BGT-binding sites after α-BGT block. At minus 20 min, five groups of six cultures each were incubated in unlabeled α-BGT (saturating conditions), the unlabeled α-BGT was washed out at time zero, and the cultures were subsequently treated as above (from Hartzell and Fambrough, 1973).

the existence of an intracellular pool of receptors which slowly feed into the surface membrane even if new receptor synthesis is blocked. It may be the general rule for plasma membrane production to involve a cytoplasmic pool of membrane components (perhaps organized as internal membranes). This appears to be true for rat liver plasma membrane synthesis. As in the case of ACh receptors, incorporation of recently made proteins into liver plasma membrane is only slowly blocked by cycloheximide, as shown in Fig. 15, which is taken from a study by Ray, Lieberman, and Lansing (1968). In the case of liver membrane synthesis, cycloheximide immediately blocked protein synthesis by 97%, and the incorporation of ^{3}H-leucyl-labeled proteins into other subcellular fractions, including internal membranes, was quickly inhibited.

Because of the specificity of α-BGT binding, we have been able to test directly for internal pools of ACh receptors in myogenic cell cultures. Table 2 summarizes data from three experiments, each involving a large number of cultures. In all these experiments we measured (a) the total number of

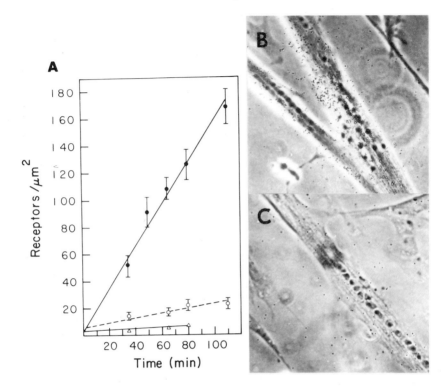

FIG. 13. Effect of inhibitors upon the incorporation of new ACh receptors into myotube surface membranes. Following a saturating exposure to unlabeled α-BGT, the appearance of new α-BGT-binding sites was determined by ^{125}I-α-BGT binding and autoradiography. ●——● = Control cells. ○----○ = Cells pretreated 3 hr in 100 μg/ml cycloheximide. △——△ = Cells incubated in 2×10^{-1}M dinitrophenol, 2×10^{-3}M iodoacetate. *B* and *C:* Autoradiographs of ^{125}I-α-BGT-treated myotubes after 90 min recovery from saturating, unlabeled α-BGT in control medium (B) and in cycloheximide-containing medium (C).

α-BGT-binding sites exposed on the cell surfaces, (b) the number of additional binding sites appearing after homogenization of the myotubes, (c) the number of internal binding sites after 3-hr incubation in cycloheximide, and, in one experiment, (d) the number of binding sites appearing on the surface during the 3 hr of cycloheximide treatment. Different criteria for α-BGT-receptor complexes were used in the experiments. In experiment 1, the internal receptor-BGT complexes were solubilized in Triton X-100 and identified as approximately 10S material by sucrose gradient centrifugation (Miledi et al., 1971; Raftery, Schmidt, Clark, and Wolcott, 1971; Berg et al., 1972; Meunier, Olsen, Menez, Fromageot, Boquet, and Changeux, 1972). In experiments 2 and 3, the DEAE-cellulose filter technique described by Klett, Fulpius, Cooper, and Reich *(this volume, personal communication)* was used to catch α-BGT-receptor complexes but to pass free α-BGT. The cytoplasmic material binding α-BGT *before* detergent extraction was

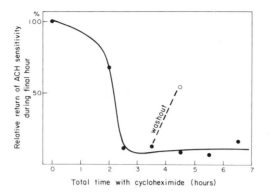

FIG. 14. ●——● Effect of 100 μg/ml cycloheximide on the return of ACh sensitivity after α-BGT block. Cycloheximide was present throughout the experiment. Myotubes were exposed to a saturating dose of α-BGT and the responses of myotubes to iontophoretic application of ACh were measured 1 hr later. Control cultures attained levels of approximately 40 mV/nC 1 hr after α-BGT block. Sensitivities are corrected for differences in resting potentials and expressed as percent of control cell recovery. ○----○ Reversibility of the cycloheximide effect. In some cultures, the cyloheximide was washed out and the ACh sensitivity measured 1 hr later. Each point is average of seven to 15 measurements.

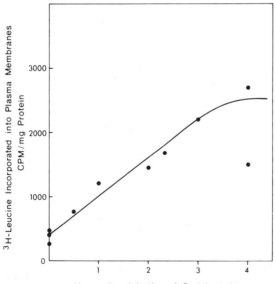

FIG. 15. Incorporation of ³H-leucine pre-labeled proteins into plasma membranes of rat liver cells *in vivo* in the absence of protein synthesis. Rats were injected intravenously with cycloheximide 5 min after ³H-leucine injection, and incorporation of ³H-leucine into proteins was quickly inhibited (redrawn from Ray et al., 1968).

TABLE 2. *Surface receptors and internal receptor pools in chick myotubes*

Experiment	Surface receptors (arbitrary units)	Internal receptors (relative to surface)	Internal receptors after 3 hr in cycloheximide	New surface receptors appearing during 3 hr in cycloheximide
1	100	32	22	—
2	100	35	28	—
3	100	38	24	10

In each experiment a large number of culture plates of cultured chick myotubes (plated at 10^5 cells/35 mm diameter culture plate, 5 days earlier) were divided into sets. Set 1 was incubated with ^{125}I-αBGT to saturate surface receptors and the number of cpm of ^{125}I bound was assayed by scintillation counting. Set 2 was incubated in unlabeled α-BGT, then washed, homogenized, and the homogenate incubated with ^{125}I-αBGT. The homogenate was centrifuged $27,000 \times g_{max}$ for 30 min, the supernatant discarded, and the pellet resuspended in 0.01 M Na_2HPO_4 + 1% Triton X-100. ^{125}I-αBGT-receptor complexes were then identified either by sucrose gradient centrifugation or by DEAE filter assay. Set 3 was pretreated 3 hr in medium containing 100 μg/ml cycloheximide and then incubated with unlabeled α-BGT in the presence of cycloheximide and homogenized, incubated with ^{125}I-αBGT, and processed further like set 2. In experiment 3 a fourth set of cultures was incubated with unlabeled α-BGT, then maintained in cycloheximide for 3 hr. The number of new binding sites appearing during 3 hr of cycloheximide treatment was determined by adding ^{125}I-αBGT to the medium during the final 20 min in cycloheximide and measuring the number of ^{125}I counts bound.

shown to be quite large, all sedimenting at $27,000 \times g$ for 30 min. This suggests that the cytoplasmic pool containing ACh receptors consists of internal membranes, a suggestion consistent with the insolubility of isolated receptors in aqueous solvents (Changeux, Meunier, and Huchet, 1971; Miledi et al., 1971).

Note that in Table 2 only approximately 30% of the internal pool of ACh receptors seems to enter the surface membrane during a 3-hr cycloheximide block of protein synthesis. Nevertheless, the cycloheximide block of return of ACh sensitivity is readily reversible (Fig. 14). We do not yet know the correct explanation for these observations: one possibility is that receptor incorporation into surface membrane after long-term cycloheximide treatment is limited by exhaustion of some other protein or other compound required for new membrane incorporation into the cell surface.

V. MEMBRANE FLUIDITY AND THE DISTRIBUTION OF ACh RECEPTORS IN EMBRYONIC MUSCLE SURFACE MEMBRANES

During rapid myotube growth, ACh receptors are rather uniformly distributed over the surface of myotubes. This is true both of total surface receptors (as in Fig. 9) and those appearing in the surface shortly after an α-BGT treatment (Fig. 13). This surface distribution of receptors is like

that in denervated muscle fibers and quite unlike that of the adult, innervated fibers or long-term cultured, spontaneously contracting fibers described in this volume by Fischbach, or some fibers contacted by neurons in
culture, described by Harris in this volume (see also Harris, Heinemann,
Schubert, and Tarakis, 1971; Kano and Shimada, 1971). There is increasing
evidence that the surface membrane at least of some cell types is best
described as a fluid mosaic (for review see Singer and Nicholson, 1972).
Following the observations of Frye and Edidin (1970) on surface antigen
mixing, Michael Edidin and I have attempted to measure the "fluidity" of
cultured myotube surface membranes. In these experiments (Edidin and
Fambrough, 1973) we used an antibody against rat muscle membranes
prepared by Criss Hartzell (Hartzell and Fambrough, 1972). The antibody
was split into monovalent Fab fragments and labeled with tetramethylrho-
damine, a fluorochrome. Then a small area of myotube surface was made
fluorescent by applying Fab with a micropipette (Fig. 16A). Then the
"spread" of the fluorescent patch was studied as a function of time (Fig.
16B–F). This spread was inhibited by low temperature but not by cyanide
or cycloheximide. Glutaraldehyde-fixed fibers which were subsequently
marked with fluorescent Fab showed no spread, and excess unlabeled
antibody did not cause rapid fading of the fluorescent patch. Thus patch
spread seems to signify translational movement of membrane antigens in the
membrane. The antigens to which the labeled Fab binds are proteins, mostly
of molecular weight slightly greater than 100,000 daltons, based on the
mobility of reduced and alkylated antigens in SDS-polyacrylamide gels
(Shapiro, Viñuela, and Maizel, 1967). We have calculated a "diffusion
constant" for Fab-antigen mobility in surface membranes: $D = 1.5 \times 10^{-9}$
cm^2/sec. This is equivalent to free diffusion of 100 Å spheres in a medium
slightly more viscous than olive oil, or if you dislike the relationship to
membrane structure implied in this analogy, slightly more viscous than
molten copper at 3,000°C.

Given the surface fluidity, it is not surprising that developing cells might
fail to generate a topology of surface functions like that eventually achieved
after hookup with other cell types. Thus we find on the one hand a developing cell apparently with little surface organization and on the other an adult,
innervated cell with an apparently relatively rigid end plate structure
different in composition and function from the bulk of the fiber surface. At
present, we know nothing concerning the possible fluidity of adult innervated
or denervated muscle surface membranes, but some speculation might be
in order. Suppose that the general case is for cells to have fluid surface
membranes except where interactions with exogenous cues result in
topological arrangements appropriate for the cell-cell interactions. Then it
may be that the end plate is unique for muscle membrane in being very
stable and nonfluid. The low level of extrajunctional sensitivity found around
innervated end plates (Miledi, 1960b; Feltz and Mallart, 1971) could even

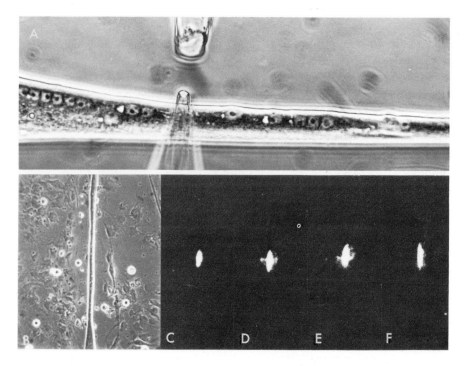

FIG. 16. *A.* Application of fluorescent Fab onto myotube by micropipetting. *B.* A cultured fiber before marking. *C–F.* The same fiber 0, 6, 12, and 165 min after marking. T ≈ 25°C.

result from the "escape" of a few ACh receptors from the end plate structure and their diffusion in the plane of the membrane. Another speculative thought is that the fluidity may be decreased by the assembly of the greater membrane or glycocalyx which covers the surface of most maturing cells. For the muscle fiber a thick extracellular layer of amorphous material covers the entire fiber surface (see Fig. 2). It seems likely that changes in the physical properties of surface membranes is a factor in synaptogenesis, and it seems likely that the ACh receptor is involved somehow in the changes.

VI. DEVELOPMENT OF OTHER MEMBRANE PROPERTIES DURING MYOGENESIS

I would like to make what will at first appear to be a digression from the biology of ACh receptors to mention some changes in membrane properties concurrent with ACh receptor production and myotube differentiation. As myotubes differentiate into cholinergic postsynaptic cells, their surface membrane properties are changing in many ways. One such change has to do with the development of a high resting transmembrane potential. As seen in Fig. 17, the transmembrane potential of cultured myogenic cells is quite low

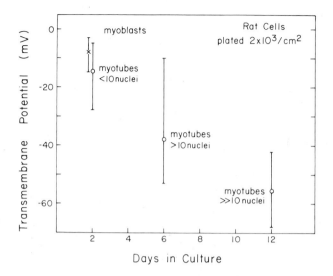

FIG. 17. Increase in transmembrane potential during differentiation and maturation of myotubes. Bars indicate total range of observed transmembrane potentials from many experiments.

in the myoblast and small, young myotube stages, and becomes progressively more inside-negative as the myotubes grow and mature. A similar trend has been reported several times from *in vivo* studies (see, for example, Hazelwood and Nichols, 1969; Boëthius and Knutsson, 1970). During this period of change, Vernadakis and Woodbury (1964) found no change in intracellular K^+ concentration and only a slow decrease in intracellular Na^+. In Fig. 18 the transmembrane potentials of three myotubes representing different developmental stages are plotted as functions of extracellular potassium ion concentration. In these experiments each curve was generated in a few minutes by passing a sodium-potassium ion gradient over the myotube while continuously recording the transmembrane potential with an intracellular microelectrode and the extracellular potassium ion concentration with a potassium ion selective electrode. Note that the curves all extrapolate to zero transmembrane potential as the extracellular potassium ion concentration approaches 150 mM. This is exactly in keeping with Vernadakis and Woodbury's finding that intracellular potassium remains at approximately 160 mM during the development of rat muscle *in vivo*. When these data are analyzed in terms of the Goldman equation (Hodgkin and Katz, 1949)

$$E_m = \frac{RT}{F} \ln\left(\frac{P_K[K^+]_o + P_{Na}[Na^+]_o}{P_K[K^+]_i + P_{Na}[Na^+]_i}\right)$$

it becomes clear that, for all reasonable values of internal sodium ion concentration, the changes in myotube resting potential are due principally to

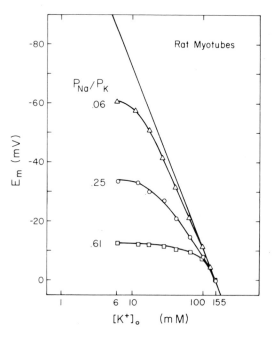

FIG. 18. Dependence of transmembrane potential (E_m) on extracellular potassium ion concentration $[K^+]_o$ for three myotubes at different developmental stages. The straight line indicates Nernstian curve for ideal potassium electrode at 37°C. A myotube was penetrated with recording electrode, a K^+-sensitive electrode (K^+-selectivity over Na^+ about 35) was placed adjacent to the myotube (within 20 μm) and then the external sodium and potassium ion concentrations were changed by perfusion so that a Na^+-K^+ gradient flowed over the myotube for about 3 to 5 min, changing $[K^+]_o$ from 6 mM to approximately 150 mM. Then the recording electrode was withdrawn. Relative permeabilities of the myotubes to sodium and potassium, calculated from the Goldman equation, are indicated on the graph.

changes in the relative permeability of the membrane to sodium ions (P_{Na}) and potassium ions (P_K). From this method of analysis (which is not universally accepted, see, for example, Hazelwood and Nichols, 1969; Hazelwood, 1972), it appears that the developing myotube surface membrane becomes more and more selectively permeable to potassium. W. F. Dryden and S. Erulkar (*personal communications* and *in press*) have studied the ionic basis of the resting potential in myogenic cells and find that the increasing potassium selectivity of the surface membrane is most readily accounted for by an increase in potassium ion permeability (analogous to the situation in several other developing cells, Steinhardt, Lunden and Mazia, 1971; Weisenseel and Jaffe, 1972) rather than a decrease in sodium ion permeability.

As myotubes develop in culture their electrical membrane constants become quite similar to those of denervated adult muscle fibers. In Table 3

TABLE 3. *Electrical membrane constants*

Fiber type	E_m (mV)	R_m (Ωcm^2)	τ_m (msec)	C_m ($\mu F/cm^2$)	λ (μm)
Cultured mouse (n = 18)	37.9	694	5.4	8.4	609
Adult rat EDL* 15-day denervated (n = 10)	54.0	805	6.4	7.9	700
Adult rat EDL*	77.0	545	1.5	2.8	530

* From Albuquerque and McIsaac (1970). Constants C_m and R_m have been recalculated by us using measured fiber radii of Albuquerque and McIsaac.

some of these constants for mouse myotubes are compared with those of denervated adult and innervated adult rat muscle fibers (Albuquerque and McIsaac, 1970). Similar data for adult mouse fibers are not available, to our knowledge.

It appears that in many respects the embryonic muscle fiber before innervation and the denervated adult muscle fiber resemble one another. The similarities between embryonic and denervated muscle fibers include similar ACh sensitivity and receptor density, similar electrical membrane constants, general inactivity, and low resting potentials. Among these similarities we may find clues to the mechanisms governing the alteration of receptor distribution during synaptogenesis.

VII. CELLULAR MECHANISMS OPERATIVE IN SYNAPTOGENESIS

At the present state of our knowledge there appear to be two somewhat interrelated control mechanisms operating in synaptogenesis and there are several very different possibilities for what each of these mechanisms might be. One mechanism seems to operate in the organization of a receptor-rich area of membrane at a point of nerve-muscle contact and in the elaboration and stabilization of this area. A second mechanism seems to operate in regulation of acetylcholine receptor density in extrajunctional membranes.

VIII. INFERENCES ABOUT THE MECHANISM OF END PLATE FORMATION

Ultrastructural studies, particularly those of Hirano (1967), Teräväinen (1968) and Kelly and Zacks (1969), indicate that the development of junctional folds occurs rather slowly, after neuromuscular junctions become functional. This suggests that the end plate structure forms in response to innervation. There is probably little direct molecular interaction between the surface of the nerve ending and the muscle fiber plasma membrane itself, due to the intervening extracellular amorphous material over the muscle fiber. Hence, nerve-muscle interaction is likely to be mediated by diffusion of some "trophic" substance from nerve ending to muscle. Such a substance could even participate directly in building the end plate membrane structure, perhaps by promoting association of ACh receptors. For further discussion of end plate formation the reader is referred to chapters by Harris and by Fischbach *(This Volume)*.

IX. INFERENCES ABOUT THE MECHANISM OF CONTROL
OF EXTRAJUNCTIONAL RECEPTORS

A. Gene-Regulation Mechanism

For the control of extrajunctional ACh receptor density there are, at present, two major candidates for a mechanism: a gene-regulation mechanism and a membrane-gating mechanism. The gene-regulation mechanism requires neuronal modulation of genetic expression in the muscle fiber. In a simple version of this model, some humoral factor is released by the functioning nerve terminal. The factor then diffuses into the muscle fiber and represses ACh receptor synthesis by blocking transcription of the gene(s) coding for ACh receptor messenger RNA(s). Paradoxically, the motor end plate at the same time becomes a site for ACh receptor accumulation, perhaps due to a secondary local derepression of the receptor gene in muscle nuclei near the end plate or collection of preexisting receptors from all over the fiber surface. Among the data marshalled in support of this mechanism are those of Luco and Eyzaguirre (1955) and Salafsky and Prewitt (1968), showing that the time of onset of fibrillation following denervation is influenced by the length of the nerve stump, suggesting that some trophic substance moving by axoplasmic flow continues to affect the muscle until its supply in the nerve stump is exhausted. There is less compelling evidence that the time of onset and the time course of development of denervation supersensitivity to ACh is similarly affected by the length of nerve stump (Emmelin and Malm, 1965). Another line of evidence for a gene-regulation mechanism comes from the studies of Guth and co-workers (Samaha, Guth, and Albers, 1970) on the neuronal regulation of myosin-ATPase type and myosin light chain species in slow and fast twitch muscles. Here the source of innervation seems to qualitatively determine the type of myosin molecules synthesized by the muscle. Further support for a neuronal mediation of gene expression comes from other nerve-target cell systems in which the neurons play an essential role in supporting development or triggering differentiation (Guth, 1968, 1969).

Until recently another major piece of evidence that a neurohumoral agent was involved in control of extrajunctional ACh sensitivity was the evidence that disused but nevertheless innervated muscle fibers failed to develop a high level of denervation sensitivity to ACh. This evidence was recently contradicted by the findings of Lømø and Rosenthal (1971, 1972) and partially confirmed by Drachman and Witzke (1972), that completely disused muscle fibers do develop "denervation supersensitivity" but that denervated fibers can be prevented from undergoing this change by continuous electrical stimulation and muscle contraction. From this data it appears that the nervous influence on ACh receptor distribution is mediated more directly by muscle fiber activity. Still unresolved is the question of mechanism, and a gene-regulation model may still serve to account for the new information. The signal governing genetic expression in this case could be a metabolite of muscle contraction, such as creatine, or could even be related to the ion fluxes of the action potential or of the excitation-contraction coupling mechanism.

The hypothesis that ACh receptor distribution is governed in part by gene regulation is a difficult one to test. Consistent with this hypothesis are the observations that the development of denervation supersensitivity can be blocked by inhibitors of RNA or protein synthesis (Fambrough, 1970; Grampp et al., 1972; Harris, *personal communication*). It seems almost certain now that denervation supersensitivity involves a great deal of new ACh receptor synthesis, but the crucial question of regulating mechanism can be phrased in this context as follows: Does ACh receptor synthesis *become activated* following denervation and disuse, or does ACh receptor synthesis continue even in the innervated, working fiber where ACh receptors are somehow excluded from entering the surface membrane as functional molecules?

Whereas the gene-regulation hypothesis would be hard to prove, it may be easier to *disprove* (providing it is incorrect) by demonstrating that ACh receptor synthesis continues in innervated adult muscle fibers even in areas of muscle cytoplasm far removed from the end plate. With a test of this sort in mind, we have tried repeatedly to find nascent cytoplasmic receptors based upon α-BGT binding to muscle polysomes. So far even when polysomes are isolated from rapidly developing embryonic muscle (from 11- or 14-day-old chick embryos) and ACh receptor synthesis is near maximal, we have found no evidence of α-BGT binding to nascent chains on polysomes. We have prepared polysomes by the method used by Heywood, Dowben, and Rich (1967) to obtain myosin-synthesizing polysomes and also by deoxycholate treatment of microsomes to obtain membrane-associated polysomes. Our test for specific binding of α-BGT to polysomes has been to test for ^{125}I-α-BGT counts sedimenting in the polysome region of sucrose gradients and shifted to a low sedimentation coefficient by treatment with ribonuclease. There are many reasons why nascent receptor chains might fail to bind α-BGT. For example, it may be that the hydrophobic nature of the receptor causes it to fold or associate correctly for α-BGT binding only after entering a lipid environment of a membrane.

Evidence less compelling but damaging to the gene-regulation model would be the demonstration of a large cytoplasmic pool of ACh receptors in innervated adult muscle fibers. Our attempts to identify such a pool have been plagued by what appears to be a high level of "nonspecific" binding of α-BGT to cytoplasmic components of adult muscle. However, it may turn out that much of the nonspecific binding is not so nonspecific.

B. Membrane-Gating Mechanism

If the gene-regulation model is not correct, then the most reasonable alternative would seem to be control at the level of surface membrane construction. A simple example of such a membrane-level control mechanism would be the incorporation of ACh receptors into surface membrane which is very sensitive to transmembrane potential. We have already mentioned that rapid receptor incorporation is occurring in developing myotubes which have low resting potentials. Albuquerque and McIsaac (1970) have shown that one of the first changes in muscle fibers following denervation is a *decrease* in the transmembrane potential by approximately 10 mV in the first 2 days. Interestingly, such a fall in transmembrane potential seems to be blocked by actinomycin D (Grampp et al., 1972; Fambrough, *unpublished observations*).

Katz and Miledi (1964) have shown that injured areas of innervated muscle also become sensitive to acetylcholine. These areas could easily be areas of reduced transmembrane potential. As yet, we do not know whether or not the inhibition or reversal of the development of supersensitivity in denervated muscles by direct electrical stimulation is associated with a high resting potential (Rosenthal, *personal communication*).

A test of the hypothesis that incorporation of ACh receptors into muscle surface membranes is gated by a sensitivity to transmembrane potential can probably be done most readily in tissue culture. In Table 4 are data on the rate of incorporation of ACh receptors into myotube surface membranes following α-BGT block of old receptors. In these experiments the transmembrane potentials were set by transferring the cultures to isotonic media of different ionic composition. As can be seen from this data, the rate of receptor incorporation is not terribly sensitive to transmembrane potential over the range 0 to −40 mV. The rate of incorporation is marginally slower at higher transmembrane potentials. However, the most interesting part of the voltage range is likely to be −55 to −80 mV. Due to the relatively high sodium ion permeability of young myotubes it is difficult, if not impossible, to push the transmembrane potentials into this range by altering external

TABLE 4. *Effect of transmembrane potential on ACh-receptor incorporation into membranes*

External medium	Transmembrane potential (mV)	Rate of incorporation (Receptors/μm^2 hr)
Standard medium Na 152 mM K 6 mM	−25	102
Low potassium medium Na 158 mM K 0.3 mM	−33	88
350 mM Sucrose medium 9:1 Na 15 mM K .06 mM	− 38	99
Low sodium medium Na 3 mM K 155 mM	− 3	115

ions. Hopefully, it will be possible to do so by voltage clamping the cells with intracellular electrodes.

X. SUMMARY

We have identified and discussed some of the properties of the neuromuscular junction postsynaptic membrane and the factors playing roles in neuromuscular junction development and in control of extrajunctional receptor density. During myogenesis, ACh receptors are synthesized and appear in the cell surface concurrently with the appearance of myofibrils in the cytoplasm. As myoblasts fuse and differentiate ACh receptors are incorporated into the membrane and the ACh receptor density increases rapidly. At this stage, unlike innervated muscle, ACh receptors are rather uniformly distributed over the myotube surface as would be expected from estimates of high-membrane fluidity in these cells. Innervation of the myotube induces the formation of the end plate, which is a very nonfluid structure, highly specialized morphologically, and containing a high concentration of ACh receptor molecules. The development and stabilization of end plate organization appear to be dependent upon innervation in a process mediated by some undefined "trophic" substance. We suggest that this neuronally derived substance might even become a structural entity in the end plate. Innervation, besides inducing end plate formation, results in a decrease in extrajunctional receptor density. Control of extrajunctional receptor density may involve changes in gene activity and/or surface membrane construction and is very likely related to transmembrane potentials or contractile activity. Two models for control of extrajunctional receptor density are discussed in relationship to observations concerning myogenesis and denervation supersensitivity.

The number of testable ideas concerning synaptogenesis and control of receptor distribution and the number of useful test systems for these ideas have greatly increased in the past several years. The time seems ripe for finally discovering answers to some of the basic questions concerning synapse formation and receptor control. We hope that in these answers will be information relevant to even broader questions of cell structure and function.

REFERENCES

Ada, G. L., Humphrey, J. H., Askonas, B. A., McDevitt, H. O., and Nossal, G. J. V. (1966): Correlation of grain counts with radioactivity (^{125}iodine and tritium) in autoradiography. *Exp. Cell Res.*, 41:557.

Albuquerque, E. X., and McIsaac, R. J. (1970): Fast and slow mammalian muscles after denervation. *Exp. Neurol.*, 26:183.

Albuquerque, E. X., Sokoll, M. D., Sonesson, B., and Thesleff, S. (1968): Studies on the nature of the acetylcholine receptor. *Eur. J. Pharmacol.*, 4:40.

Axelsson, J., and Thesleff, S. (1959): A study of supersensitivity in denervated mammalian skeletal muscle. *J. Physiol.*, 147:178.

Barnard, E. A., Wieckowski, J., and Chiu, T. H. (1971): Cholinergic receptor molecules and cholinesterase molecules at mouse skeletal junctions. *Nature*, 234:207.

Bauer, W. C., Blumberg, J. M., and Zacks, S. I. (1962): Short and long-term ultrastructural changes in denervated mouse motor endplates. In: *Proc. IV Int. Congr. Neuropathology*, edited by Georg Thieme, pp. 16–18. Stuttgart.

Berg, D. K., Kelly, R. B., Sargent, P. B., Williamson, P., and Hall, Z. (1972): Binding of α-bungarotoxin to acetylcholine receptors in mammalian muscle. *Proc. Natl. Acad. Sci. U.S.A.*, 69:147.

Betz, W., and Sakmann, B. (1971): "Disjunction" of frog neuromuscular synapses with proteolytic enzymes. *Nature New Biology*, 232:94.

Birks, R., Katz, B., and Miledi, R. (1960): Physiological and structural changes at the amphibian myoneural junction in the course of nerve degeneration. *J. Physiol.*, 150:145.

Blasie, J. K., and Worthington, C. R. (1969): Planar liquid-like arrangement of photopigment molecules in frog retinal receptor disk membranes. *J. Mol. Biol.*, 39:417.

Boëthius, J., and Knutsson, E. (1970): Resting membrane potential in chick muscle during ontogeny. *J. Exp. Zool.*, 174:281.

Chang, C. C., and Lee, C. Y. (1963): Isolation of neurotoxins from the venom of *Bungarus multicinctus* and their modes of neuromuscular blocking action. *Arch. Int. Pharmacodyn. Ther.*, 144:241.

Changeux, J.-P., Kasai, M., and Lee, C. Y. (1970): Use of a snake venom toxin to characterize the cholinergic receptor protein. *Proc. Natl. Acad. Sci. U.S.A.*, 67:1241.

Changeux, J.-P., Meunier, J.-C., and Huchet, M. (1971): Studies on the cholinergic receptor protein of *Electrophorus electricus*. 1. An assay for the cholinergic site and solubilization of the receptor protein from electric tissue. *Mol. Pharmacol.*, 7:538.

Crevier, M., and Bélanger, L. F. (1955): Simple method for histochemical detection of esterase activity. *Science*, 122:556.

del Castillo, J., and Katz, B. (1955): On the localization of acetylcholine receptors. *J. Physiol.*, 128:157.

Drachman, D. B., and Witzke, F. (1972): Trophic regulation of acetylcholine sensitivity of muscle: Effect of electrical stimulation. *Science*, 176:514.

Edidin, M., and Fambrough, D. (1973): Fluidity of the surface of cultured muscle fibers: Rapid lateral diffusion of marked surface antigens. *J. Cell Biol.*, 57:27.

Emmelin, N., and Malm, L. (1965): Development of supersensitivity as dependent on the length of degenerating nerve fibers. *Quart. J. Exp. Physiol.*, 50:142.

Fambrough, D. M. (1970): Acetylcholine sensitivity of muscle fiber membranes: Mechanism of regulation by motoneurons. *Science*, 168:372.

Fambrough, D. M., and Hartzell, H. C. (1972): Acetylcholine receptors: Number and distribution at neuromuscular junctions in rat diaphragm. *Science*, 176:189.

Fambrough, D. M., and Rash, J. E. (1971): Development of acetylcholine sensitivity during myogenesis. *Dev. Biol.*, 26:55.

Feltz, A., and Mallart, A. (1971): An analysis of acetylcholine responses of junctional and extrajunctional receptors of frog muscle fibers. *J. Physiol.*, 218:85.

Fischman, D. A. (1970): The synthesis and assembly of myofibrils in embryonic muscle. *Curr. Top. Develop. Biol.*, 5:235.

Frye, L. D., and Edidin, M. (1970): The rapid intermixing of cell surface antigens after formation of mouse-human heterokaryons. *J. Cell Sci.*, 7:319.

Grampp, W., Harris, J. B., and Thesleff, S. (1972): Inhibition of denervation changes in skeletal muscle by blockers of protein synthesis. *J. Physiol.*, 221:743.

Guth, L. (1968): "Trophic" influence of nerve on muscle. *Physiol. Rev.*, 48:645.

Guth, L. (1969): Trophic effects of vertebrate neurons. *Neurosci. Res. Prog. Bull.*, 7:1.

Hall, Z. W. (1973): Multiple forms of acetylcholinesterase and their distribution in end plate and non-end plate regions of rat diaphragm muscle. *J. Neurobiol.*, 4:343.

Hall, Z. W., and Kelly, R. B. (1971): Enzymatic detachment of end plate acetylcholinesterase in muscle. *Nature New Biology*, 232:62.

Harris, A. J., Heinemann, S., Schubert, D., and Tarakis, H. (1971): Trophic interaction between cloned tissue culture lines of nerve and muscle. *Nature*, 231:296.

Hartzell, H. C., and Fambrough, D. M. (1972): Acetylcholine receptors: Distribution and extrajunctional density in rat diaphragm after denervation correlated with acetylcholine sensitivity. *J. Gen. Physiol.*, 60:248.

Hartzell, H. C., and Fambrough, D. M. (1973): Acetylcholine receptor production and incorporation into membranes of developing muscle fibers. *Dev. Biol.*, 30:153.

Hazelwood, C. F. (1972): Pumps or no pumps. *Science*, 177:815.

Hazelwood, C. F., and Nichols, B. L. (1969): Changes in muscle sodium, potassium, chloride, water and voltage during maturation in the rat: An experimental and theoretical study. *Johns Hopkins Med. J.*, 125:119.

Heitzmann, H. (1972): Rhodopsin is the predominant protein of rod outer segment membranes. *Nature New Biology*, 235:114.

Heywood, S. M., Dowben, R. M., and Rich, A. (1967): The identification of polysomes synthesizing myosin. *Proc. Natl. Acad. Sci. U.S.A.*, 57:1002.

Hirano, H. (1967): Ultrastructural study on the morphogenesis of the neuromuscular junction in the skeletal muscle of the chick. *Z. Zellforsch.*, 79:198.

Hodgkin, A. L., and Katz, B. (1949): The effect of sodium ions on the chemical activity of the giant axon of the squid. *J. Physiol.*, 108:37.

Holtzer, H. (1970): Myogenesis. In: *Cell Differentiation*, edited by O. Schjeide and J. deVellis, pp. 476–503. Van Nostrand Reinhold Co., New York.

Hunter, W. M., and Greenwood, F. C. (1962): Preparation of iodine-131 labelled human growth hormone of high specific activity. *Nature*, 194:495.

Jacobson, M. (1970): *Developmental Neurobiology.* Holt, Rinehart and Winston, New York.

Kano, M., and Shimada, Y. (1971): Innervation and acetylcholine sensitivity of skeletal cells differentiated *in vitro* from chick embryo. *J. Cell. Physiol.*, 78:233.

Katz, B., and Miledi, R. (1964): The development of acetylcholine sensitivity in nerve-free segments of skeletal muscle. *J. Physiol.*, 170:389.

Kelly, A. M., and Zacks, S. I. (1969): The fine structure of motor end plate morphogenesis. *J. Cell. Biol.*, 42:154.

Koelle, G. B., and Horn, R. S. (1968): Acetyldisulfide ($CH_3COS)_2$, a major active component in the thiolacetic acid histochemical method for acetylcholinesterase. *J. Histochem. Cytochem.*, 16:743.

Lee, C. Y., Tseng, L. F., and Chiu, T. H. (1967): Influence of denervation on the localization of neurotoxins from elapid venoms in rat diaphragm. *Nature*, 215:1177.

Leuzinger, W., Goldberg, M., and Cauvin, E. (1969): Molecular properties of acetylcholinesterase. *J. Mol. Biol.*, 40:217.

Lømø, T., and Rosenthal, J. (1971): Development of acetylcholine sensitivity in muscle following blockage of nerve impulses. *J. Physiol.*, 216:52P.

Lømø, T., and Rosenthal, J. (1972): Control of ACh sensitivity by muscle activity in the rat. *J. Physiol.*, 221:493.

Luco, J. V., and Eyzaguirre, C. (1955): Fibrillation and hypersensitivity to ACh in denervated muscle: Effect of length of degenerating nerve fibers. *J. Neurophysiol.*, 18:65.

Massoulie, J., and Rieger, F. (1969): L'acetylcholinestérase des organes électriques de poissons (torpille octgymnote); complexes membranaires. *Europ. J. Biochem.*, 11:441.

Meunier, J.-C., Olsen, R. W., Menez, A., Fromageot, P., Boquet, P., and Changeux, J.-P. (1972): Some physical properties of the cholinergic receptor protein from *Electrophorus electricus* revealed by a tritiated α-toxin from *Naja nigricollis* venom. *Biochemistry*, 11:1200.

Miledi, R. (1960*a*): The acetylcholine sensitivity of frog muscle fibers after complete and partial denervation. *J. Physiol.*, 151:1.

Miledi, R. (1960*b*): Junctional and extrajunctional acetylcholine receptors in skeletal muscle fibers. *J. Physiol.*, 151:24.

Miledi, R., Molinoff, P., and Potter, L. (1971): Isolation of the cholinergic receptor protein of *Torpedo* electric tissue. *Nature*, 229:554.

Miledi, R., and Potter, L. T. (1971): Acetylcholine receptors in muscle fibers. *Nature*, 233:599.

Miledi, R., and Slater, C. R. (1968): Electrophysiology and electron-microscopy of rat neuromuscular junctions after nerve degeneration. *Proc. Roy. Soc. B*, 169:289.

Nickel, E., and Waser, P. G. (1968): Elektronen mikroskopische Untersuchungen am Diaphragma der Maus nach einseitiger Phrenikotomie. I. Die degenerierende motorische End platte. *Z. Zellforsch.*, 88:278.

Padykula, H. A., and Gauthier, G. F. (1970): The ultrastructure of the neuromuscular junctions of mammalian red, white and intermediate skeletal muscle fibers. *J. Cell Biol.*, 46:27.

Raftery, M. A., Schmidt, J., Clark, D. G., and Wolcott, R. G. (1971): Demonstration of a specific α-bungarotoxin binding component in *Electrophorus electricus* membranes. *Biochim. Biophys. Res. Comm.*, 45:1622.

Ray, T. K., Lieberman, I., and Lansing, A. I. (1968): Synthesis of the plasma membrane of the liver cell. *Biochim. Biophys. Res. Comm.*, 31:54.

Rieger, F., Bon, S., and Massoulie, J. (1972): Conversion spontanée des formes acetylcholinestéraseiques natives de l'organe électrique de gymnote, en forme globulaire. *C. R. Acad. Sci. Série D*, 274:1753.

Rogers, A. W., Darzynkiewicz, Z., Salpeter, M. M., Ostrowski, K., and Barnard, E. A. (1969): Quantitative studies on enzymes in structures in striated muscles by labeled inhibitor methods. I. The number of acetylcholinesterase molecules and of other DFP-reactive sites at motor endplates, measured by radioautography. *J. Cell Biol.*, 41:665.

Salafsky, J. B., and Prewitt, M. A. (1968): Development of fibrillation potentials in denervated fast and slow skeletal muscle. *Am. J. Physiol.*, 215:637.

Samaha, F. J., Guth, L., and Albers, R. W. (1970): The neuronal regulation of gene expression in the muscle cell. *Exp. Neurol.*, 27:276.

Shapiro, A. L., Viñuela, E., and Maizel, Jr., J. V. (1967): Molecular weight estimation of polypeptide chains by electrophoresis in SDS-polyacrylamide gels. *Biochim. Biophys. Res. Comm.*, 28:815.

Singer, S. J., and Nicholson, G. L. (1972): The fluid mosaic model of the structure of cell membranes. *Science*, 175:720.

Steinhardt, R. A., Lundin, L., and Mazia, D. (1971): Bioelectric responses of the echinoderm egg to fertilization. *Proc. Natl. Acad. Sci. U.S.A.*, 68:2426.

Teräväinen, H. (1968): Development of the myoneural junction in the rat. *Z. Zellforsch.*, 87:249.

Vernadakis, A., and Woodbury, D. M. (1964). Electrolyte and nitrogen changes in skeletal muscle of developing rats. *Am. J. Physiol.*, 206:1365.

Warren, L., and Glick, M. C. (1968): Membranes of animal cells. II. The metabolism and turnover of the surface membrane. *J. Cell Biol.*, 37:729.

Weisenseel, M. H., and Jaffe, L. F. (1972): Membrane potential and impedance of developing fucoid eggs. *Dev. Biol.*, 27:555.

Woodward, D. J., Hoffer, B. J., Siggins, G. R., and Bloom, F. E. (1971): The ontogenetic development of synaptic junctions, synaptic activation and responsiveness to neurotransmitter substances in rat cerebellar Purkinje cells. *Brain Res.*, 34:73.

Yaffe, D. (1969): Cellular aspects of muscle differentiation *in vitro. Curr. Top. Develop. Biol.*, 4:37.

Synaptic Transmission and Neuronal Interaction
Raven Press, New York 1974

Role of Acetylcholine Receptors in Synapse Formation

A. John Harris

Department of Physiology, University of Otago Medical School, Dunedin, New Zealand

One of the most obvious questions regarding the nervous system is: How are nerve cells and effector cells connected together so that the system can function? Despite more than 100 years of experimentation there has been little progress toward any fundamental answer to this question. Probably the most important advance has been the recognition that the arrangements and interconnections of nerve cells are very orderly, and, even at a fine level, very much the same from animal to animal.

Since many of these connections develop before the animal has had a chance to use the nervous system, it is necessary to postulate the existence of mechanisms which allow neurons to recognize the cells on which they should form synapses. The ways in which these mechanisms operate are largely unknown.

I. THE USE OF MODEL SYSTEMS

Few studies of the physiology of synapse formation during embryonic development have been made directly, mainly because of the technical difficulties involved. Most of our present knowledge of the phenomena and mechanisms involved in the development of synaptic connections comes from experiments on model systems, either employing adult synapses, which are denervated and allowed to regenerate in the animal, or by the use of culture techniques, with either tissue explants or disaggregated cells.

The principal difficulties encountered when working with embryonic materials are the limited possibilities of visualizing single cells and watching their development over a period of time; the lack of homogeneity of the tissues, with concomitant problems in biochemical analysis; and the limited number of experimental procedures that are compatible with the life of the organism. Ideally, the best preparation would be one with a homogenous population of cells arranged so that individual cells could be visualized and available for study for an extended period of time. Tissue culture seems to offer the best hope of providing systems of this kind. More than 60 years ago R. G. Harrison showed that it was possible to maintain nerve cells in primary culture (Harrison, 1907) and his experiment has been repeated in many different forms since then, including in recent years the maintenance of disaggregated single nerve cells under conditions where they extend axons and enter into synaptic relations with one another (Crain and Bornstein, 1972). However, primary cultures such as these are not really satisfactory for many of the questions we would like to ask. They are not homogenous, and the nerve cells do not undergo mitosis, so that the possibilities both of biochemical analysis and of the study of development are limited. The best system would use permanent tissue culture lines of cells, which could be maintained by serial transfer for an indefinite length of time, and which would retain their full normal set of developmental potentialities. An attempt to derive such a system is now in progress, and the experiments described below give some indication of the present state of the project.

II. ACETYLCHOLINE SENSITIVITY AND SYNAPSE FORMATION

Although little is known about how synapses are arranged on nerve cells during embryonic development, some information is available from studies on the nerve-muscle junction, a preparation that has provided much relevant information on the development and function of neural synapses (Katz, 1966). This junction has the advantage of experimental accessibility for electrophysiological, histological, and biochemical investigations, but has the limitation that unlike most central nervous system neurons there is usually only one synapse received on each cell.

Before receiving innervation, the embryonic skeletal muscle cell is sensitive to neurotransmitter (acetylcholine) all over its surface (Diamond and Miledi, 1962). Near the time when nerve-muscle interaction is beginning there is a gradient of sensitivity from the center to the ends of the muscle fibers, but it is not known whether this gradient is present before the initial approach of the nerves. Initially, several motor nerve terminals make contact with each muscle cell (Redfern, 1970), and acetylcholine sensitivity begins to become restricted to these points of contact. Eventually one of these nerves takes control of the whole muscle fiber, and the other contacts are lost. Acetylcholine sensitivity becomes restricted to the close vicinity of the nerve-muscle junction (Peper and McMahan, 1972). There is some evidence that this junction is never completely stable, and that the nerve terminal is continually sending out new sprouts and retracting old ones throughout life (Barker and Ip, 1966; Tuffery, 1971). If another motor nerve is implanted into the muscle, it will grow and send ramifications throughout the muscle, but will make few or no functional synapses so long as the original innervation is maintained (Aitken, 1950; Fex, Sonesson, Thesleff and Zelena, 1966). Cutting the original nerve allows the implanted nerve to form functional synapses as soon as 3 days later (Fex and Thesleff, 1967). From the results of experiments such as these it is necessary to assume a mechanism whereby the possession of a normal innervation restricts the ability of a muscle fiber to accept contacts from other nerves, and that a denervated muscle becomes attractive to new innervation.

There are circumstances under which this restriction can be overcome. If a muscle fiber is locally damaged, the damaged portion will accept the formation of a new synapse despite the continued presence and function of the original innervation (Miledi, 1963). Poisoning a muscle with botulinus toxin has a similar effect; the poisoned muscle will accept new innervation, despite the presence, although not in this case the function, of the original nerve (Fex et al., 1966). A denervated muscle, as indicated previously, will accept new innervation. New synapses form preferentially at the sites of the old end plates (Miledi, 1960b; Aitken, 1965; Bennett, McLachlan, and Taylor, 1973a) but they may form elsewhere (Guth and Zalewski, 1963; Gwyn and Aitken, 1966).

The common factor in these experiments is that the region of muscle accepting the new synapse is sensitive to acetylcholine. A muscle fiber normally possesses acetylcholine receptors at the end plate (Peper and McMahan, 1972; Hartzell and Fambrough, 1973) and sometimes at the muscle-tendon junctions (Katz and Miledi, 1964a) but not elsewhere. A damaged portion of a muscle fiber develops acetylcholine sensitivity during the course of repair (Katz and Miledi, 1964b); a denervated muscle acquires the well-known denervation hypersensitivity (Cannon and Rosenblueth, 1949) which involves, among other things, the spread of acetylcholine sensitivity over the whole surface of each muscle fiber (Axelsson and Thesleff, 1959; Miledi, 1960a). A botulinus-poisoned muscle behaves in many respects as a denervated one, and becomes hypersensitive to acetylcholine (Thesleff, 1960).

Denervation of nerve cells, both in the central nervous system and the autonomic nervous system, also gives rise to hypersensitivity (Cannon and Rosenblueth, 1949) and in the case of parasympathetic ganglion cells in the heart the mechanism leading to hypersensitivity has been shown to be the same as in muscle (Kuffler, Dennis, and Harris, 1971). Sensitivity to neural transmitter (acetylcholine) is restricted to the close vicinity of individual synaptic boutons on the ganglion cell surface (Harris, Kuffler, and Dennis, 1971b) but, after section of the vagosympathetic nerve to the heart, the cells become sensitive over their whole surface. Regeneration of the preganglionic nerve leads to the removal of this diffuse sensitivity at an early stage in reinnervation, leaving very discrete sensitive spots associated with the new synaptic boutons (M. J. Dennis and A. J. Harris, *unpublished results*). This type of experiment has not been done in any direct way with central nervous system cells, but it is known that denervated neurons within the CNS will accept new innervation from neighboring nerve cells (Raisman, 1969). It seems reasonable to assume that the basis of denervation hypersensitivity in the CNS is the same as in the periphery.

This general association between regions of a cell that will accept synapses and the localization on the cell surface of receptors for neurotransmitter substances has never been shown to be causal. It remains an interesting question whether the receptors themselves are involved in the communication process between an ingrowing nerve and its presumptive postsynaptic connection, or whether their presence is coincident with some other membrane property of more direct relevance to synapse formation.

We asked this question directly by blocking the acetylcholine receptors on the surface of developing muscle fibers with snake venom before they had had an opportunity to become innervated, letting nerves grow toward the muscles, and then looking for signs of interaction between the two tissues. The experiment was done with a model system, using cloned cell lines in tissue culture, and taking the raised acetylcholine sensitivity near the nerve-muscle contact point as a marker for interaction. The presynaptic element in the model system is a mouse neuroblastoma, and the postsynaptic tissue is a cloned line of rat skeletal muscle myoblasts (Harris, Heinemann, Schubert, and Tarakis, 1971a).

III. EXPRESSION OF DIFFERENTIATED FUNCTIONS BY NEUROBLASTOMA

Neuroblastoma in man is a tumor most frequently seen in young children. The tumor is often made up of a mass of rapidly growing round cells, but these may sometimes form rosettes, or even differentiate further into nerve-like cells with axons (ganglioneuroma) (Stout, 1947). Cells from human tumors, when placed in tissue culture with a surface to which they can attach, extend neurites and take on a nerve-like appearance (Murray and Stout, 1947; Goldstein, Burdman, and Journey, 1964). Recently, cloned tissue culture lines of neuroblastoma cells have been derived from a mouse tumor (C1300, the Jackson Laboratories) (Augusti-Tocco and Sato, 1969; Schubert, Humphreys, Baroni, and Cohn, 1969; Olmstead, Carlson, Klebe, Ruddle, and Rosenbaum, 1970; Seeds, Gilman, Amano, and Nirenberg, 1970).

The usefulness of neuroblastoma as a model for studying the development and function of the nervous system depends on the extent to which the properties of nerve cells in general can be studied in it. Most nerve cells have a specialized region (dendrites and/or cell body) which receives synapses from other cells; they have a long process (axon) which transmits nerve impulses to other cells; they have specialized areas for the synthesis, storage, and release of neural transmitter substances (synaptic terminals); and they may have long-term (trophic) effects on the expression and maintenance of differentiation in the tissues they innervate. All these properties are at least partially present in clones from the C1300 tumor, although they are not all equally accessible to study. Some can be demonstrated even in rapidly growing and dividing round cells from suspension culture; others are expressed only if the cells can be maintained for some time under adequate conditions without cell division (Augusti-Tocco and Sato, 1969; Schubert et al., 1969; Nelson, Ruffner, and Nirenberg, 1969; Harris and Dennis, 1970; Nelson, Peacock, and Amano, 1971*a;* Nelson, Peacock, Amano, and Minna, 1971*b;* Rosenberg, Vandeventer, de Francesco, and Friedkin, 1971; Amano, Richelson, and Nirenberg, 1972).

The different clones from the C1300 neuroblastoma may be grown in suspension culture as round cells, which often aggregate into large floating clumps, but if they are plated on a suitable substrate they will extend processes (Fig. 1), which are briefly retracted during mitosis and then re-extended. Three types of process can be recognized: short hairlike extensions that anchor cells to the substrate; small neurites, usually less than 50 μm long, often with many branches, which in the electron micrograph appear as simple extensions of cytoplasm and contain ribosomes as well

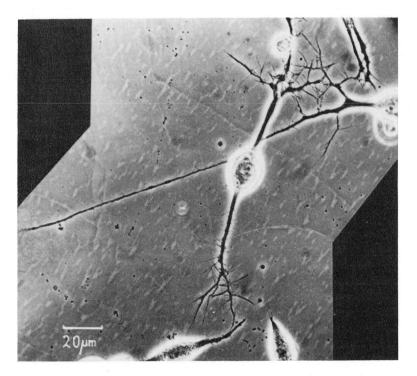

FIG. 1. Neuroblastoma cells extending processes. (Clone N12, plated 7 days at 32°C in medium with 10% fetal calf serum.)

as other normal intracellular inclusions; and longer, 50 μm to several mm, axon-like processes, which contain neurotubules (Schubert, Humphreys, de Vitry, and Jacob, 1971*a*).

Whereas some nerve-like properties of neuroblastoma may be expressed even in the round cells from suspension culture (e.g., action potential generation and synthesis of neurotransmitters), both these and the other nerve-like properties are best seen when the cells have gone for some time without mitosis, while maintained on a surface to which they can attach, under appropriate culture conditions. One easy way of achieving this state is to grow the cells in their normal medium, with 10 or 20% fetal serum, but to keep them at 32°C, which greatly slows cell division. Cells can then be maintained at relatively low density for a month or more without sub-culturing, and during this time they undergo an extensive morphological differentiation, many of the cells extending processes several millimeters long.

There are differences between cells even when cloned cells grown in the same dish are compared, but, in general, the well-differentiated cells possess a vigorous action potential mechanism (Fig. 2) and have passive membrane properties similar to those of normal sympathetic ganglion cells. Parts of the cell surface develop a sensitivity to acetylcholine, and small pulses of this drug when delivered through an iontophoretic pipette so as to affect only a few square microns of cell surface cause a brief depolarization of the cell, which, if of sufficient magnitude, may initiate an action potential (Fig. 2). The cell surface is not always uniformly sensitive to acetylcholine.

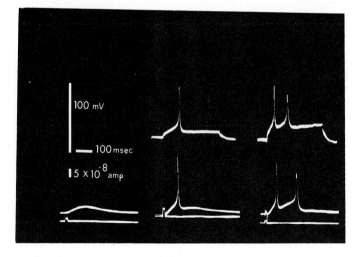

FIG. 2. Action potentials invoked in a neuroblastoma cell by an intracellular current pulse *(top traces)* or by applying a pulse of acetylcholine to the cell body with an iontophoretic pipette *(bottom traces).* The acetylcholine current pulse is monitored below the bottom traces. (Clone C1A, plated for 1 month at 32°C in medium with 10% fetal calf serum.)

A few days after initiation of the culture, a low-level sensitivity may be found on the cell body or at the tips of the growing processes. After a longer period, a variety of patterns is seen. Some cells seem uniformly sensitive. Others can be found where only the cell body and one process are sensitive, although another process may be sensitive only on its growing tip (Fig. 3).

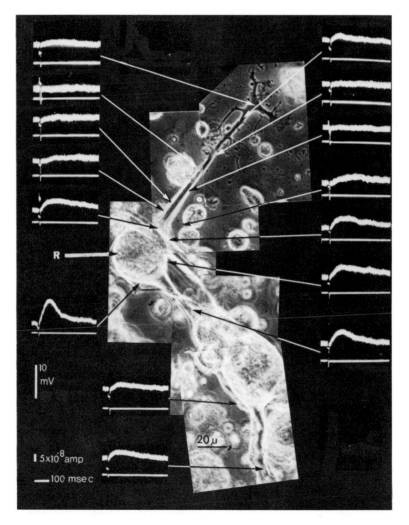

FIG. 3. Distribution of acetylcholine sensitivity on the surface of a neuroblastoma cell with two processes. The top process is insensitive except near the growth cone at its tip, whereas the bottom process is sensitive along its length. The top of each pair of traces shows the response to the pulse of acetylcholine released from the iontophoretic pipette by the current pulse monitored in each lower trace. The position of the recording electrode is shown by the arrow (R). (Clone C1A, plated for 1 month at 32°C in medium with 10% fetal calf serum.)

These differences suggest an analogy with normal axons and dendrites (assuming that the evidence from muscle, where the distribution of acetylcholine sensitivity provides a marker for places where synapses may form, is relevant to phenomena in nerve cells).

The differentiated cells, from some clones at least, may show an increase in content of choline acetyltransferase, the enzyme used for synthesis of the neurotransmitter acetylcholine (Rosenberg et al., 1971). Acetyl-

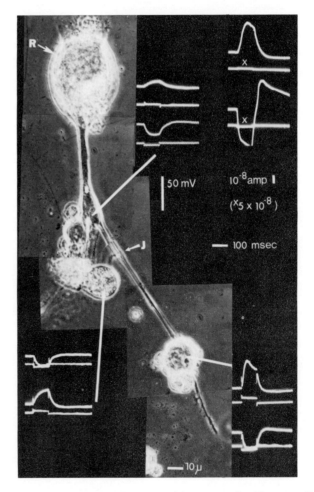

FIG. 4. Electrical coupling between four neuroblastoma cells. The recording electrode *(R)* was inserted in the top cell, and a current-passing electrode inserted into each of the three lower cells in turn. Each set of traces shows the voltage response recorded from the top cell in response to depolarizing and hyperpolarizing current pulses delivered to the other three cells. The current pulse is monitored below each voltage record. The point where the middle cell sent its process to join the others is marked *(J)*. (Clone C1A, plated 1 month at 32°C in medium with 10% fetal calf serum.)

cholinesterase also increases, but its relevance as an indicator of nerve-like differentiation is unclear as various tissue culture cell lines that definitely are not of neural origin, e.g., plasmacytoma, also show an increase in their content of this enzyme in aging cultures (Schubert, Tarakis, Harris, and Heinemann, 1971*b*).

Cultured neuroblastoma cells have not been seen to form synapses with one another, although a small proportion may become electrically coupled (Fig. 4). Structural evidence for synapse formation has been reported from studies of human neuroblastomas (Greenberg, Rosenthal, and Falk, 1969). Another nerve-like property of neuroblastoma cells is their exertion of a trophic effect on cultured muscle cells; and it is this effect that we study in our model system (Harris et al., 1971*a*).

IV. EXPRESSION OF DIFFERENTIATION IN CULTURED MYOBLASTS

The postsynaptic element in our model system is a permanent cell line of rat skeletal muscle myoblasts, originally derived from primary cultures of rat skeletal muscle (Yaffe, 1968). We maintain a cloned line of these cells, L6, by serial subculture of mononucleate myoblasts. Preparations of myotubes are obtained by letting the myoblasts grow to confluence, at which time they fuse to form a network of large multinucleate cells. The further development of the cultures is variable; some spontaneously develop into striated muscle cells, while others remain in the myotube stage. Physiological properties of the cells during the earlier phases of this sequence have recently been described in detail (Harris et al., 1971*a;* Patrick, Heinemann, Lindstrom, Schubert, and Steinbach, 1972; Kidokoro, 1973).

When electrically stimulated at their normal resting potential, which lies in the range −60 to −70 mV, the mononucleate myoblasts do not produce action potentials, nor can they be depolarized by acetylcholine. If they are hyperpolarized to approximately −100 mV, a very small regenerative electrical response can be induced (Kidokoro, 1973). The mononucleate cells do respond to acetylcholine, but the response is a long-lasting hyperpolarization (Fig. 5) and it is not inhibited by curare.

After fusion of the myoblasts to form multinucleate myotubes there is a marked increase in electrical excitability, even in binucleate cells, so that, if the resting potential is adequate, action potentials can be evoked. Delayed rectification is not seen in the myoblasts, but it develops after fusion, so that an action potential is followed by a long-lasting hyperpolarization. At a later time a stage is reached where most cells in a dish spontaneously discharge action potentials at a steady rate.

The development of a depolarizing response to acetylcholine is not so clearly associated with cell fusion. Binucleate myotubes or even cells with up to seven nuclei may be seen where the only response to acetylcholine

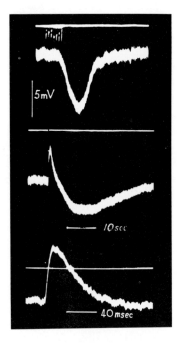

FIG. 5. Responses to iontophoretic application of acetylcholine to developing muscle cells. *(Top):* Slow hyperpolarization seen after delivery of a series of pulses of acetylcholine to a mononucleate myoblast. Similar responses may be seen in some myotubes shortly after fusion has begun. *(Center):* Dual response, depolarization followed by hyperpolarization seen in a myotube with four nuclei. Other myotubes in this dish with similar numbers of nuclei could give purely depolarizing or purely hyperpolarizing responses. *(Bottom):* Depolarizing response to acetylcholine seen in a mature myotube. The acetylcholine pulse is monitored above each voltage record. Note the large difference in time scale between the top two records and the bottom one.

is the hyperpolarization seen in unfused myoblasts. Other cells examined shortly after fusion give a biphasic response to acetylcholine, a fast depolarization followed by the slow hyperpolarization (Fig. 5). However, once a substantial degree of cell fusion has taken place in a culture dish, all the cells examined give the fast rising depolarizing response to acetylcholine that is seen near the end-plate regions of normal rat muscle cells (del Castillo and Katz, 1954; Krnjević and Miledi, 1958). Cells examined shortly after fusion sometimes have marked differences in degree of acetylcholine sensitivity at different parts of their surface. This usually occurs at two distinct regions, with a sharp boundary between them, and presumably is the result of the recent fusion of two myotubes with different levels of sensitivity. A few days later the acetylcholine sensitivity is uniformly distributed over the surface of all the individual myotubes in the culture dish, with regional differences greater than twofold on any one cell being uncommon.

V. EFFECTS OF INTERACTION BETWEEN
NEUROBLASTOMA AND MUSCLE

When neuroblastoma cells are added to a culture of fused muscle cells, they settle on the myotubes and begin to extend neurites. If the neuroblastoma cells come from a rapidly growing culture and if the muscle cells are in their normal medium, the neuroblastoma cells continue to divide, so that in a few days the culture becomes overgrown with neuroblastoma. For this reason it has been necessary to devise procedures to limit the growth of neuroblastoma cells. A number of different methods have been worked out, the simplest being to "predifferentiate" the neuroblastoma cells. This is done by maintaining the neuroblastoma cells for several days in medium with low serum (1 to 2%) in which case they go through only one or two cell divisions and then extend long neurites (Seeds et al., 1970; Schubert et al., 1971*a*). The cells are then lifted off the culture dish by treatment with viokase and added to a muscle culture, preferably one that has gone for 4 or 5 days without a change of medium. Under these conditions a large proportion of the neuroblastoma cells extend processes immediately, without cell division. Some of these processes may then contact muscle cells. Time-lapse cinemicrography shows that these extending neurites are very mobile, with the neuroblastoma cell continually sending out and retracting numerous extensions as if exploring its environment. However, some points at which a neurite contacts a muscle cell seem relatively stable, at least for periods of a day or two, and it is this type of contact that we look for when mapping the distribution of acetylcholine sensitivity on myotubes. Such contacts are recognized by looking for points where a process ends on a myotube, or where it makes an abrupt change in direction as it overlies the myotube.

The most striking effect of interaction between neuroblastoma processes and myotubes is a raised acetylcholine sensitivity on the surface of the myotube close to the point of contact. Acetylcholine sensitivity is measured by impaling a cell with a recording microelectrode, and then bringing another microelectrode filled with a concentrated solution of acetylcholine close to the surface of the cell and passing a pulse of current through it. The sensitivity is expressed as the ratio of depolarization evoked to the amount of electric charge passed through the pipette, the units being mV/nC. Typically, myotubes have sensitivities of the order of 100 mV/nC, regardless of which point on their surface is stimulated. If, however, a neuroblastoma process touches the cell, a greater sensitivity can be measured close to the contact point (Figs. 6 and 7). When cells are examined 2 days after interaction, differences in sensitivity are already apparent, contact points being two to four times more sensitive than the extrajunctional area; 5 days after interaction differences in the range of four to 10 times are commonly seen; and several weeks after interaction (Fig. 7) differences greater than 20 times have been found.

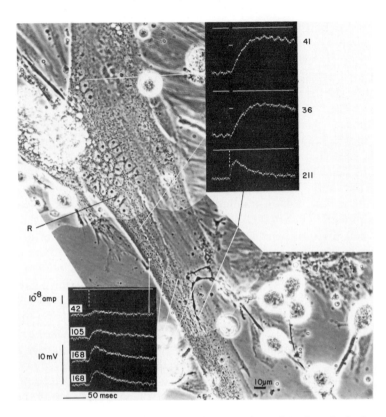

FIG. 6. Localization of acetylcholine sensitivity near the point of contact of a neuro-blastoma cell process with a myotube, 7 days after mixing the cells. In the region of contact, acetylcholine sensitivity is approximately 200 mV/nC, whereas by 50 μm away it has fallen to the background level of 40 mV/nC. The acetylcholine current pulses are monitored above each voltage record (1 msec pulses marked with dotted lines). Numbers are acetylcholine sensitivity in mV/nC.

The raised sensitivity is closely restricted to the vicinity of the contact and is not detectable more than 50 μm away; sensitivity often reaches background levels within 10 μm of a contact. We have argued (Harris et al., 1971a) that this raised acetylcholine sensitivity at the contact point may involve the same mechanisms that operate during the early stages of synapse formation in an animal. The most pertinent evidence for this view is that when primary cultures of spinal cord neurons are mixed with the cloned muscle line the first indication of interaction is a raised sensitivity near the contact point (A. J. Harris, *unpublished results*). In 17-day-old rat embryos, a stage when the first signs of nerve muscle contact can be detected physiologically, Diamond and Miledi (1962) noted that acetylcholine sensitivity tended to be greater near the middle of the diaphragm muscle, in the region where the mature synapse is later found, than near the ends.

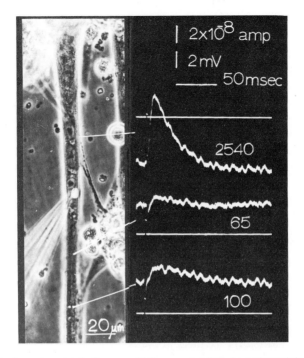

FIG. 7. Localization of acetylcholine sensitivity examined 27 days after mixing the different cell types. Representative traces are given, showing the difference between sensitivities at the contact point and elsewhere of approximately 25 ×. Fine mapping near the contact point showed that sensitivity fell by more than 10-fold over a distance of 10 μm from the junction *(not shown)*. Numbers are acetylcholine sensitivity in mV/nC.

The other evidence concerns the specificity of the effect. Clearly the phenomena seen with the model system should depend on the nerve-like character of the neuroblastoma, and would be less likely to be of relevance to the normal process of synapse formation if they could be shown to occur with cells that definitely were not of neural origin. We have so far been able to test this point with only one type of cell. This occurred when interacting primary cultures of spinal cord cells with the myotubes; not only did nerve cell processes contact the muscle cells, but some glial cells did also. Glial cells were identified by their higher resting potentials and their inability to produce an action potential; in no case could we find any difference in sensitivity on the myotube surface associated with a point of contact (A. J. Harris, *unpublished results*).

VI. INTERACTION IN THE PRESENCE OF *NAJA NAJA* α-NEUROTOXIN

We used the model system of L6 myoblasts and N18 neuroblastoma to find whether the presence of functional acetylcholine receptors is a necessary prerequisite for nerve-muscle recognition and interaction. Acetylcholine sensitivity was abolished by adding *Naja naja* α-neurotoxin to the myoblasts before adding the neuroblastoma cells.

Patrick et al. (1972) have shown that this toxin, a protein of known sequence with 71 amino acid residues (Nakai, Sasaki, and Hayashi, 1971), specifically binds to acetylcholine receptors on the surface of L6 myotubes. The specific binding site is defined by the ability of agents such as curare to protect it from inactivation by toxin. Binding is reversible, but toxin dissociates very slowly, with a half-life of binding of approximately 7 hr. Patrick et al. (1972) have shown that, after adding toxin to L6 myotubes, the decrement with time in the response to iontophoretic application of acetylcholine parallels the increase in amount of labeled toxin bound to myotubes, thus demonstrating that the iontophoretic assay for acetylcholine sensitivity gives a good indication of the relative number of acetylcholine receptors available on the myotube surface.

Our initial experiment was to add toxin to a muscle culture at a concentration of 2 μg/ml (3×10^{-7} M) 30 min before adding neuroblastoma. All detectable response to iontophoretic application of acetylcholine was lost less than 30 min after adding the toxin, and no response could be obtained from cells maintained for 10 days in the continued presence of toxin, showing that it remained stable under these conditions.

After adding predifferentiated neuroblastoma cells, the cultures were maintained for 4 days or more and then examined with microelectrodes. Neuroblastoma clone N18 was used for these experiments due to its very low content of choline acetyltransferase (Amano et al., 1972). Each culture dish was washed 10 times with normal tissue culture medium in order to remove unbound toxin, and dishes were then examined at various times after washing. Initially, no response to iontophoretically applied acetylcholine could be seen, but within 2 hr after the wash a small response could be evoked from most cells. By approximately 12 hr after the wash, sensitivity had returned to normal levels.

As soon as any sensitivity could be detected, a difference between junctional and extrajunctional sensitivity was clearly apparent. If the experiment was done 2 hr after the wash, larger than normal acetylcholine pulses had to be applied in order to produce a measurable effect, but regions of myotube membrane close to neuroblastoma contacts were consistently two to 10 times more sensitive than any other area of the muscle.

The results of a series of such experiments are presented in Fig. 8. In this figure we compare the sensitivity of junctional spots with the mean sensitivity of from two to 20 other spots (means seven spots per cell) elsewhere on the cell. In Fig. 9 typical records made during such an experiment are presented. Not only were junctional spots more sensitive than spots elsewhere on the same cell, but also they were more sensitive than spots on myotubes in the same dish that did not receive contacts from neuroblastoma cells.

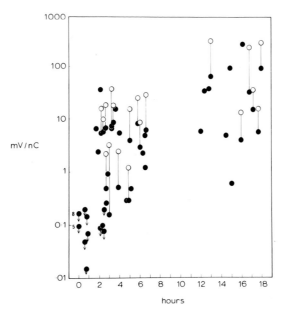

FIG. 8. Sensitivity to acetylcholine on myotubes at various times after washing off *Naja* toxin with normal medium. The open circles are sensitivities at points of contact with neuroblastoma processes; the filled circles are the mean sensitivity of a number of randomly chosen spots elsewhere on the cells. The vertical lines join junctional and extra-junctional measurements from the same cell. The arrows indicate limits of detection in cases where no response was seen.

Because the binding of toxin is reversible there are two possible reasons for the appearance of acetylcholine sensitivity after washing off the toxin. Receptors may have become available due to dissociation of previously bound toxin, or they may have been newly incorporated into the cell membrane. Either way, the process of communication between neuroblastoma and muscle that preceded the appearance of a neuroblastoma contact and associated localization of sensitivity on the muscle appears to have taken place in the absence of functional receptors. When function was detectable, nerve-muscle contact and localization of sensitivity had already occurred.

These preliminary experiments have now been extended in much greater detail by J. H. Steinbach, as a Ph.D. thesis project. His results (Steinbach, Harris, Patrick, Schubert, and Heinemann, 1973) show that the majority of receptors seen shortly after a simple wash are newly synthesized. If the experiment is done in the presence of an inhibitor of protein synthesis (added to the preparation some time in advance of removing toxin from the medium), sensitivity takes much longer to appear, although localization is still apparent once it does. His definitive experiment is to compete

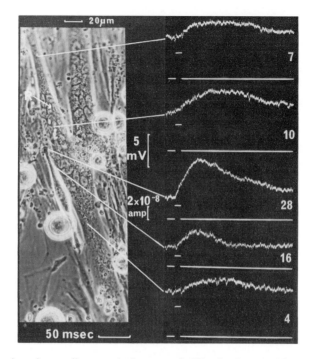

FIG. 9. Examples of recordings made from a cell 190 min after washing off toxin. Mean background sensitivity was 7.3 mV/nC, while recordings made from different spots within 10 μm of one another close to the neuroblastoma contact gave values of 47, 38, 33, and 28 mV/nC respectively. The top trace in each pair is the depolarizing response due to a pulse of current through the acetylcholine pipette, monitored in the bottom trace. Numbers are acetylcholine sensitivities in mV/nC.

the toxin off rapidly with a high concentration of curare, while suppressing protein synthesis. This procedure activates receptors that were on the muscle during the period of incubation in toxin, and his results show that interaction had taken place during this time.

A possible difficulty with these experiments is that the results may have been due to the release of acetylcholine from the tips of growing neuroblastoma processes, so that toxin was competed off small areas of muscle, and functional receptors made available. A second possibility is that the interaction requires the release of acetylcholine, but that this reacts with sites on the muscle distinct from those that are blocked by the *Naja* toxin. In designing the experiment, these difficulties were approached in two ways: a clone of neuroblastoma with a very low level of choline acetyltransferase was employed, and free toxin was present throughout the incubation, so that the chance of a receptor remaining unblocked for more than a few seconds was very low. Experiments performed by Steinbach have made these possible difficulties appear even less likely. He finds that the interaction between nerve and muscle in the presence of toxin is not affected by performing the whole experiment in the presence of a drug that inhibits the synthesis of acetylcholine.

We therefore conclude that neuroblastoma neurites were able to recognize and form attachments to muscle cells in the presence of *Naja* toxin, at a time when acetylcholine sensitivity was undetectable with the ionto-phoretic technique. Patrick et al. (1972) estimated the density of acetyl-choline receptors on L6 myotubes to be approximately $100/\mu^2$. With the dose of toxin used in the present experiments, less than one receptor/1 μ^2 would remain available at a given time. Accordingly, if active receptors are a prerequisite for recognition of the muscle surface by the growing nerve, fewer than one receptor/μ^2 must be enough. As nerve-muscle contacts were as easily found in toxin-treated as in control cultures, it seems more reasonable to accept the alternative hypothesis, that receptors are not necessary for recognition of the muscle by the nerve.

VII. RELATIONSHIP OF THE MODEL SYSTEM TO SYNAPSE FORMATION *IN VIVO*

The results described above indicate that the formation of nerve-muscle contacts with associated localization of acetylcholine sensitivity in the model system is not in any important way dependent on the availability of functional acetylcholine receptors on the muscles, nor on the synthesis of acetylcholine in the neuroblastoma cells. This conclusion is independent of whether the localization of receptors is induced by contact or whether they are present as local "hot spots" on the myotubes before contacts are made.

The important question remains as to the relevance of these findings to the development of nerve-muscle contacts during embryogenesis. There are two aspects to this question: one concerns the applicability of the model system to the *in vivo* process; the other, the nature of the communication of the trophic information between nerve and muscle if this is not mediated by acetylcholine release or by recognition of acetylcholine receptors.

The validity of the model cannot firmly be assumed at this time, but some relevant points can be discussed. The first is that we do not at present have evidence for the development of true chemical synaptic transmission in this system. Early attempts to see whether or not it developed were limited by the technical problems of overgrowth with neuroblastoma, but now that these problems are largely overcome we are again examining this question.

An interspecies difference does not interfere with the formation of functional synapses in primary tissue cultures (Crain, 1970). The C1300 neuro-blastoma is assumed to be of sympathetic origin, and sympathetic nerves do not normally innervate skeletal muscles. However, cross-innervation experiments have shown that the vagus nerve can form functional synaptic connections with skeletal muscles in frogs (Landmesser, 1971) and in rabbits (Bennett, McLachlan, and Taylor, 1973*b*). Furthermore, although Fischbach (1972) found that only about one in 20 spinal cord neurons that contacted muscle cells in primary cultures was capable of synaptic transmission, we found (A. J. Harris, *unpublished results*) that the localization of acetylcholine sensitivity to junctional regions in a similar system was more commonly seen. Thus it would seem that in these respects at least, the model system is not obviously inappropriate. Given our present knowledge, it would seem an unlikely coincidence if the mechanisms that underlie the localization of acetylcholine sensitivity in the model system were to be distinctly different from those that produce a similar effect during the early stages of synapse formation in primary cultures or *in vivo*.

Experimental work with *in vivo* systems indicates that there are a number of separable trophic effects of nerves on muscles. Some of these effects are the raising of the level of acetylcholine sensitivity at the end plate, the lowering of extrajunctional acetylcholine sensitivity, the induction of subsynaptic folds at the end plate, the induction of synaptic acetylcholinesterase, and the general maintenance of muscle weight and function. Only the first of these effects occurs in this model system, and the only comment that can presently be made about the communication mechanism is that it is independent of the cholinergic nerve-muscle communication mechanism. We do not have evidence for or against the existence of preferred spots for innervation on the muscles. We have seen no "hot spots" of acetylcholine sensitivity similar to the raised sensitivity that is retained at denervated end plates in normal muscle, but if we make a conservative estimate of the number of such spots in a dish, e.g., one per myotube, the probability of detecting these with the iontophoretic technique is low. Also, our experiment with toxin does not eliminate the possibility that whereas functional acetylcholine receptors are not prerequisites for the initiation of synapse formation they still may in some way attract growing or regenerating nerves to preferred spots on a muscle surface. This would be a simple explanation for the marked tendency for regenerating nerves to grow to old end plates in a denervated muscle, particularly as it is estimated (Fambrough and Hartzell, 1972) that acetylcholine receptors form the majority of protein molecules in end-plate membrane.

The localized sensitivity in the postjunctional membrane could have two origins; it could be due to maintenance of the noninnervated level of sensitivity while that in extrajunctional areas decreased; or it could be a heightened sensitivity due to the incorporation of additional receptors following nerve contact. Both *in vivo* and *in vitro* the second of these alternatives seems to be the important factor; extrajunctional sensitivity may or may not decline, depending perhaps on the degree of activation of the muscle (Lømø and Rosenthal, 1972), but junctional sensitivity becomes much higher than on any noninnervated muscle fiber, both in the model system (Fig. 7) and at the end plate of an adult skeletal muscle fiber in an animal.

VIII. THE USE OF CLONED CELL LINES

As was mentioned above, studying the development of the nervous system in an animal is technically very difficult, and it has long been thought that tissue culture offered great promise as a means of evading many of these technical problems. Tissue culture may take a number of different forms. Perhaps the simplest technique is to maintain small explants of tissue. These retain much of their normal tissue architecture, and explants of nervous tissue have been shown to exhibit "organotypic bioelectric properties" and to support the outgrowth of axons that can functionally innervate nearby muscle explants (Crain, 1970). On the other hand, it is difficult to visualize individual cells, and the tissue mass is heterogenous in its cell composition.

Some of these difficulties may be overcome by disaggregating the tissue into single cells. The cells may then be subject to fractionation or selection procedures, and, because they form monolayers in the culture chamber, single cells may easily be visualized. Disaggregated nervous tissue will survive in culture, and the nerve cells may grow axons and form functional synaptic contacts with other cells (Fischbach, 1970, 1972; Crain and Bornstein, 1972). Such cultures still pose problems due to the heterogeneity of cell types, and the lack of reproducibility between different preparations.

In recent years a number of permanent cell lines that exhibit differentiated features have become available. These cells multiply in tissue culture and can be maintained for an indefinite number of cell generations. Because of this property they are relatively easily cloned, so that cell cultures of great genetic homogeneity can be maintained. Cloned cell lines now available include pituitary (Tashjian, Yasumura, Levine, Sato, and Parker, 1968), hepatic (Thompson, Tomkins, and Curran, 1966), endoreticular (Cohn, 1967), and teratoma (Rosenthal, Wishnow, and Sato, 1970; Kahan and Ephrussi, 1970).

The fact that most permanent cell lines, such as the neuroblastoma lines used in the present study, are derived from tumors raises the problem of the extent to which they can be considered "normal." They are clearly abnormal in that they fail to regulate cell division in the way that normal cells should, but, without further evidence, it is unlikely that the rare event, whether it was a mutation or an expression of viral genes, that produced the neoplasm should at the same time be associated with mutations in the genetic material controlling the differentiated functions under study.

The clonal system used in the present study offers a number of particular advantages over model systems employing primary cultures or regenerating nerve fibers *in vivo*. The cells used develop through a full cycle from mitosis onward while in the culture dish, and accordingly offer a much closer analogy with normal development than do cells in primary culture. There neurons are essentially undergoing a process of regeneration, and even muscle cells, which divide in culture, may be derived from myotubes that were innervated and perhaps underwent a neurally invoked induction before they were broken down into mononucleate fragments and placed in culture. The clonal system provides homogenous material, which both gives potential for biochemical studies (e.g., Patrick et al., 1972) and aids in the reproducibility of experiments. The availability of clonal lines with different properties, such as the different C1300 clones isolated by Amano et al. (1972) with their different contents of enzymes for neurotransmitter synthesis, provides opportunities for well-controlled analyses of the relevance of the expression of particular cell functions to the phenomenon being studied. The fact that it is a tissue culture system provides the associated advantages of visibility and experimental accessibility, and allows the application of drugs and procedures which would be incompatible with life in an *in vivo* system.

The major disadvantage of the clonal system is the constant need to correlate phenomena seen in the model system with the same phenomena as they occur in primary culture and *in vivo*. Provided that this is done, systems such as the one described here may provide information about the mechanisms underlying the normal process of embrylogical development of the brain and other body tissues that could be obtained in no other way. This volume provides a clear example of how use of the several different approaches toward understanding these problems is both necessary and complementary if our knowledge of the development and function of synaptic connections is to be extended further.

ACKNOWLEDGMENTS

Much of the original impetus behind this project came from Mel Cohn at the Salk Institute. The experiments described here were done in collaboration with Steve Heinemann, Jim Patrick, David Schubert, and Joe Henry Steinbach, who are part of the neurobiology group at the Salk Institute. The work was supported by grants from the New Zealand Medical Research Council, the Muscular Dystrophy Associations of America, National Institutes of Health, National Science Foundation, and the Sloan Foundation.

REFERENCES

Aitken, J. T. (1950): Growth of nerve implants in voluntary muscle. *J. Anat.*, 84:38–49.
Aitken, J. T. (1965): Problems of reinnervation of muscle. In: *Degeneration Pattern in the Nervous System: Progress in Brain Research*, Vol. 14, edited by M. Singer and J. P. Schade, pp. 232–262. Elsevier, Amsterdam.
Amano, T., Richelson, E., and Nirenberg, M. W. (1972): Neurotransmitter synthesis by neuroblastoma clones. *P.N.A.S.*, 69:258–263.
Augusti-Tocco, G., and Sato, G. (1969): Establishment of functional clonal lines of neurons from mouse neuroblastoma. *P.N.A.S.*, 64:311–315.

Axelsson, J., and Thesleff, S. (1959): A study of supersensitivity in denervated mammalian skeletal muscle. *J. Physiol.,* 147:178–193.

Barker, D., and Ip, M. C. (1966): Sprouting and degeneration of mammalian motor axons in normal and de-afferentated skeletal muscle. *Proc. Roy. Soc. B,* 163:538–554.

Bennett, M. R., McLachlan, E. M., and Taylor, R. S. (1973a): The formation of synapses in reinnervated mammalian striated muscle. *J. Physiol.,* 233:481–500.

Bennett, M. R., McLachlan, E. M., and Taylor, R. S. (1973b): The formation of synapses in mammalian striated muscle reinnervated with autonomic preganglionic nerves. *J. Physiol.,* 233:501–518.

Cannon, W. B., and Rosenblueth, A. (1949): The supersensitivity of denervated structures. A law of denervation. *Experimental Biology Monographs,* Macmillan, New York.

Cohn, M. (1967): Natural history of the myeloma. *Symp. Quant. Biol.,* 32:211–221.

Crain, S. M. (1970): Bioelectric interactions between cultured fetal rodent spinal cord and skeletal muscle after innervation *in vitro. J. Exp. Zool.,* 173:353–369.

Crain, S. M., and Bornstein, M. B. (1972): Organotypic bioelectric activity in cultured reaggregates of dissociated rodent brain cells. *Science,* 176:182–184.

del Castillo, J., and Katz, B. (1954): The membrane change produced by the neuromuscular transmitter. *J. Physiol.,* 125:546–565.

Diamond, J., and Miledi, R. (1962): A study of foetal and new-born rat muscle fibres. *J. Physiol.,* 162:393–408.

Fambrough, D. M., and Hartzell, H. C. (1972): Acetylcholine receptors: Number and distribution at neuromuscular junctions in rat diaphragm. *Science,* 176:189–191.

Fex, S., Sonesson, B., Thesleff, S., and Zelena, J. (1966): Nerve implants in botulinum poisoned mammalian muscle. *J. Physiol.,* 184:872–882.

Fex, S., and Thesleff, S. (1967): The time required for innervation of denervated muscles by nerve implants. *Life Sci.,* 6:635–639.

Fischbach, G. D. (1970): Synaptic potentials recorded in cell cultures of nerve and muscle. *Science,* 169:1331–1333.

Fischbach, G. D. (1972): Synapse formation between dissociated nerve and muscle cells in low density cultures. *Devel. Biol.,* 28:407–429.

Goldstein, M. N., Burdman, J. A., and Journey, L. H. (1964): Long-term tissue culture of neuroblastomas. II. Morphological evidence for differentiation and maturation. *J. Nat. Cancer Inst.,* 32:165–199.

Greenberg, R., Rosenthal, I., and Falk, G. S. (1969): Electron microscopy of human tumors secreting catecholamines: Correlation with biochemical data. *J. Neuropath. Exp. Neurol.,* 28:475–500.

Guth, L., and Zalewski, A. A. (1963): Disposition of cholinesterase following implantation of nerve into innervated and denervated muscle. *Exp. Neurol.,* 7:316–326.

Gwyn, D. G., and Aitken, J. T. (1966): The formation of new motor endplates in mammalian skeletal muscle. *J. Anat.,* 100:111–126.

Harris, A. J., and Dennis, M. J. (1970): Acetylcholine sensitivity and its distribution on mouse neuroblastoma cells. *Science,* 167:1253–1255.

Harris, A. J., Heinemann, S., Schubert, D., and Tarakis, H. (1971a): Trophic interaction between cloned tissue culture lines of nerve and muscle. *Nature,* 231:296–301.

Harris, A. J., Kuffler, S. W., and Dennis, M. J. (1971b): Differential chemosensitivity of synaptic and extrasynaptic areas on the neuronal surface membrane in parasympathetic neurons of the frog, tested by microapplication of acetylcholine. *Proc. Roy. Soc. B,* 177:541–553.

Harrison, R. G. (1907): Observations on the living developing nerve fiber. *Anat. Rec.,* 1:116–118.

Hartzell, H. C., and Fambrough, D. M. (1973): Acetylcholine receptor production and incorporation into membranes of developing muscle fibers. *Devel. Biol.,* 30:153–165.

Kahan, B. W., and Ephrussi, B. (1970): Developmental potentialities of clonal *in vitro* cultures of mouse testicular teratoma. *J. Nat. Cancer Inst.,* 44:1015–1036.

Katz, B. (1966): *Nerve, Muscle and Synapse.* McGraw-Hill, New York.

Katz, B., and Miledi, R. (1964a): Further observations on the distribution of acetylcholine reactive sites in skeletal muscle. *J. Physiol.,* 170:379–388.

Katz, B., and Miledi, R. (1964b): The development of acetylcholine sensitivity in nerve-free segments of skeletal muscle. *J. Physiol.,* 170:389–396.

Kidokoro, Y. (1973): Development of action potentials in a clonal rat skeletal muscle cell line. *Nature New Biol.*, 241:158–159.

Krnjević, K., and Miledi, R. (1958): Acetylcholine in mammalian neuromuscular transmission. *Nature*, 182:805–806.

Kuffler, S. W., Dennis, M. J., and Harris, A. J. (1971): The development of chemosensitivity in extrasynaptic areas of the neuronal surface after denervation of parasympathetic ganglion cells in the heart of the frog. *Proc. Roy. Soc. B*, 177:555–563.

Landmesser, L. (1971): Contractile and electrical responses of vagus-innervated frog sartorius. *J. Physiol.*, 213:707–725.

Lømø, T., and Rosenthal, J. (1972): Control of ACh sensitivity by muscle activity in the rat. *J. Physiol.*, 221:493–513.

Miledi, R. (1960a): The acetylcholine sensitivity of frog muscle fibres after complete or partial denervation. *J. Physiol.*, 151:1–23.

Miledi, R. (1960b): Properties of regenerating neuromuscular synapses in the frog. *J. Physiol.*, 154:190–205.

Miledi, R. (1963): Formation of extra nerve-muscle junctions in innervated muscle. *Nature*, 199:1191–1192.

Murray, M. R., and Stout, A. P. (1947): Distinctive characteristics of the sympathicoblastoma cultivated *in vitro*. *Am. J. Path.*, 23:429–441.

Nakai, K., Sasaki, T., and Hayashi, K. (1971): Amino acid sequence of toxin A from the venom of the Indian cobra *(Naja naja)*. *Biochem. Biophys. Res. Comm.*, 44:893–897.

Nelson, P. G., Peacock, J. H., and Amano, T. (1971a): Responses of neuroblastoma cells to iontophoretically applied acetylcholine. *J. Cell Physiol.*, 77:353–362.

Nelson, P. G., Peacock, J. H., Amano, T., and Minna, J. (1971b): Electrogenesis in mouse neuroblastoma cells *in vitro*. *J. Cell Physiol.*, 77:337–352.

Nelson, P., Ruffner W., and Nirenberg, M. (1969): Neuronal tumor cells with excitable membranes grown *in vitro*. *P.N.A.S.*, 64:1004–1010.

Olmstead, J., Carlson, K., Klebe, R., Ruddle, F., and Rosenbaum, J. (1970): Isolation of microtubule protein from cultured mouse neuroblastoma cells. *P.N.A.S.*, 65:129–136.

Patrick, J., Heinemann, S. F., Lindstrom, J., Schubert, D., and Steinbach, J. H. (1972): Appearance of acetylcholine receptors during differentiation of a myogenic cell line. *P.N.A.S.*, 69:2762–2766.

Peper, K., and McMahan, U. J. (1972): Distribution of acetylcholine receptors in the vicinity of nerve terminals on skeletal muscle of the frog. *Proc. Roy. Soc. B*, 181:431–440.

Raisman, G. (1969): Neuronal plasticity in the septal nuclei of the adult rat. *Brain Res.*, 14:25–48.

Redfern, P. A. (1970): Neuromuscular transmission in new-born rats. *J. Physiol.*, 209:701–709.

Rosenberg, R. N., Vandeventer, L., de Francesco, L., and Friedkin, M. E. (1971): Regulation of the synthesis of choline-o-acetyltransferase and thymidylate synthetase in mouse neuroblastoma in cell culture. *P.N.A.S.*, 68:1436–1440.

Rosenthal, M. D., Wishnow, R. M., and Sato, G. H. (1970): *In vitro* growth and differentiation of clonal populations of multipotential mouse cells derived from a transplantable testicular teratocarcinoma. *J. Nat. Cancer Inst.*, 44:1001–1014.

Schubert, D., Humphreys, S., Baroni, C., and Cohn, M. (1969): *In vitro* differentiation of a mouse neuroblastoma. *P.N.A.S.*, 64:316–323.

Schubert, D., Humphreys, S., de Vitry, F., and Jacob, F. (1971a): Induced differentiation of a neuroblastoma. *Devel. Biol.*, 25:514–546.

Schubert, D., Tarakis, H., Harris, A. J., and Heinemann, S. (1971b): Induction of acetylcholine esterase activity in a mouse neuroblastoma. *Nature New Biology*, 233:79–80.

Seeds, N. W., Gilman, A. G., Amano, T., and Nirenberg, M. W. (1970): Regulation of axon formation by clonal lines of a neural tumor. *P.N.A.S.*, 66:160–167.

Steinbach, J. H., Harris, A. J., Patrick, J., Schubert, D., and Heinemann, S. (1973): Nerve-muscle interaction *in vivo*: The role of acetylcholine. *J. Gen. Physiol.*, 62:255–270.

Stout, A. P. (1947): Ganglioneuroma of the sympathetic nervous system. *Surg., Gynec. and Obst.*, 84:101–110.

Tashjian, A. H., Yasumura, Y., Levine, L., Sato, G. H., and Parker, M. C. (1968): Establishment of clonal stains of rat pituitary tumor cells that secrete growth hormone. *Endocrinology*, 82:342–352.

Thesleff, S. (1960): Supersensitivity of skeletal muscle produced by botulinum toxin. *J. Physiol.*, 151:598–607.

Thompson, E. B., Tomkins, G. M., and Curran, J. F. (1966): Induction of tyrosine α ketoglutarate transaminase by steroid hormones in a newly established tissue culture cell line. *P.N.A.S.*, 56:296–303.

Tuffery, A. R. (1971): Growth and degeneration of motor end-plates in normal cat hind limb muscles. *J. Anat.*, 110:221–247.

Yaffe, D. (1968): Retention of differentiation potentialities during prolonged cultivation of myogenic cells. *P.N.A.S.*, 61:477–483.

Synaptic Transmission and Neuronal Interaction
Raven Press, New York 1974

Synaptic Analysis of the Interrelationships Between Behavioral Modifications in *Aplysia*

Thomas J. Carew and Eric R. Kandel

Department of Neurobiology and Behavior, Public Health Research Institute of the City of New York, and Department of Physiology and Psychiatry, New York University Medical School, New York, New York 10016

I. INTRODUCTION

During the last two decades it has become evident that many chemical synapses can undergo changes in functional effectiveness lasting minutes and even hours in response to repeated or patterned presynaptic stimulation. Some synapses show facilitation, some depression, and some facilitation at one frequency of stimulation and depression at other frequencies (for review see Eccles, 1964). These plastic capabilities of chemical synapses may be important for behavior. A central question in the neural analysis of behavior is how neuronal functioning is modified by learning. The abundance of chemical synapses in the nervous system makes it attractive to think that certain types of synaptic plasticity may mediate specific forms of behavioral modifications. This rationale has encouraged a number of workers to try to extend the study of synaptic physiology to behavior and to learning in order to examine what relationships, if any, exist between different behavioral modifications and synaptic plasticity. To bridge the gap between synaptic mechanisms and behavioral modifications, it is first necessary to develop suitable preparations in which behavior can be studied at the cellular level. One needs to identify the specific nerve cells that control the various components of a behavior and to determine how these cells are synaptically interconnected with each other. This task has now been partially accomplished for a few simple behaviors in the leech, the crayfish, and several opisthobranch molluscs (Willows, 1968; Kupfermann and Kandel, 1969; Nicholls and Purves, 1970; Zucker, 1972; Kupfermann, Carew, and Kandel, 1974).

Because the nervous system of opisthobranch molluscs is favorable for identifying nerve cells and for studying central synaptic transmission (for reviews see Tauc, 1967; Kandel and Gardner, 1972; Gerschenfeld, 1973), these animals may prove particularly useful for synaptic analyses of behavioral problems. Although little was known about opisthobranch behavior until recently, a number of reflex and instinctive behaviors have now been described in *Aplysia, Navanax, Pleurobranchaea,* and *Tritonia* (Paine, 1963; Willows, 1968; Kupfermann and Kandel, 1969; Davis and Mpitsos, 1971; Koester, Mayeri, Liebeswar, and Kandel, 1974; Bennett, *this volume*). For instance, in *Aplysia,* the reflex responses and instinctive behaviors (fixed-action patterns) of the respiratory and the cardiovascular systems have been analyzed and found to be controlled by a single ganglion, the abdominal ganglion. Much of the neural circuitry controlling each of these systems has been delineated on the cellular level (Kupfermann and Kandel, 1969; Kupfermann et al., 1974; Mayeri, Koester, Liebeswar, Kupfermann, and Kandel, 1973; Koester et al., 1974). One behavior, the defensive withdrawal reflex of the respiratory complex (gill, siphon, and mantle shelf), has been found to be capable of undergoing a variety of modifications that vary in complexity from habituation to sensitization and in duration from short-term changes lasting minutes and hours to prolonged changes lasting weeks.

In earlier work Kupfermann, Castellucci, Pinsker, and Kandel (1970) and Castellucci, Pinsker, Kupfermann, and Kandel (1970) examined the neurophysiological mechanisms underlying the short-term behavioral modifications of the defensive withdrawal reflex and found that these involve plastic changes in the functional effectiveness of preexisting excitatory synaptic connections. Here we will describe the wider range of behavioral modifications which can now be achieved in this reflex and examine the interrelated synaptic mechanisms mediating these different behavioral modifications.

In the first part of this chapter we describe our preliminary attempts to develop an adequate behavioral methodology in *Aplysia,* comparable to that which has long been available for vertebrates. Controlled behavioral studies were needed to test the range of modifiability of a given behavior. But they were also necessary to define the parameters that one needs to use in cellular neurophysiological experiments to examine effectively the plastic capabilities of synapses that mediate the behavioral modifications. In the second part of the chapter we describe studies that have examined the neural circuit of the gill-withdrawal reflex during the establishment of different behavioral modifications in an attempt to specify the functional changes underlying each of them and the relationships between them.

II. A DEFENSIVE WITHDRAWAL REFLEX IN *APLYSIA:* METHODOLOGICAL PROBLEMS IN STUDYING MOLLUSCAN BEHAVIOR

The behavior we will consider is a defensive withdrawal reflex of the external organs of the mantle cavity (Fig. 1). Analogous defensive escape and withdrawal responses are found in all major invertebrates as well as

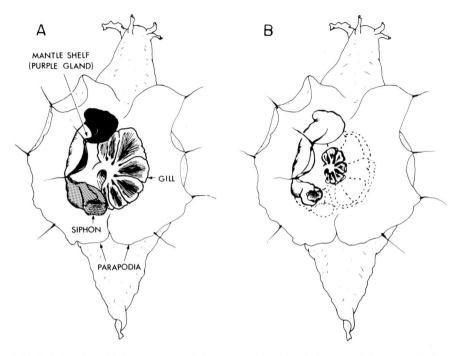

FIG. 1. Defensive withdrawal reflex of siphon and gill. Dorsal view of an intact *Aplysia*. The parapodia and mantle shelf have been retracted to reveal the gill. *(A):* Position of organs in unstimulated condition illustrating the excitatory receptive field for the withdrawal reflex. The most sensitive area of the receptive field consists of two regions, the edge of the mantle shelf containing the purple gland and the siphon. The surrounding area is less sensitive. *(B):* Comparison of the position of the mantle organs at rest *(dashed lines)* and during withdrawal reflex following tactile stimulation of the siphon (modified from Kupfermann and Kandel, 1969).

vertebrates. The mantle cavity is a respiratory chamber containing a gill. The chamber is covered by a fold of skin, the mantle shelf, whose posterior edge forms an exhalant funnel, the siphon. When the siphon or the mantle shelf is touched, the siphon, the gill, and the mantle shelf contract and withdraw into the mantle cavity. The function of this reflex is obvious: the gill is a delicate structure, and when endangered it withdraws under the mantle shelf for protection. This response has short latency and is graded, depending on the intensity of the stimulus. Two features of this behavior are relevant for subsequent analysis. First, the excitatory receptive field of this reflex to weak tactile stimuli involves two anatomically distinct areas: (1) the siphon and (2) the mantle shelf which contains the purple gland on its margin (Fig. 1A). One can elicit the reflex independently from either area of the receptive field. Second, there are two main motor components of the reflex: siphon withdrawal and gill withdrawal. An effective tactile stimulus invariably elicits both components so that either can be used as an index of reflex responsiveness (Figs. 1B and 2C). This is important because gill withdrawal is best studied in restrained animals (Fig. 2A), whereas siphon withdrawal can be studied in freely moving animals (Fig. 2B, C). The gill is normally covered by the mantle shelf and parapodia, and measurement of gill withdrawal requires that the animal be restrained and the mantle shelf be retracted. Although restrained animals survive well for up to 24 hr, they cannot be maintained well beyond this. Long-term studies thus require

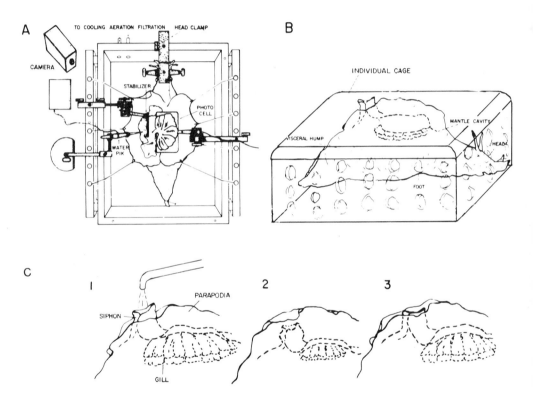

FIG. 2. Restrained and unrestrained animals for studying different components of the defensive withdrawal reflex. *(A):* Restrained preparation for studying the gill-withdrawal component. The animal is immobilized in a small aquarium containing cooled (15°C) and aerated circulating seawater. Gill contractions are monitored with a photocell placed under the gill. In addition, a 16-mm movie camera can be employed for a cinematographic analysis of gill contraction (modified from Pinsker, Kupfermann, Castellucci, and Kandel, 1970). *(B):* Unrestrained animal for studying the siphon-withdrawal component. The animal is permanently housed and fed in an individual perforated cage kept in a large, cooled (15°C) seawater aquarium. The siphon can be stimulated and its withdrawal measured in freely moving animals. *(C):* The siphon-withdrawal component in an unrestrained animal. Enlarged view of siphon as it normally protrudes between parapodia. *(C₁):* Stimulation of siphon by 800-msec jet of seawater from a Water Pik. *(C₂):* Withdrawal of siphon *(dashed lines)* between the parapodia and out of view. *(C₃):* Return of siphon to view. The duration of siphon-withdrawal response is timed from the offset of the stimulus until the experimeter can unambiguously visualize the siphon between the parapodia.

unrestrained animals. Because the siphon normally protrudes between the parapodia, it is readily visualized and its withdrawal can be studied in unrestrained animals in long-term experiments (Fig. 2B, C).

To study the behavior of molluscs and certain other invertebrates it is essential to delineate central control of behaviors from that mediated by peripheral neurons and nerve nets (for discussion see Bullock and Horridge, 1965; Kandel and Spencer, 1968). Both the gill- and siphon-withdrawal components of the defensive withdrawal reflex are mediated by motor neurons located in the abdominal ganglion (see Fig. 13). However, direct stimulation of either organ recruits a peripheral system that mediates local responses (Kandel and Spencer, 1968; Peretz, 1970). An advantage of the gill component is that the stimulus which elicits it is applied to the siphon or purple gland, structures distant from the gill. As a result, mild or moderate intensity stimuli elicit gill withdrawal without involving peripheral pathways (Kupfermann and Kandel, 1969; Kupfermann, Pinsker, Castellucci, and Kandel, 1971).[1] Siphon withdrawal is also under central control, but stimulation of the siphon invariably also recruits a peripherally mediated siphon contraction which adds to the centrally mediated response (Lukowiak and Jacklet, 1972; Kupfermann et al., 1974).

Because the siphon component of the reflex is useful for studying long-term behavioral processes, it was essential to examine to what degree the peripherally mediated withdrawal contributed to the total response. Siphon-withdrawal responses to siphon stimulation were therefore examined in two groups of animals: an experimental group that had the abdominal ganglion removed and a control group which underwent a similar surgical procedure except for the actual removal of the ganglion (Pinsker, Hening, Carew, and Kandel, 1973). Prior to surgery, control (mock-operated) and experimental (deganglionated) animals were matched on the basis of their response to a single test stimulus. On the day following surgery, all animals were coded and siphon withdrawal to repeated stimulation was measured (using a blind procedure). The time during which the siphon disappeared from view between the parapodia was used as a measure of siphon withdrawal (Fig. 2C2). Deganglionated animals showed significantly less siphon withdrawal following surgery (Wilcoxin signed-ranks, matched-pairs test, for two independent replications, $p < 0.025$ and $p < 0.005$) and also significantly less withdrawal than the postoperative control animals (Mann-Whitney U test, $p < 0.013$ and $p < 0.001$; see Table 1). The median postoperative response of the mock-operated control groups was 98 sec, whereas that of the deganglionated experimental groups was 0 sec (Table 1). These experiments suggest that, despite the activation of peripheral pathways, the

---

[1] This gill-withdrawal reflex is to be distinguished from the withdrawal of individual gill pinnules to direct stimulation (the pinnule response) which is not dependent on the central nervous system (Peretz, 1970; Kupfermann et al., 1971).

TABLE 1. *Median duration (seconds) of siphon withdrawal, sum of trials 1 to 10**

Condition	Not sensitized**			Sensitized		
	N	Preop	Postop	N	Preop	Postop
Mock-operated	13	78	98		61	268
		(40–118)	(45–151)	11	(42–116)	(124–429)
Deganglionated	14	83	0		54	0
		(53–141)	(0–4)	6	(24–103)	(0–0)

* The values in parentheses are first and third quartiles.
** Data are pooled from two independent experiments, each with deganglionated and mock-operated animals. In both experiments deganglionated animals showed significantly lower postoperative responses than the mock-operated animals (Exp. 1, $p < 0.013$; Exp. 2, $p < 0.001$) and their own preoperative scores (Exp. 1, $p < 0.025$; Exp. 2, $p < 0.005$). In both experiments surgery produced no significant change in mock-operated scores.

siphon-withdrawal reflex in the intact animal is mediated in great part by the central nervous system. This is not to suggest that all siphon-withdrawal is centrally mediated. In the absence of the abdominal ganglion, the siphon can move when stimulated, but the movement is usually small and deganglionated animals typically are unable to perform an integrated withdrawal reflex that actually removes the siphon between the parapodia and out of view (Fig. 2C2). We will consider below (Section III C) other controls for central mediation.

III. BEHAVIORAL MODIFICATIONS OF THE DEFENSIVE WITHDRAWAL REFLEX

A. Short-Term Habituation and Dishabituation

As is the case for defensive withdrawal reflexes of vertebrates, gill and siphon withdrawal in *Aplysia* can be modified to undergo both short- and long-term habituation and dishabituation. Habituation, perhaps the most rudimentary form of learning, is a decrease in a behavioral response that occurs when an initially novel stimulus is repeatedly presented without reinforcement. It is usually specific to the form and the site of stimulation and it is relatively enduring (Thorpe, 1963).

Once a response has been habituated, two processes can lead to its restoration. By withholding the stimulus to which the animal has been habituated, *spontaneous recovery* occurs after varying periods of time. An almost immediate restoration or *dishabituation* can be produced by changing the stimulus pattern or by presenting another stronger stimulus to another part of the animal. Habituation and spontaneous recovery have been demonstrated for a wide variety of behavioral responses in all animals examined. Dishabituation is a more complex process and is not found in certain types of invertebrate behavior (Thorpe, 1963).

Instances of habituation abound in daily life. A common example is the habituation of orienting behavior. When a novel stimulus, such as a sudden noise, is presented for the first time, one reacts to it both with a somatic response, an investigatory or target reflex, and an autonomic response. One turns toward the stimulus and, concomitantly, one's heart rate and respiratory rate increase. If the same noise is repeated, however, one's attention, as well as one's autonomic responses, gradually diminishes. Thus a novel sound initially produces vasoconstriction of the blood vessels of fingers, but fails to do so after 10 to 15 stimulus presentations (Sokolov, 1960). As a result of habituation one can become accustomed to initially distracting sounds and can work effectively in a noisy environment. One even becomes habituated to the clothes he wears and to his own bodily sensations. These enter our awareness rarely, only under special circumstances. In this sense habituation is learning to ignore recurrent external or internal stimuli which have lost novelty or meaning.

Besides being a behavioral modification in its own right, habituation is thought to be involved in more complex learning, which often consists not only in acquiring new responses but also in learning to reduce errors by eliminating responses to inappropriate stimuli. The ability of an animal to attend to and perceive a particular stimulus event often depends upon its ability not to attend to other sources of stimulation. In its most general sense, habituation is important for perception and is thus relevant for understanding how the brain abstracts, stores, and retrieves sensory information.

The exact relationship of habituation to more complex learning is not well understood. Habituation is generally defined as a "relatively permanent waning of a response as a result of repeated stimulation" (Thorpe, 1963). Learning is commonly defined as a "relatively permanent change in behavior resulting from conditions of practice" (Kling, 1971) that is not due to maturation, fatigue, or other short-term effects (Hilgard and Bower, 1966). Both definitions specify that repeated stimulation (training) leads to prolonged behavioral change (Petrinovich, 1973). Habituation and learning are also similar in some of their parametric features: the kinetics of acquisition, the long time course until spontaneous recovery (memory), stimulus discrimination, and generalization. Furthermore, as we consider below, both learning and habituation can vary as a function of the spacing of training trials. In each case spaced training is more effective than massed training. The major difference between habituation and learning is probably the greater temporal specificity to pairing of stimuli or of stimulus to response, characteristic of learning (Miller, 1967). It is often stated that habituation also differs from learning in that habituation only produces a decrease in response strength whereas learning can produce increases or decreases (see, for example, Petrinovich, 1973). But this difference no longer applies when dishabituation is included in the habituation paradigm.

The gill- and siphon-withdrawal components of the defensive withdrawal reflex readily habituate to repeated tactile stimuli. For instance, in restrained animals a single training session of 10 or more tactile stimuli (jets of seawater) delivered either to the siphon or purple gland, produces short-term

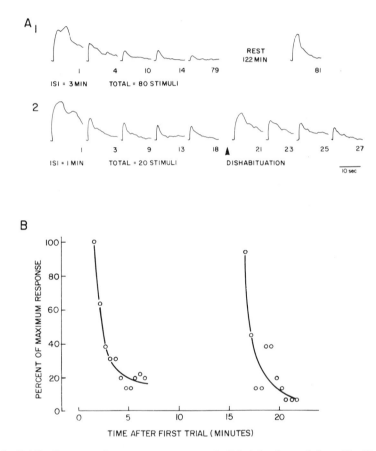

FIG. 3. Habituation, spontaneous recovery, and dishabituation of the gill-withdrawal reflex. (A): Photocell records (see Fig. 2A) from two habituation sessions in a single preparation. The interval between stimuli (ISI) and total number of habituating stimuli are indicated. A_1 shows decrement of the response with repetition of the stimulus. Following a 122-min rest the response was almost fully recovered. A_2 shows a later experiment from the same preparation. After rehabituation of the response, a dishabituating stimulus consisting of a strong and prolonged tactile stimulus to the neck region was presented at the arrow. Successive responses were facilitated for several minutes (from Pinsker et al., 1970). (B): The kinetics of two consecutive habituation training sessions. The gill-withdrawal reflex was habituated by delivering 10 tactile stimuli to the siphon (30-sec ISI) in a restrained preparation. Ten min later, gill withdrawal had almost completely recovered, and the reflex was rehabituated (modified from Kupfermann et al., 1971).

habituation of gill withdrawal (Fig. 3A, B) that recovers spontaneously only after a period of rest ranging from minutes to several hours (Fig. 3A, B). However, a strong tactile or electrical stimulus to the head or neck of the animal produces immediate dishabituation of an habituated response that lasts several minutes (Fig. 3A2).

Because it is an easily produced behavioral modification in a reflex whose neural circuit is well understood (Fig. 13), habituation and dishabituation of gill withdrawal in *Aplysia* have been useful for examining the mechanisms of short-term memory. If these behavioral modifications could be prolonged, one might be able to use this system to study long-term memory. In addition, by examining the conversion from one stage of habituation to the other, it may be possible to gain insights into the relationship of short- to long-term memory.

By repeating the training sessions, we have found that both habituation and dishabituation could be extended into a long-term form (Carew, Pinsker, and Kandel, 1972; Pinsker et al., 1973.)

B. Long-Term Habituation

To establish long-term habituation, we presented an experimental group of animals 10 habituation trials per day for 4 days (days 1 to 4). On this schedule, the animals showed, on each day, the expected within-session habituation. In addition, the animals showed progressive buildup of habituation across days so that on the fourth day of training their reflex responsiveness was only 20 to 30% of that which they had exhibited on the first day (Fig. 4A, B). One day (day 5), 1 week (day 12), and 3 weeks (day 26) after training, both the experimental group and a control group were coded, randomly mixed, and given 10 habituation trials using a blind procedure. The sum of 10 trials (the net amount of time spent responding during the entire habituation training session) was then used as a single score for each animal in the statistical analyses[2] (Fig. 4B, C). On the first day of training (day 1), the habituation scores of the experimental and control groups were not statistically different from each other. After training, however, the experimental animals showed significantly greater habituation (lower net response tendency) than the control group on the retention tests given 1 day ($p < 0.001$), 1 week ($p < 0.01$), and 3 weeks ($p < 0.02$) later. These data indicate that the retention of habituation acquired by the experimental group during 4 days of training lasted for at least 3 weeks.

In addition to comparing experimentals and controls, we did an intragroup

---

[2] After an overall statistical difference between groups was determined by means of a Kruskal-Wallis one-way analysis of variance, between-group statistical comparisons were made by means of a Mann-Whitney U test. Within-group comparisons were made by means of Wilcoxin signed-ranks matched-pairs tests (Siegel, 1956).

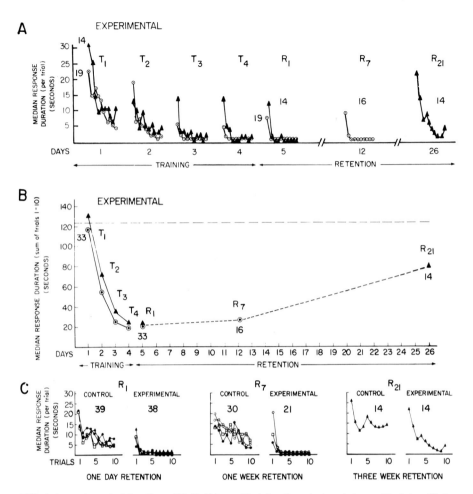

FIG. 4. Long-term habituation. *(A):* Buildup of habituation during 4 days of training (T_1 to T_4) and retention of 1 day (R_1), 1 week (R_7), and 3 weeks (R_{21}) after training. Data from three experiments are presented: two independent, identical replications in which retention was tested 1 day and 1 week after training have been pooled (⊙——⊙); in the third experiment, retention was tested at 1 day and 3 weeks (▲——▲). Each data point for each trial is the median duration of siphon withdrawal for the entire group. The number of animals contributing scores for each curve is indicated. *(B):* Time course of habituation. Habituation within each daily session is expressed as a single score, the sum of 10 trials. Retention tested at both 1 day (R_1) and 1 week (R_7) after training (⊙——⊙), and retention at both 1 day and 3 weeks (R_{21}) (▲——▲) is compared with control (day 1) habituation *(upper dashed line).* The number of animals in each retention test is indicated. *(C):* Comparison of experimental and control habituation on each of the 3 retention days. Retention 1 day (R_1) and 7 days (R_7) after training are based on data from two independent replications, which were pooled in *(A),* and are presented separately [(●——●): experimental, n = 9; control, n = 10; and (○——○): experimental, n = 10; control, n = 10]. An additional control [(○-----○), n = 7] received no habituation training until the 1-week retention test. A third independent replication is also shown [(□——□): experimental spaced training, n = 5; control, n = 5] and forms part of the massed as compared to spaced-training data (see Fig. 6B). Three-week retention is based on 14 experimental and 14 control animals (▲——▲) in which retention was tested at 1 day and 3 weeks after training (from Carew et al., 1972).

analysis using each animal as its own control. This revealed that the control group exhibited the same habituation 1 day and 1 week after training as they did on the first day of training. In contrast the experimental group exhibited significantly greater habituation 1 day after training than on the first day of training ($p < 0.005$), and this was unchanged 1 week later ($p < 0.005$). Even 3 weeks later the experimental animals still exhibited significantly greater habituation than on the first day of training ($p < 0.005$) although they now also showed significantly less habituation than they exhibited in the retention test 1 day after training ($p < 0.005$). Therefore, at 3 weeks the experimental animals exhibited partial recovery of reflex responsiveness compared to their performance on the first day after training, but they still exhibited significant retention of habituation compared to their initial performance on the first day of training. The control group showed responses at 3 weeks that were comparable to that of the first day of training.

The kinetics and time course of long-term habituation of this reflex resemble certain aspects of higher learning (Fig. 5). For example, when a human subject is asked to tap a Morse code key and hold it down for 0.7 sec (Fig. 5B), his performance improves with repeated trials within a session and also progressively improves across days (Macpherson, Dees, and Grindley, 1949). Although a comparison of a few parametric features are by themselves not very meaningful, it is interesting to note that with long-term habituation, as with learning, there is a slight "forgetting" between the last performance of one day and the first performance the next day, despite the progressive improvement over days (Fig. 5A, B).

In view of these similarities, it became interesting to inquire whether long-term habituation in *Aplysia* shared other features with more complex

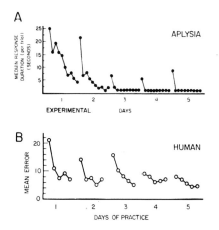

FIG. 5. Comparison of long-term habituation in *Aplysia* to human learning. *(A):* Buildup of habituation in *Aplysia* during 5 days of training. Data replotted from experiment illustrated in Fig. 4A [(⊙——⊙), n = 19]. *(B):* Buildup of learning (reduction of errors) in human subjects during 5 days of training. The subjects were asked to depress a Morse code key for 0.7 sec (from Macpherson et al., 1949).

learning and in particular whether the development of the long-term process
is influenced by the temporal pattern of stimulation. In vertebrates, tem-
porally spaced, or distributed, training often produces much better long-term
retention than massed training (Kling, 1971). To investigate the effects of
massed as compared to spaced habituation training on the retention of
habituation, we randomly divided 25 animals into three groups: a spaced-
training group (N = 5), a massed-training group (N = 15), and a control
group (N = 5) (Fig. 6A, B). Animals receiving massed training were given
no stimulation on days 1 to 3 and then given 40 consecutive habituation
trials on day 4 (Fig. 6A). Animals receiving spaced training were given 10
habituation trials per day for 4 days (days 1 to 4) (Fig. 6B). One day and 1
week after training, all animals, including the controls, were coded and were

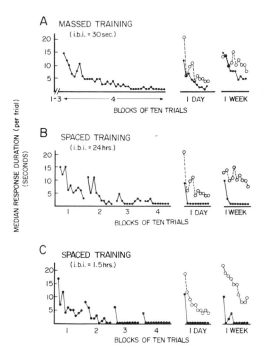

FIG. 6. Comparison of massed and spaced habituation training in *Aplysia*. *(A):* Experimental massed animals [n = 15, (●——●)] received no stimulation for 3 days. On day 4
they were given 40 consecutive training trials (intertrial interval = 30 sec). The controls
[n = 5, (○——○)] received no training. Retention was tested 1 day and 1 week after
training. *(B):* Experimental spaced animals [n = 5, (●——●)] were given four blocks
(10 trials/block) of habituation training, with each block separated by 1 day. Controls
(○——○) are the same as in *A*. Retention of habituation was tested 1 day and 1 week after
training. Studies illustrated in *A* and *B* were carried out concurrently and used the same
control population. *(C):* Experimental spaced animals [n = 9, (●——●)] were given four
blocks of training separated by 1.5 hr. Controls [n = 9, (○——○)] received no training.
Retention was tested 1 day and 1 week after training. (*A* and *B* are from Carew et al.,
1972; *C* is from Carew and Kandel, 1973).

given 10 habituation trials. The animals receiving spaced training exhibited significantly greater habituation 1 day and 1 week after training than did the animals receiving massed training ($p < 0.01$), despite the fact that both groups had received the same number of training trials (Fig. 6A, B). Animals in the massed-training group did show a significantly lower response tendency 1 day after training than they showed on trials 1 to 10 of day 4 ($p < 0.01$). But, on the 1-week retention test, the massed-training group was no longer significantly lower than its initial performance indicating that this group showed no retention of training 1 week later, whereas the spaced training group still exhibited significant retention of habituation ($p < 0.01$).

Thus, massing 40 habituation trials in one session is not as effective as spacing the 40 trials (10 per day) over four daily sessions. Although both massed- and spaced-training groups showed identical short-term habituation in the first 10 trials, the habituation of the massed-training groups is not retained as long as that of the spaced-training group. An interesting question now arises: what feature of the training procedures leads to the conversion from short- to long-term retention? If spacing is important, must the training sessions be separated by a complete day or can shorter intervals also be effective?

To examine this question we repeated the training procedures for spaced training but now separated the four sessions by only 90 min (Carew and Kandel, 1973). With this procedure, experimental animals also showed a buildup of habituation across sessions (Fig. 6C) and significantly greater habituation than controls 1 day and 1 week after training ($p < 0.001$). An intragroup analysis revealed that the experimental animals showed significantly greater habituation both 1 day and 1 week after training ($p < 0.005$ in each case) than they did in the first 10-trial session of acquisition. Thus, training sessions do not have to be separated by a full day to obtain effective long-term habituation: separations of as little as 90 min are sufficient (Figs. 6C and 7).

These behavioral experiments indicate that the conversion from short-term to long-term habituation seems critically dependent upon the temporal patterning of training sessions, but they do not provide direct insights into the mechanism of the conversion. An important aspect of the distributed training procedure might be interruptions, even ones as brief as 90 min, that permit partial recovery of reflex responsiveness. Rehabituation of a partially recovered response may be crucial for the development of long-term habituation.

Although long-term habituation has been described for some vertebrate behaviors (see Farel, 1971, for studies in frogs; and Glaser, 1966, for studies in man), most studies of habituation have not examined massed versus spaced training. In the few instances in which this has been examined, the results are similar to those obtained in *Aplysia*. For example, the mobbing response of chaffinches to models of a predator (owls), undergoes both

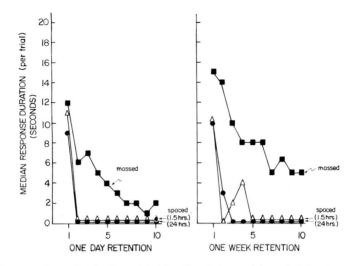

FIG. 7. A comparison of retention of habituation 1 day and 1 week following massed or two types of spaced habituation training. Superimposed graphs based on data illustrated in Fig. 6. Massed group [n = 15, (■———■)] received 40 consecutive training trials with an intertrial interval of 30 sec. The spaced training groups had either 1.5 hr, n = 9, (△———△) or 24 hr, n = 5, (●———●) between training sessions. Both groups which received spaced training show retention of habituation which is superior to that shown by the massed training group. Filled symbols indicate data from the same experiment (see Figs. 6A–B), open symbols are from Fig. 6C.

short- and long-term habituation, and spaced training results in more prolonged habituation than massed training (Hinde, 1954).

C. Central Mediation of Long-Term Habituation

We have used the siphon-withdrawal component of the defensive withdrawal reflex to study long-term habituation, because it can be studied in unrestrained animals. Although siphon withdrawal is largely centrally mediated, it invariably also contains a peripherally mediated component (Kandel and Spencer, 1968; Lukowiak and Jacklet, 1972). In contrast, siphon stimulation activates the gill component without involving peripheral pathways. Since a cellular analysis of long-term habituation is currently only feasible in the central circuits, we examined whether long-term habituation of the siphon-withdrawal component of the defensive reflex was also accompanied by long-term habituation of the gill-withdrawal component. If this were so, one could be confident that the cellular changes underlying long-term habituation of at least the gill component were central (Kupfermann et al., 1970).

Thirty-three animals were divided into an experimental group (N = 17) that received 4 days of habituation training and a control group (N = 16), that received no habituation training. Either 1 day or 1 week after training

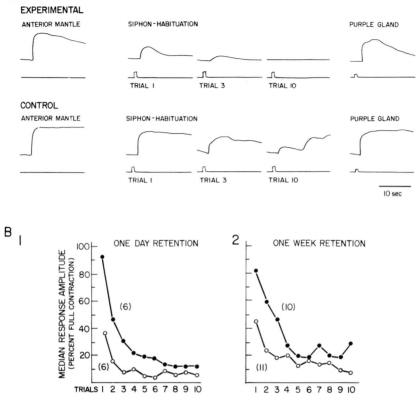

FIG. 8. Long-term habituation of gill withdrawal following siphon habituation training. *(A):* Gill-withdrawal reflex of an experimental and a control animal (see Fig. 2A). One week previously, experimental animals had exhibited significant 24-hr retention of habituation of siphon withdrawal as compared to controls. Seven days later, retention of habituation of gill withdrawal, produced by the previous siphon habituation training, was measured. A single test gill contraction was first produced by vigorous tactile stimulation of the anterior mantle region. After a brief period of rest, habituation of gill withdrawal was produced by repetitive siphon stimulation with a jet of seawater (10 trials; interstimulus interval, 30 sec), and was followed by another single test stimulus to the purple gland. Anterior mantle and purple gland stimulation produced comparable contractions in both experimental and control animals. However, siphon stimulation produced a significantly greater habituation of the gill-withdrawal reflex in experimental than in control animals (compare trials 1, 3, and 10 of both experimental and control records). Time calibration, 10 seconds. *(B):* Comparison of experimental and control habituation of gill withdrawal at 1 day and 1 week. Median amplitude of gill responses is expressed as a percentage of a full contraction. The number of animals in each group is indicated in parentheses. (B_1): Gill withdrawal 24 hr after siphon habituation training. Experimental animals (O———O) exhibited significantly greater habituation ($p < 0.001$) of gill withdrawal (sum of trials 1 to 10) than controls (●———●) and were significantly lower than controls on nine out of 10 trials. (B_2): Gill withdrawal 1 week after siphon habituation training. Experimental animals again exhibited significantly greater habituation ($p < 0.001$) and were significantly lower than controls on eight out of 10 trials. These data indicate that long-term habituation of siphon withdrawal also produces long-term habituation of gill withdrawal (from Carew et al., 1972).

the experimental animals were mixed with controls, and habituation of the gill-withdrawal reflex of both groups was measured in restrained animals (Fig. 2A), using a blind procedure (Fig. 8). Both 1 day and 1 week after training, experimental animals exhibited significantly greater habituation of gill withdrawal than controls ($p < 0.001$). Experimental animals also showed a significantly decremented reflex responsiveness compared to controls on the first trial and throughout the habituation training session ($p < 0.001$). The finding that siphon training also gives rise to long-term habituation of gill withdrawal provided the opportunity for a neural analysis considered below.

D. Long-Term Dishabituation[3]

In collaboration with Pinsker and Hening, we also examined whether dishabituation might be prolonged (Pinsker et al., 1973). Whereas habituation simply involves a decreased responsiveness due to repeated activity in a single pathway, dishabituation involves an altered (heightened) responsiveness in one reflex pathway due to the facilitatory influence of another pathway. In this sense dishabituation is similar to associative conditioning. It is different from conditioning, however, in that it does not require a temporal association of activity in the two pathways. Classical conditioning is dependent on the pairing of two stimuli in a precise sequence; sensitization is not dependent on paired presentation.

Thirty-eight animals were matched on the basis of a pretraining habituation session of 10 trials and divided into experimental and control groups (Fig. 9A). Thirteen days after matching, experimental animals were given an electric shock to the head four times per day for 4 days. Control animals received no shock. Retention of dishabituation was measured 1 day, 1 week, and 3 weeks after the last day of dishabituation training (Fig. 9B, C, D). We found that dishabituated animals showed significantly longer siphon withdrawal than controls both 1 day and 1 week after training ($p < 0.01$ in each case). The dishabituated groups also showed significantly longer siphon withdrawal 1 day and 1 week after training compared to their own initial values in the matching sessions ($p < 0.005$ on both days); the control group's scores were not changed from their previous matching scores. In the 3-week retention test, the dishabituated animals no longer were significantly different from controls, indicating that they had largely recovered. However, some effects of dishabituation were still evident even at 3 weeks when the experimental animals were compared with their own initial matching scores. Since the within-group comparison is statistically more powerful than the between-group comparison, a significantly greater amount of

---

[3] In this section we arbitrarily refer to all enhancements of reflex response preceded by a strong stimulus as dishabituation. In Section VI below we will distinguish further between dishabituation and sensitization.

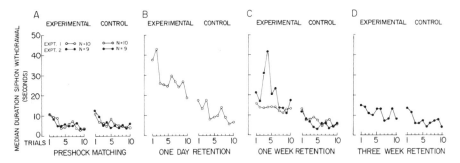

FIG. 9. Long-term dishabituation of siphon withdrawal. The median duration of siphon withdrawal is shown for each trial of a 10-trial block. A minimum intertrial interval of 30 sec was used. The results of two independent experiments are shown, but they are pooled for discussion in the text. In experiment 1 (O——O) n = 20, and in experiment 2 (●——●) n = 18; in both experiments, animals were divided into experimental and control groups. Animals were matched on the basis of the initial amount of siphon withdrawal during a pretraining habituation session of 10 trials. Thirteen days after matching, the experimental animals were given four shocks/day for 4 days, whereas the controls received no shocks. In experiment 1, retention of dishabituation was tested 1 day *(B)* and 1 week *(C)* after the last shock. In experiment 2, retention was tested 1 week *(C)* and 3 weeks *(D)* after the last shock. Significant dishabituation was evident in the 1-day and the 1-week retention tests, whereas there was almost complete recovery in the 3-week retention test (from Pinsker et al., 1973).

siphon withdrawal ($p < 0.005$) compared to the matching scores was still detectable in the dishabituated animals at 3 weeks. Therefore, 4 days of exposure to the stressful environment of repeated shocks produces significantly elevated reflex responsiveness in these animals which persisted for weeks.

We also examined whether the amplitude or duration of reflex responsiveness could be further enhanced by spacing the training sessions over 10 days. In addition, we increased the number of noxious stimuli from 16 to 20 and omitted the initial habituation session on the day prior to training. Animals which received this more distributed training showed greater and more prolonged dishabituation than those which only received 4 days of training (Fig. 10). Furthermore, the kinetics of test habituation exhibited by these animals was different from that shown by the animals in the earlier dishabituation experiments. Rather than showing the usual exponential decline in responsiveness, the animals exhibited a progressive buildup of responsiveness in the first few trials (comp. Figs. 10A and 9B). Thus, as is the case for habituation, dishabituation can be prolonged for days and even weeks, and distributed training appears effective in prolonging dishabituation.

The experiments also provide some insight into the relation of long-term dishabituation to habituation. In both experiments the dishabituating stimulus produced reflex responsiveness that exceeded control levels (Figs. 9 and 10). Moreover, in the second experiment, "dishabituation"

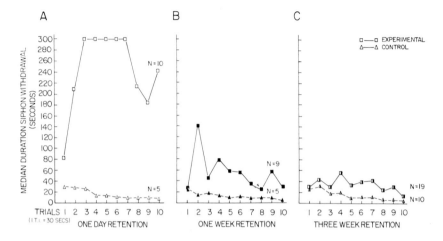

FIG. 10. Long-term dishabituation of siphon withdrawal. As in Fig. 9 the median duration of siphon withdrawal is shown for each trial of a 10-trial block. Of a total of 29 animals, 19 were assigned to the experimental dishabituation group (□——□) and 10 to the control group (△——△). The initial preshock matching (not shown) was based on only two trials separated by about 1 hour. Beginning 5 days after matching, the dishabituation group was given two shocks/day for 10 days. During training, all animals were given a single siphon test stimulus each day and, on the basis of their overall responsiveness to the test stimuli, subjects in each group were matched and assigned at the end of the 10 days to either the 1-day or the 1-week retention group. Half of the animals in each group were tested for retention of dishabituation 1 day after the last shock (A), whereas the other half were tested at 1 week (B). Three weeks after the last shock, all animals were tested for retention (C). In all comparisons, the dishabituated animals showed significantly greater siphon withdrawal than controls. Note the difference in the duration of siphon withdrawal in these animals compared to those illustrated in Fig. 9. The flat peak of the dishabituation group on the 1-day retention test results from the fact that more than half of the animals exceeded a predetermined 300-sec limit on those trials (from Pinsker et al., 1973).

occurred without prior habituation (Fig. 10). These results suggest that dishabituation is not merely a removal of the habituating process but is an independent facilitation superimposed upon habituation. This type of facilitatory process is generally called sensitization (Kling, 1971). In Section VI below we consider, in more detail, the relation of dishabituation to habituation and of dishabituation to sensitization.

To summarize, the siphon- and gill-withdrawal reflex in *Aplysia* show considerable capacity for modification including short- and long-term habituation and short- and long-term dishabituation. In each case repeated training sessions produce a long-term process which lasts up to 3 weeks. The degree to which this seemingly simple behavior can be modified is surprising. This finding results from the use of unrestrained animals that allows one to examine many subjects rapidly in a given session and to test the same subject and matched controls repeatedly over several weeks. This methodology is not restricted to the paradigms examined here. It would be interesting, and possible, to examine how long-term habituation and dishabituation interact. Does one process override the other? Or is there a recency-primary effect? It should also be possible to determine how motivational variables (hunger, satiety, arousal) affect the acquisition of habituation and dishabituation.

IV. METHODOLOGICAL PROBLEMS IN RELATING NEURONAL MECHANISMS TO BEHAVIOR

To relate cellular function to behavior it is necessary to use progressively simpler preparations, each of which retains critical effector and sensory structures but allows one to analyze in greater detail the underlying neuronal processes. Toward this end Kupfermann et al. (1970) and Castellucci et al. (1970) have used three types of preparations. The first preparation (Fig. 11A) is an intact animal restrained in a small chamber (illustrated in Fig. 2A) with a small slit in the neck that permits one to externalize the abdominal ganglion while it is still attached to its sensory receptors and effector organs by its four peripheral nerves, and to the remainder of the central nervous system by its two pleuroabdominal connectives. In this preparation the

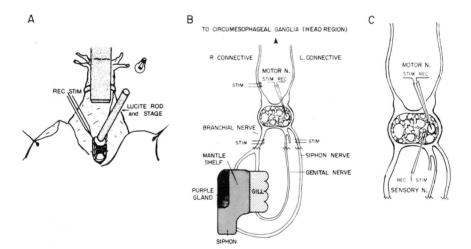

FIG. 11. Three preparations used in cellular studies of gill withdrawal. *(A):* Top view of anterior portion of the intact preparation. The abdominal ganglion was externalized through a small slit made in the skin above the ganglion. The Lucite rod and stage acted as a light guide, so that a strong light directed at the top of the rod transilluminated the ganglion. The body wall had a tendency to tighten around the Lucite stage, thereby slowing blood loss (from Kupfermann et al., 1970). *(B):* Composite diagram of the isolated ganglion test system either with or without (∼) the gill, siphon, and mantle shelf still attached to the ganglion by their respective peripheral nerves. The siphon or branchial nerves are stimulated electrically and the responses of one of the motor neurons, usually L7, is recorded intracellularly. *(C):* Further simplified test system in which the monosynaptic connection of individual mechanoreceptor neurons onto motor neurons can be investigated (modified from Castellucci et al., 1970).

response of gill and siphon can be correlated with the activity of single nerve cells (Kupfermann et al., 1970). In the second preparation (Fig. 11B) the abdominal ganglion is removed from the animal with or without its sensory connection to the siphon skin and its motor connection to siphon and gill. By recording from appropriate motor neurons and electrically stimulating appropriate sensory pathways, one can use this preparation as a test system of the behavior (Castellucci et al., 1970). We have usually worked with cell L7, one of the major motor cells of the gill (Fig. 12A). Stimulating an afferent pathway produces a complex EPSP in L7 that stimulates the EPSP produced by natural tactile stimuli (Fig. 12B). This system is therefore useful for examining how different patterns or combinations of afferent stimuli modify synaptic transmission between afferent pathways and the motor neurons (Fig. 12A). The third preparation (Fig. 11C) is

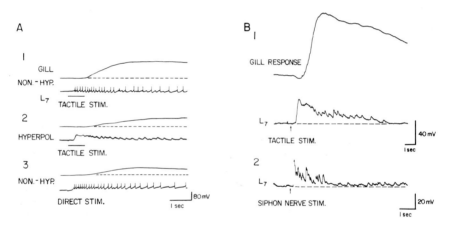

FIG. 12. Test system for gill-withdrawal reflex. *(A):* Contribution of motor neuron L7 to the total gill-withdrawal reflex. The top trace of each pair is a photocell record of gill contraction, the bottom trace is an intracellular record from L7. The gill-withdrawal reflex was elicited every 5 min by a jet of seawater (indicated by solid line under L7 record) applied to the siphon and, on alternate trials, L7 was hyperpolarized so that the excitatory input could not discharge it. Comparisons of nonhyperpolarized (1) to hyperpolarized (2) trials showed that the gill contraction was reduced by about 40%. This reduction was approximately equal to the size of the gill contraction produced by L7 when it was directly fired by a long depolarizing pulse (3) that caused L7 to fire in a pattern comparable to that produced by the normal excitatory input (compare A_1 to A_3) (from Kupfermann et al., 1972). *(B):* Comparison of EPSP produced in L7 in response to a tactile stimulus to the siphon in an intact preparation, and the EPSP produced in L7 in the isolated ganglion in response to a brief electrical stimulus to the siphon nerve. *(B_1):* Simultaneous record of gill contraction and of an EPSP in L7 in response to a jet of seawater applied to the siphon. Cell L7 was hyperpolarized about 50 mV to prevent spike generation. The gill contraction is due to the activity of the other motor neurons in the reflex. When L7 fired, the reflex gill response was about twice as large. *(B_2):* EPSP produced in L7 by a 1.5 msec electrical shock to the siphon nerve. The cell was hyperpolarized about 30 mV to prevent firing. The general configuration and time course of the EPSPs produced with natural and artificial stimulation was roughly comparable. Note the difference in time calibration in B_1 and B_2 (from Carew et al., 1971).

similar to the second, but the test system is further simplified by recording from individual sensory elements and reducing the afferent test pathway to its most elementary component, the monosynaptic connection from mechanoreceptor neurons in the siphon skin and a gill or siphon motor neuron (Castellucci et al., 1970).

Although we will refer to work carried out with all three preparations, most of the experiments we will discuss here are based on the second preparation (Figs. 11B and 12).

V. CELLULAR ANALYSIS OF BEHAVIORAL MODIFICATIONS

A. Synaptic Analysis of Short-Term Habituation and Dishabituation

In earlier work Kupfermann et al. (1969, 1974) and Castellucci et al. (1970) analyzed the neural elements of both the gill and siphon components of the defensive withdrawal reflex and described a wiring diagram of the behavior, indicating how the elements are interconnected (Fig. 13A). They found the motor component of the reflex to consist of at least 10 cells organized in a hierarchical pattern (Fig. 13A). Five motor cells produce movements largely limited to the gill, four cells produce movements limited to the siphon, and one cell (L7) produces movements of the gill, the siphon, and the mantle shelf. In this discussion we will focus on the gill component of this system (Fig. 13B). But we have carried most of our studies out on cell L7, a major motor cell for the gill which is also a motor cell for the siphon and mantle shelf.

During reflex actions, cell L7 (and each of the other gill motor cells) receives a large complex excitatory postsynaptic potential (EPSP) that consists of monosynaptic and polysynaptic contributions (Fig. 12A2). The EPSPs are mediated by a group of sensory neurons and interneurons that form distinctive clusters near the motor cells. The sensory cells make chemical excitatory synaptic connections to different motor neurons. In addition, they make excitatory chemical connections to at least three classes of interneurons: two types of excitatory interneurons and one inhibitory interneuron, cell L16 (Fig. 13; Castellucci et al., 1970; Castellucci and Kandel, 1974).

By examining the functional properties of the wiring diagram during habituation and dishabituation, Kupfermann et al. (1970) and Castellucci et al. (1970) found that the electrical properties of the neurons were not altered. No apparent changes occurred in the input resistance of the motor neurons during stimuli that produced habituation and dishabituation (Fig. 14A). These measurements are not completely conclusive because they do not rule out resistance changes at sites electrically remote from the microelectrode in the cell body. But the measurements are quite sensitive to resistance changes occurring in at least some parts of the synaptic region

A DEFENSIVE WITHDRAWAL REFLEX

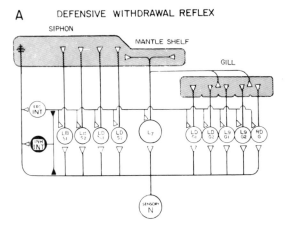

B GILL WITHDRAWAL REFLEX

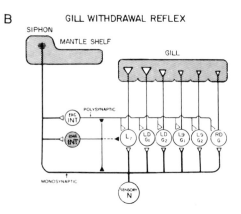

FIG. 13. Neural circuit of the defensive withdrawal reflex. *(A):* Schematic wiring diagram indicating the sensory, interneuronal, and motor neuron components of the total defensive withdrawal reflex. The population of mechanoreceptor sensory neurons connect to the motor neurons directly and indirectly via excitatory and inhibitory interneurons. The excitatory interneurons and the sensory neurons represent small groups of cells. The inhibitory interneuron and the motor cells are unique individuals. *(B):* Schematic wiring diagram of gill-withdrawal component of the defensive withdrawal reflex (from Kupfermann et al., 1974).

in the neuropil (Fig. 14B) and thus tend to rule out gross changes in input resistance occurring in the neuropil region near the cell body.

By examining the changes in the synaptic drive onto the motor neuron at both the level of the complex EPSP, produced by stimulation of the entire afferent input (Fig. 14A), and at the level of the elementary EPSP, produced by stimulating single sensory neurons (Fig. 15), Castellucci et al. (1970) found that the major change produced in the neural circuit by these behavioral modifications was in the functional effectiveness of certain synaptic connections. One class of synapses, that made by the sensory neuron onto interneurons and motor neurons, proved to be endowed with

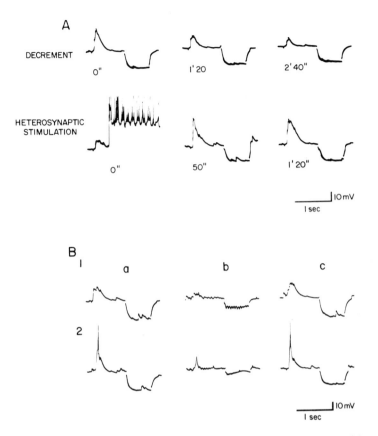

FIG. 14. EPSP decrement and heterosynaptic facilitation in the absence of input resistance change in the soma of motor neuron L7. *(A):* Decrement of the complex EPSP in L7. The siphon nerve was stimulated every 10 sec and the EPSP recorded. A constant current hyperpolarizing electrical pulse was applied through another intracellular electrode and the resulting hyperpolarizing electrotonic potential was recorded concomitantly with the synaptic activity. During EPSP decrement, there was no significant change in soma input resistance in L7 as indicated by the relative constancy of the electrotonic potential. The heterosynaptic stimulation (left connective: 6/sec for 6 sec) produced facilitation of the decremented EPSP, and the facilitation was also not accompanied by a change in soma input resistance. *(B):* Resistance changes (measured by an electrotonic potential) produced in the cell body of L7 as the result of synaptic activity attributed to Interneuron II. Three successive traces (10 sec apart) in two experiments (B_1 and B_2). A spontaneously occurring burst of IPSPs attributed to Interneuron II produced a large decrease in the input resistance as measured in the cell body (compare a and c to b in parts B_1 and B_2) (from Carew et al., 1971).

considerable plastic properties so that transmission across these synapses was greatly decreased during habituation and recovered only after a period of rest. However, transmission could be returned immediately to a normal or even a larger value as a result of the presentation of a dishabituatory stimulus (Fig. 15). Because the EPSP produced by stimulating a single

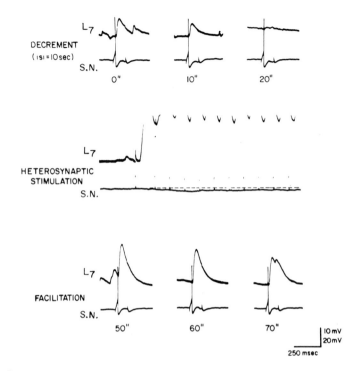

FIG. 15. Decrement and facilitation of an elementary, presumably monosynaptic EPSP in the gill motor neuron L7. The intracellular stimulation of the sensory neuron (S.N. = lower trace of each pair) was repeated every 10 sec. After 3 stimuli *(top trace)*, heterosynaptic stimulation was applied to the left connective (7/sec for 5.5 sec). In the middle set of traces the heterosynaptic stimulus to the left connective is illustrated. Rather than firing the sensory neuron the heterosynaptic stimulus (note stimulus artifacts in S.N. trace) caused a sustained hyperpolarization of the sensory neuron. After the heterosynaptic stimulation, the EPSP produced by the sensory neuron in L7 was facilitated for several minutes (third set of traces). All indicated times are referred to the first stimulus (0″) (from Carew et al., 1971).

sensory neuron undergoes decrement that parallels habituation (Fig. 15) and will do so even in high Ca^{++} high Mg^{++} seawater solutions that increase the threshold of interneurons (Castellucci et al., 1970; Castellucci and Kandel, *in preparation*), the likelihood is reduced that the EPSP decrement is due to presynaptic inhibition resulting from the activation of parallel elements which act upon and inhibit the presynaptic terminals of the primary sensory neurons. These findings rather suggest that the decrease in the EPSP during habituation is the result of a homosynaptic (low frequency) depression of the excitatory synapse and that the increase in the EPSP during dishabituation is due to heterosynaptic facilitation at the same synapse. The mechanisms underlying these changes are not yet known but could be either an alteration in the mechanisms of transmitter release or a change in the sensitivity of the postsynaptic receptor.

More recently, Castellucci and Kandel *(in preparation)* have found that habituation produces a similar decrement in the EPSPs produced by the sensory neurons on the interneurons, and the motor neurons to the siphon. These results indicate that the major loci of habituation of the withdrawal reflex are the central synapses made by the different branches of the sensory neurons. A similar locus and synaptic mechanism have now also been proposed by Zucker (1972) for habituation of the crayfish tail-flip response.

These results are therefore consistent with the idea that genetic and developmental processes determine the basic properties of the individual cells and the anatomical interconnections between cells. These processes leave unspecified the degree of effectiveness of certain of these connections. Environmental factors such as habituation and dishabituation express themselves through the plastic capabilities of these connections.

VI. THE RELATIONSHIP OF HABITUATION TO DISHABITUATION AND OF DISHABITUATION TO SENSITIZATION

Pavlov, who discovered habituation of the orienting reflex at the beginning of this century, attributed it to the building up of an inhibitory process. He also observed that a decremented reflex could be restored by a period of rest and attributed the restoration to disinhibition, the removal of the inhibitory process (for review see Pavlov, 1927). These theoretical notions have continued to influence current thinking, as is evident in the work of Konorski (1948, 1967), Sokolov (1963), Wickelgren (1967a,b), and Wall (1970).

The cellular analysis of habituation of the flection reflex of the spinal cat (Spencer, Thompson, and Neilson, 1966b) and that in *Aplysia* which we described are, however, best explained by a decreased excitatory drive. A corollary to these findings is that disinhibition is an unlikely mechanism for dishabituation.

The first clear suggestion that dishabituation might not be due to disinhibition was made by Sharpless and Jasper (1956), who proposed that dishabituation is not specifically related to habituation but is a separate process, a form of sensitization, whereby a strong stimulus enhances the responsiveness of a variety of reflexes. A similar conclusion was reached by Hagbarth and Kugelberg (1958) in studying human abdominal reflexes. Further behavioral evidence in support of this notion was provided by Spencer, Thompson, and Neilson (1966a) while studying dishabituation of the flection reflex in the cat. Spencer et al. found that a "dishabituatory" stimulus could also facilitate nonhabituated responses (sensitized) and that habituated responses could be facilitated beyond their control values. Neither of these findings can be explained by disinhibition; that could only restore decremented responses to their initial value.

The anatomical features of the gill-withdrawal reflex make it useful for

examining further the interrelationship between habituation and dishabituation. The siphon, innervated by the siphon nerve, and the anterior third
of the purple gland, innervated by the branchial nerve, provide two anatomically distinct afferent pathways for the reflex response (Fig. 16). The
two pathways are relatively independent; habituation of gill withdrawal by
one pathway does not alter responsiveness by the other (Fig. 17). We will
refer to these two pathways as "siphon" and "purple gland," respectively.

To examine the relationship of dishabituation to sensitization, we compared the effects of a common "dishabituating" stimulus on habituated
and nonhabituated responses using the two reflex pathways (Carew,
Castellucci, and Kandel, 1971). If the dishabituation is due to a removal
of habituation, the "dishabituating" stimulus should facilitate only the
habituated pathway and restore it to its original value. If, however, dishabituation is a special manifestation of sensitization, then one would
predict that: (1) a "dishabituating" stimulus might facilitate a nonhabituated
response as well as a habituated one, and (2) the habituated response might
be capable of being facilitated beyond its control value.

Using restrained animals (Fig. 2A), we presented a single test stimulus

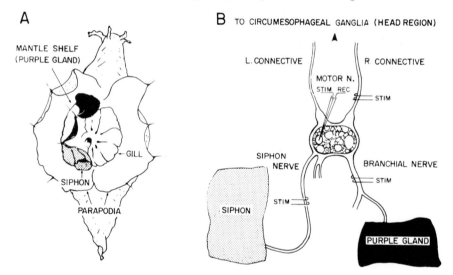

FIG. 16. Two pathways for gill withdrawal. *(A):* The anterior part of the mantle shelf and
its edge, the purple gland, are indicated in *solid black*. This area of the receptive field for
the gill-withdrawal reflex was used in the behavioral experiments and is referred to as the
purple gland. The siphon and the posterior part of the mantle shelf and of the purple
gland are *stippled*. This region is referred to as the *siphon*. *(B):* Diagram illustrating
innervation of siphon by the siphon nerve and purple gland by the branchial nerve. In the
neurophysiological studies, the siphon nerve, which innervates the siphon, and the
branchial nerve, which innervates the anterior part of the mantle shelf and purple gland,
were electrically stimulated. Stimulation of either the right or left connective provided a
pathway for heterosynaptic facilitation (from Carew et al., 1971).

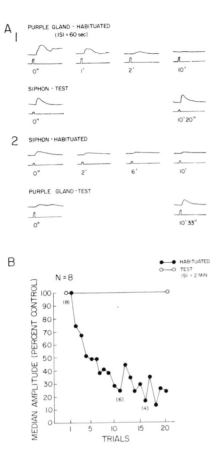

FIG. 17. Lack of generalization of habituation from the purple gland to siphon. *(A):* Stimuli were applied to the siphon and to the purple gland to produce a gill-withdrawal reflex which was recorded with a photocell (top trace of each pair; bottom trace is stimulus monitor). *(A₁):* A single test stimulus was first presented to the siphon (0″). Repetitive stimuli were then applied to the purple gland which produced habituation of the reflex response (0″ to 10′). A second test stimulus now applied to the siphon (10′20″) produced an undecremented response, similar to the reflex withdrawal to the first test stimulus (0″), indicating that no generalization of habituation occurred from the purple gland to the siphon. *(A₂):* After a 40-min rest, the experimental procedure was reversed. The first test stimulus to the purple gland (0″) produced a response which is still partially habituated, indicating incomplete recovery from the previous repetitive stimulation (compare purple gland habituated 0″ to purple gland test 0″). Even though the reflex was then habituated by repetitive stimulation to the siphon (0″ to 10′), a second test stimulus to the purple gland (10′33″) produced a response that was further recovered, indicating that no generalization of habituation occurred from the siphon to the purple gland (time calibration = 5 sec). *(B):* Summary of eight runs in four experiments designed to examine generalization of habituation between the habituated and test pathways. As indicated in parentheses, all runs had at least 10 trials; six had 15 trials, and four had 20 trials. A sign test revealed that there was no significant difference between the second and first test stimulus (median amplitude = 100% in each case) even though significant habituation ($p < 0.001$ was obtained (from Carew et al., 1971).

which produced a gill-withdrawal reflex to either the siphon or the purple gland, and then habituated the reflex by repeated stimulation of the other pathway. Following a second test stimulus to the nonhabituated pathway, a strong tactile stimulus was presented to the head. This type of stimulus produced dishabituation in every preparation; the mean percent dishabituation, obtained by measuring the amplitude of the dishabituated responses minus the amplitude of the last habituated response, was 65%. Sometimes dishabituation was larger than the initial control value (Fig. 18). These results are similar to those obtained in long-term dishabituation experiments in unrestrained animals (Figs. 9 and 10). Sensitization of nonhabituated responses was also observed (Fig. 18), and in every instance in which the head stimulus produced sensitization of the nonhabituated response it also produced dishabituation of the habituated response. However, sensitization was only observed in one-third of the experiments. Why it was not produced more consistently in the restrained animals is not clear, particularly since it is readily demonstrable in unrestrained animals (Figs. 9 and 10). Perhaps the head clamp restraint provides a chronic sensitizing influence on reflex responsiveness that makes further facilitation difficult to produce. Further experiments are necessary to clarify this point.

We next examined how the neuronal correlates of dishabituation relate to those of sensitization. These can be studied in a test system of the isolated

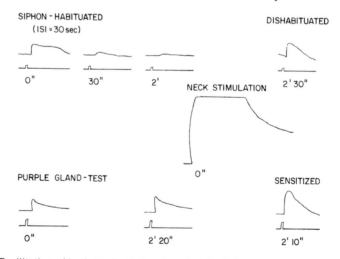

FIG. 18. Facilitation of both habituated and nonhabituated responses following presentation of a single "dishabituatory" stimulus. After a single test stimulus to the purple gland (0"), repetitive stimuli were delivered to the siphon, producing habituation of gill withdrawal. After a second test to the purple gland (2'20"), indicating that no generalization of habituation had occurred, a series of vigorous brush strokes was presented to the neck region, producing a prolonged gill contraction. Subsequent presentation of a stimulus first to the purple gland and then to the siphon revealed facilitation of both nonhabituated responses (sensitization) and habituated responses (dishabituation) (from Carew et al., 1971).

ganglion (Fig. 11B). In this system the siphon and branchial nerves, containing the main afferent nerves from the siphon and anterior portion of the purple gland (see Fig. 16B), are stimulated electrically and intracellular recordings are obtained from gill motor neuron L7. Brief (1.5 msec) electrical pulses applied to one of these nerves produced complex EPSPs in L7 that are quite similar to those produced by natural stimulation to siphon or purple gland in an intact preparation (compare Fig. $12B_1$ and $12B_2$). As was the case with natural stimuli in the intact preparation (Fig. 11A), repeated electrical stimulation of a peripheral nerve in the isolated ganglion produced a decrement of the EPSP which paralleled the behavioral habituation (Fig. 19). Moreover, as in the behavioral experiment, EPSP decrement produced by repetitive stimulation of the siphon nerve does not generalize to the branchial nerve or vice versa (Figs. 19 and 20).

In one series of four experiments (N = 9 runs), we delivered two test stimuli, separated by 10 min, to the control nerve to assess the amount of EPSP decrement that could be produced by presentation of the test stimulus alone (mean = 7%) (Fig. 20A). We then delivered 20 stimuli (isi = 30 sec) to the other (experimental) nerve, which produced significant decrement of the EPSP ($p < 0.005$). A third test stimulus was then delivered to the

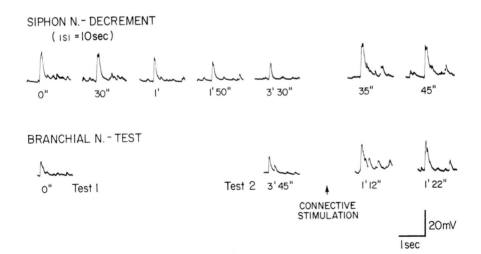

FIG. 19. Facilitation of both decremented and nondecremented EPSPs following a single train of stimuli to the connective. A single test stimulus was delivered to the branchial nerve (Test 1, line 2), and produced an EPSP in L7. Repetitive stimulation was then applied to the siphon nerve to produce EPSP decrement (line 1). After a second test to the branchial nerve (Test 2, line 2) revealed that no generalization of EPSP decrement had occurred from the siphon nerve to the branchial nerve, a single train of stimuli (6/sec for 6 sec) was delivered to the left connective. Subsequent presentation of a stimulus, first to the siphon nerve (line 1) and then to the branchial nerve (line 2) revealed facilitation of both decremented and nondecremented EPSPs (from Carew et al., 1971).

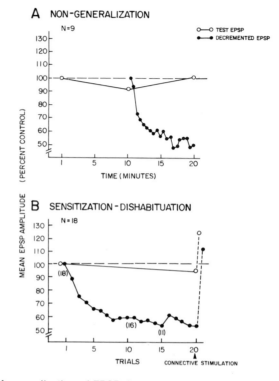

FIG. 20. Lack of generalization of EPSP decrement and facilitation of both decremented EPSPs (analogous to behavioral dishabituation) and nondecremented EPSPs (analogous to behavioral sensitization). *(A):* Summary graph of nine runs from four preparations indicating that there is no generalization of EPSP decrement between decremented and test inputs to the motor neuron (L7). Although repeated stimulation of the experimental nerve produced a significant decrement of the EPSP ($p < 0.005$), there was no significant difference between any of the three test EPSPs produced from stimulation of the control nerve (from Carew et al., 1971). *(B):* Pooled data from 18 runs in five experiments using two interstimulus intervals: 30-sec interstimulus interval ($N = 9$) and 10-sec interstimulus interval ($N = 9$). All 18 runs had at least 10 trials, 16 had 15 trials, and 11 had 20 trials, as indicated in parentheses. A single test EPSP was produced by stimulation to the control nerve, followed by significant decrement of the EPSP ($p < 0.005$) produced by repeated stimulation of the experimental nerve. A second test stimulus produced a test EPSP which was not significantly different from the first test EPSP, showing that no generalization of decrement to the test nerve had occurred. After a single train of stimuli (6/sec for 6 sec) to the connective, both decremented and nondecremented EPSPs were significantly facilitated ($p < 0.031$ in each case). Because the facilitation data had a normal distribution, they are presented in terms of mean percent EPSP amplitude rather than median percent.

control nerve. There was no significant difference between the first, second, and third test EPSPs, indicating that no generalization of EPSP decrement had occurred (mean test EPSP = 101% control; Fig. 20A).

Castellucci et al. (1970) had found that a decremented complex EPSP could be facilitated following a strong stimulus to the connectives, and at times the facilitated EPSP was even larger than control (Fig. 14A). We extended this study by comparing the facilitation produced by connective stimulation on decremented and nondecremented EPSPs.

Connective stimulation significantly facilitated the decremented EPSP ($p < 0.031$, N = 5);[4] the mean percent facilitation was 110.4% (Fig. 20B). In 67% of cases, the facilitation was greater than control. The same stimulus also significantly facilitated the nondecremented EPSPs ($p < 0.031$),[4] sometimes by greater than 200% (mean percent facilitation = 123.8%; Figs. 19 and 20B). Both decremented and nondecremented EPSPs showed similar increases compared to their initial controls. The decremented EPSPs obviously showed proportionately more facilitation when the last observed (decremented) response was used as control. These data suggest that the facilitating stimulus augments all responses toward a common ceiling and that decremented EPSPs were proportionately more facilitated because they were smaller (see also Kandel and Tauc, 1965).

In summary, a strong stimulus capable of producing dishabituation of a habituated pathway in the intact but restrained animal was also capable of producing sensitization of a nonhabituated pathway, at least part of the time. Similar and more consistent effects were seen in unrestrained animals. In the neurophysiological experiments, the same strong stimulus which produced facilitation of a decremented EPSP usually also produced facilitation of a nondecremented EPSP. Taken together, these data support the notion that dishabituation of the gill-withdrawal reflex is not simply the removal of habituation, but is an independent process, a special case of sensitization. Dishabituation differs from sensitization only in involving a previously habituated response. These and other neurophysiological findings (see Castellucci et al., 1970) suggest that the neuronal correlates of habituation and dishabituation (sensitization) involve two separate regulatory mechanisms acting on a common set of synapses. Habituation leads to a prolonged decrease in synaptic efficacy which is limited to the stimulated pathway; sensitization leads to a briefer but more widespread heterosynaptic facilitation of synaptic efficacy involving both stimulated and unstimulated pathways (Fig. 21). The differences in the spatial extent of the pathways mediating habituation and sensitization (dishabituation) explains the lack of generalization of habituation as well as the evident generalization of sensitization to nonhabituated pathways.

Available evidence from behavioral studies in vertebrates also indicates that habituation and dishabituation are separate processes, suggesting that this interrelationship may be quite general (see, for example, Hagbarth and

---

[4] Data were pooled for presentation (Fig. 20) from five experiments in which two different interstimulus intervals were used: in three experiments, 30 sec (N = 8 runs); in one experiment, 30 sec (N = 1 run) and 10 sec (N = 7 runs); and in one experiment, 10 sec (N = 2 runs). Statistical comparison of EPSP facilitation was made by means of a sign test. For each experiment a single score (the mean percent facilitation for all runs) was computed for both decremented and nondecremented EPSPs. In every experiment facilitation of decremented EPSPs was observed ($p < 0.031$), and facilitation of nondecremented EPSPs exceeded 100% ($p < 0.031$).

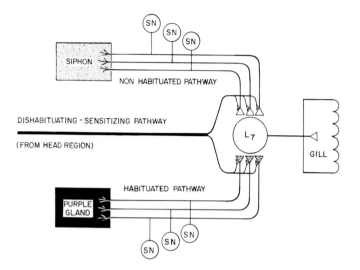

FIG. 21. Schematic model of habituation and dishabituation. Following stimulation of the purple gland, the habituation is restricted to that pathway because of a homosynaptic decrement at the synapses between the sensory neurons and the motor neuron (L7). By contrast, dishabituation affects both the habituated pathway (purple gland) and the non-habituated one (siphon). The difference in spatial extent of the pathways mediating habituation (shaded synapses) and sensitization (dishabituation) explains the lack of generalization of habituation as well as the evident generalization of sensitization (dis-habituation). The model postulates that the sensitizing pathway (which is not necessarily monosynaptic) mediates presynaptic facilitation on the synapse between the primary sensory neurons (SN) and the motor neuron L7. The model deals only with the mono-synaptic components of the reflex. The polysynaptic components have not been analyzed but apparently do not contribute significantly to generalization (from Carew et al., 1971).

Kugelberg, 1958; Spencer et al., 1966*a*). Thus, in studies of human ab-dominal reflexes, Hagbarth and Kugelberg (1958) found that habituation was restricted to the stimulated site and there was very little generalization. Habituation of the reflex by stimulating one abdominal site had no effect on the response elicited by a neighboring region 3 to 4 cm away. This distance represents the approximate limit of a subject's capacity for two-point discrimination (Fig. 22). Although detailed psychological studies were not done, Hagbarth and Kugelberg report that during habituation subjects sometimes perceived an illusion of declining stimulus intensity and that during sensitization they sometimes perceived the illusion of increasing intensity of the test stimulus. They also found that a strong stimulus enhanced habituated abdominal reflexes beyond control value (Fig. 23) and could also facilitate nonhabituated responses. They write:

> Sensitization also increases the spatial irradiation of the reflex in the musculature of the abdominal wall. . . . It often irradiates to the flexor muscles of the extremities and causes general crouching of the

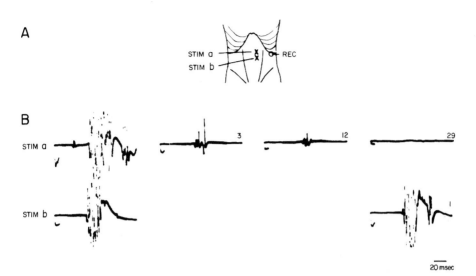

FIG. 22. Lack of generalization of habituation of human abdominal reflexes. *(A):* Electrical stimuli are applied at sites *a* and *b* of the abdomen 4 to 5 cm apart. Recordings are obtained by inserting electrodes in the left external oblique muscles (Rec). Stimuli were applied every 5 to 10 sec. *(B):* A single stimulus was first applied to sites *a* and *b*. Then site *a* was repeatedly stimulated for 29 trials (of which trials 3, 12, and 29 are illustrated) and dishabituation of the abdominal reflex was produced. A single stimulus now applied to site *b* still showed full reflex responsiveness, indicating specificity of habituation to the stimulated pathway. Repeated stimulation at site *b* also did not generalize to *a* (from Hagbarth and Kugelberg, 1958).

body . . . with increasing strength of sensitization the abdominal skin reflex gradually emerges into a more widespread reaction which has a striking resemblance not only to startle responses . . . but also to the pathological abdominal mass reflexes sometimes encountered in spinal man. . . . (p. 311)

The proposed relationship of sensitized abdominal responses to pathological mass reflexes is interesting. In a sense the heightened responsiveness of the sensitized siphon-withdrawal reflex in *Aplysia* also resembles, in its inappropriateness a pathological reflex, because it persists for many days after the noxious stimulation has stopped (Figs. 9 and 10). A heightened reflex responsiveness was appropriate for the animal as long as it lived in a dangerous environment in which it was exposed to daily stressful stimuli, but the heightened responses are inappropriate for the neutral environment in which the animal lives after training. These observations raise the possibility that prolonged sensitization might serve as a model for behavioral abnormalities.

This possibility is consistent with the idea recently proposed by Groves and Thompson (1970) that sensitization is an instance of a more general

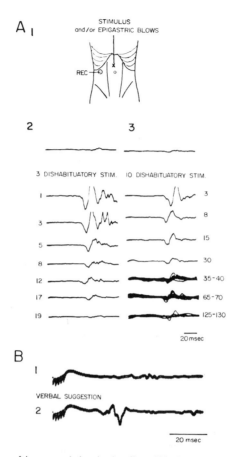

FIG. 23. Sensitization of human abdominal reflex. *(A):* Skin stimulus applied to epigastrium. *(A₁):* Recordings obtained from right external oblique. *(A₂):* Repeated mechanical stimuli (at 5 to 10 sec intervals) are applied to the epigastrium and produce habituation of reflex response (top trace). Three dishabituating stimuli are then applied (blows to the epigastrium). These produce sensitization of the decremented response that last for the next 17 trials. *(A₃):* Following the 19th stimulus in *A₂*, 10 dishabituating stimuli were applied and produced more prolonged sensitization that lasted for the next 125 trials. *(B):* Sensitization by verbal suggestion. *(B₁):* A weak electrical stimulus applied to the epigastrium produced no response but became effective *(B₂)* after subject was told that the next stimulus would be painful (from Hagbarth and Kugelberg, 1958).

state, i.e., behavioral "arousal." From an analytic point of view, it may be useful to divide behavioral "arousal" into at least two components: (1) orientation, and (2) general, heightened responsiveness to stimuli. Sensitization is analogous to this second component of arousal. Both sensitization and arousal lead to increased responsiveness, and in each case the heightened responsiveness is generalized. Insofar as arousal may include sensitization, it provides an opportunity to substitute a somewhat vague, albeit useful behavioral concept (arousal) for one that is more restricted and more testable (sensitization). For example, "arousal" produced by a high level of background stimulation impairs reflex habituation in vertebrates. Thus, Hagbarth and Kugelberg found that in man attention, expectancy, and apprehension can sensitize habituated responses (Fig. 23B). Long-term sensitization following noxious stimulation in *Aplysia* is crudely analogous to chronic arousal or – to be even more loosely anthropomorphic – may be analogous to chronic fear. It would therefore be of interest to see whether other factors, besides noxious stimuli, known to affect arousal level in vertebrates, such as background sensory stimulation or alterations in level of motivation, can affect the rate of habituation in *Aplysia*.

VII. RELATION OF SHORT- TO LONG-TERM HABITUATION

One of the major issues in the investigation of the neural basis of behavior concerns the relationship between short- and long-term memory. A key question is: are the processes which underlie long-term memory the same as those which underlie short-term memory, or are there unique processes which characterize the different stages of memory formation?

That there are different processes of memory formation for short- and long-term memory was first suggested by William James in 1890, and soon supported by Müller and Pilzecker's experiments in 1900. They found that a subject would forget recently learned material if he engaged in "vigorous mental activity." They called this forgetting "retroactive interference" and suggested that the memory was impaired because the subsequent disruptive mental activity interfered with the still-persisting neural events which underlie short-term memory. A number of both animal and human learning studies subsequently confirmed Müller and Pilzecker's observation that a newly formed memory was susceptible to disruption for a short period of time after the formation; later the memory became more stable and less capable of being disrupted (Minami and Dallenbach, 1946; Postman and Alper, 1946; for review see McGoech and Irion, 1952).

Early thinking about memory was also influenced by the clinical observation that head trauma or convulsions could produce amnesia for events which recently preceded the trauma, and yet could leave more permanent memories relatively intact. This phenomenon called "retrograde amnesia" was common in epileptics who frequently had amnesia for the events which immediately preceded their seizure. McDougall (1901) suggested that the retroactive interference found by Müller and Pilzecker might explain retrograde amnesia.

In 1949 retrograde amnesia was experimentally produced in animals by Duncan. Using electroconvulsive shock to produce an epileptic-like grand mal seizure, he found that short-term memory appeared to be differently affected than long-term memory by the seizure. In the same year, Hebb (1949) developed a dual-trace hypothesis based on two different memory processes (see also Gerard, 1949). Hebb suggested that short-term memory consisted of a labile and easily disrupted reverberating electrical activity in closed neuronal circuits in the brain. Long-term memory reflected a more permanent structural change in the brain.

During the next 20 years, many experiments attempted to examine conditions under which both short-term and long-term memories could be impaired or facilitated (for review see McGaugh and Herz, 1972). In addition to convulsions, a variety of other methods, all usually injurious to brain function, were used to interfere with the short-term process: spreading depression, hypothermia, anoxia. Puromycin, cycloheximides, and other antibiotics that inhibit protein synthesis were found to interfere with long-term learning (Flexner, Flexner, and Stellar, 1963; Agranoff, Davis, Casola, and Lim, 1967; Barondes and Cohen, 1966, 1968).

A picture that emerged from these studies was that short-term memory involved a labile process which converted to a more stable neural process if allowed to run its course (see Russell, 1959; McGaugh, 1966). This simplified picture has been criticized on several points. The time course of short-term memory as based on studies of retrograde amnesia can vary from seconds (Chorover and Schiller, 1965; Quartermain, Paolino, and Miller, 1965) to hours or even days (Kopp, Bohdanecky, and Jarvik, 1966) depending upon the disruptive procedure and upon the learning task. In some experiments the recently learned material, which at first appeared to be lost as a result of retrograde amnesia, was found to return days or even weeks later (Weiskrantz, 1966). Also, most of the procedures that are used to interfere with memory are traumatic, some devastatingly so, and the data obtained by different memory-blocking agents are not consistent. This led Weiskrantz (1970) to suggest that what appears as short-term memory is only an early sensitive phase of long-term memory.

In an attempt to clarify the relationship between short- and long-term memory, we have examined the conversion from short- to long-term habituation (Carew and Kandel, 1973). For this purpose we used four training sessions, consisting of 10 trials per session, separated by 90 min. This shortened training period leads to satisfactory acquisition of long-term habituation (Figs. 6 and 7) and has the advantage that it allows one to monitor, during a single 5-hr period, the cellular changes that accompany the entire acquisition process.

Using the test system of the isolated ganglion we carried preparations in organ cultures containing streptomycin (0.1 mg/ml), penicillin (20 μ/ml), and glucose (0.1%), and then electrically stimulated an afferent nerve while monitoring the synaptic input it produced in L7. Since the response decrement is limited to the stimulated pathway (Fig. 20), each ganglion contained its own control. This is essential for distinguishing a real decrease in synaptic effectiveness due to repeated stimulation, from deterioration of the preparation due to prolonged isolation. In approximately half of the experiments the siphon nerve was used as the experimental nerve and the branchial nerve as the control; in the remaining experiments the branchial nerve served as the experimental nerve and siphon as control. Stimulus parameters were chosen for both nerves which produced EPSPs of roughly comparable amplitude in L7. The parameters were then held constant throughout both acquisition and retention phases. Input resistance of the motor cell was monitored continuously by injecting hyperpolarizing current pulses into the soma.

In parallel with the behavioral experiments (Fig. 25A), four blocks of 10 stimuli each (interstimulus intervals of 30 sec) were presented to the experimental nerve during acquisition, with 90 min separation between blocks. Following the first block of stimuli to the experimental nerve, a block of 10 stimuli were also delivered to the control nerve at the same interval. Since EPSP decrement produced from stimulation of one nerve does not generalize to the other nerve, repeated stimulation of the control nerve produced comparable decrement (Figs. 24 and 25B). In the second, third, and fourth blocks of 10 stimuli, only the experimental nerve was stimulated and the EPSP decrement built up across blocks, reaching 90% decrement (10% of initial experimental EPSP) in the fourth block (Figs. 24 and 25B). A single test stimulus was presented to the control nerve at the end of the fourth block and occasionally also at the end of the third block (Figs. 24 and 25B). The same statistical tests were used as in the behavioral experiments. The first experimental EPSP of block four was found to be significantly more decremented than the test EPSP from the control nerve ($p < 0.001$). There was also greater decrement of the EPSP to experimental nerve stimulation in block four than in block one. The sum of the responses of trials 1 to 10 of the experimental nerve in block four was significantly less than the sum of responses of the experimental EPSP in block one ($p < 0.005$).

Although some deterioration may have occurred during the experiments, the buildup of EPSP decrement across blocks cannot be accounted for by deterioration or by nonspecific changes that could have occurred in organ culture. Test stimuli to the control nerve produced EPSPs which had recovered to 84.5% of the initial control EPSP. Some portion of even this 15.5% change in that control EPSP is probably not due to deterioration but to the decrement produced by the 10 stimuli delivered to the control nerve in the first block of acquisition 4.5 to 5 hr before. Also, the input resistance of the neuron did not vary by more than 7% throughout the experiments. The buildup of EPSP decrement was therefore chiefly due to the four sessions of 10 stimuli each to the experimental nerve. This buildup (Figs. 24 and 25B) parallels the buildup of behavioral habituation produced in the intact animal with an identical temporal sequence of stimulus presentation (Fig. 25A).

At the end of acquisition, we removed the microelectrode from cell L7, maintained the ganglion for another 24 hr in organ culture, and then re-

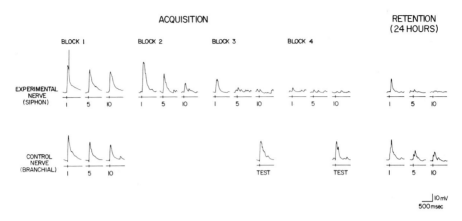

FIG. 24. Acquisition and 24-hr retention of EPSP decrement. Sample records from responses in L7 following stimulation of experimental nerve (siphon) and control nerve
(branchial). Records for the experimental nerve are taken from 1st, 5th, and 10th stimulus
of each of the 10-trial training blocks and 24 hr later during the test for retention. The
control nerve was only stimulated for block 1 of 10 trials. Single test stimuli were applied
to the control nerve at the end of acquisition blocks 3 and 4. A 10-trial block was used
24 hr later to compare retention of EPSP decrement in the experimental nerve to that of
the control nerve. In the 24-hr retention test both experimental and control EPSPs have
partially recovered. The experimental EPSP, however, showed significantly greater ($p <$
0.001) and more rapid decrement than the control EPSP (from Carew and Kandel, 1973).

impaled the motor neuron to test for 1-day retention of EPSP decrement.
We hyperpolarized the membrane to approximately the same level as during
acquisition and stimulated the same nerves with identical parameters
used on the previous day. We found that stimulating the experimental nerve
on the first trial produced a significantly smaller EPSP than the EPSP from
the control nerve ($p < 0.01$). The 10 repeated stimuli to the experimental
nerve also produced significantly greater EPSP decrement than the same
stimulation to the control nerve ($p < 0.01$) (Figs. 24 and 25). The control
nerve also showed decrement but it was much less profound.

Thus the acquisition of long-term habituation involves a gradual but
profound decline in the synaptic potential produced in the gill motor neuron
L7 by stimulation of the afferent nerve. These changes persist for more
than 24 hr. That such limited training (a total of 40 stimuli) should lead to
such prolonged plastic changes in neuronal function is interesting in view
of the generally reported difficulty in both vertebrates and invertebrates
in producing 24-hr long changes in acute experiments even following
thousands of stimuli (Eccles, 1964; Spencer and April, 1970). The ease
with which prolonged neuronal changes were produced in our experiments
is probably attributable to the selection of a stimulus pattern of known
behavioral effectiveness and the use of a synaptic pathway known to be
involved in a modifiable behavioral reflex.

In the test system of the gill-withdrawal reflex in the isolated ganglion,

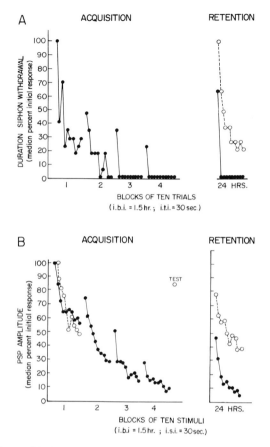

FIG. 25. Comparison of behavioral response decrement and EPSP decrement. *(A):* Acquisition and retention of long-term habituation of siphon withdrawal following four training sessions separated by 1.5 hr. All scores are expressed as a percentage of the median of each group's initial response (block 1, trial 1). The median duration of the initial response was 17 sec for the experimentals and 19 sec for the controls (see Fig. 6C). *(B):* Acquisition and retention of EPSP decrement. The EPSP amplitudes from both experimental (●———●) and control (○———○) nerves (n = 10) are expressed as a percentage of the initial amplitude. In Acquisition, six experiments were run with the siphon nerve as experimental, and four experiments with the branchial nerve as experimental. In block 1, 10 stimuli were first applied to the experimental nerve and then to the control nerve, and produced in L7 comparable EPSP decrement from both nerves, indicating lack of EPSP generalization. Repeated blocks of stimuli to the experimental nerve produced progressive buildup of EPSP decrement. A single test to the control nerve produced an EPSP which was recovered to 84.5% control, indicating that deterioration cannot account for experimental EPSP decrement. In Retention, the cell was reimpaled 24 hr later and repolarized to the membrane potential maintained for Acquisition. The ordinate in Retention was redrawn to indicate that, even though the repolarization can be closely approximated, it cannot be considered to be exact. In the retention test, stimulation of the experimental nerve produced significantly greater EPSP decrement (*p* < 0.001) than stimulation of the control nerve (from Carew and Kandel, 1973).

these synaptic changes obviously occurred centrally and did not involve sensory adaptation or motor fatigue. The alterations also did not result from a change in the soma input resistance, but we cannot exclude more remote resistance changes. Thus these long-term synaptic changes in the complex EPSP resemble, superficially, those found with short-term habituation. Similar appearing synaptic changes in the complex EPSP can be produced by a number of different cellular mechanisms, however. Only after these changes are analyzed on a monosynaptic level will one be able to determine whether short- and long-term habituation results from similar or different cellular mechanisms.

It is interesting to note that the buildup of behavioral habituation across blocks of trials seems to asymptote by the third block, so that except for the first trial, the curves are generally flat by the third block of training (Figs. 4A, 5A, and 25A). One might therefore assume that, because there are no further changes in the behavioral responses after the first trial in blocks three and four, there are no further changes occurring in the nervous system. Yet if one examines the synaptic potential in the gill motor neuron, further decrement occurs throughout the third and fourth blocks of stimulation (compare Figs. 24 and 25B). During these experiments the motor neuron was hyperpolarized to prevent spike discharge. Had the cell not been polarized, the excitatory synaptic input to the cell would have produced action potentials and a concomitant gill contraction until the synaptic potential had decremented to the point where it no longer brought the motor cell to threshold. At this point the behavior it produced would have dropped out. However, even after the behavior was no longer triggered, the synaptic potential would have continued to decrement with continued stimulation. Although undetectable behaviorally, this continued decrement might affect the duration of the habituation or the ease with which rehabituation might occur. Such a mechanism probably underlies the "subzero" effect that has been described as a common feature of habituation, whereby continued stimulation of a completely habituated response prolongs the retention of habituation (Thompson and Spencer, 1966). The point at which the synaptic input is no longer capable of triggering the motor cell provides a behavioral threshold. As long as the EPSPs are above this threshold, decrements in EPSP amplitude produce a concomitant decrement in behavioral response. However, synaptic decrement below this threshold produced no further observable change at the time, even though continual changes in synaptic transmission might still be occurring. Thus, what appears behaviorally to be an all-or-none process may be a continuous one at the level of synaptic transmission.

VII. SUMMARY AND CONCLUSIONS

Because of its simplicity, there has been a long-standing controversy among students of behavior as to whether habituation can be considered learning, even in its most elementary form (see, for example, Miller 1967; Kling, 1971). Often not appreciated in these discussions is that there are restricted and extended forms of the habituation paradigm. In its restricted form, habituation consists of a short-term response decrement lasting minutes or hours. The decremented response recovers spontaneously but cannot be dishabituated or shows only homonymous dishabituation. In its extended form habituation consists of a decrement that is capable of being prolonged to last days and weeks, and the duration of habituation is dependent upon the pattern of stimulation. In addition, the response can be dishabituated heteronymously for hours or days by stimulating an entirely different site or pathway.

Independent of one's definition of learning, what intuitively separates the more interesting forms of learning from the less interesting ones are three features: (1) time course or duration of the memory, (2) specificity to pattern of stimulation, and (3) that ability of the response to be manipulated to cause both an increase and a decrease in response strength. Thus what distinguishes the extended form of the habituation paradigm from the restricted form are features that generally distinguish more interesting learning from less interesting forms. As a result, an effective argument can be made that the extended form of the habituation paradigm blends, almost imperceptibly, with other learning paradigms. As analyses of the neural mechanisms of associative forms of learning become available, a more direct appraisal of their interrelationships to habituation will become possible.

Independent of its relationship to other forms of learning, the extended form of the habituation paradigm provides an unusually powerful tool for studying how behavior becomes modified. For the ability to habituate to non-noxious stimuli is not simply a laboratory paradigm but is fundamental to modifications in most instinctive, reflex, and perceptual processes. An understanding of the cellular basis of the extended form of the habituation paradigm is thus likely to provide principles of behavioral and neural plasticity which are of wide generality.

Studies of habituation are particularly useful for studying memory. Here these studies might answer the question: is the long-term form of habituation different from the short-term form? Does the long-term form require a structural change in the nervous system that is dependent on new macromolecular synthesis? This idea has been tested in more complex types of learning in vertebrates by examining the effects of protein and RNA synthesis inhibitors on long-term memories (Flexner et al., 1963; Barondes and Cohen, 1966, 1968; Agranoff et al., 1967). The results obtained suggest that long-term memory requires the synthesis of new protein and perhaps even of new RNA. The interpretation of these results is difficult, however, because the inhibitors produce other physiological side effects and because most of the studies rely solely on behavioral criteria for the assessment of memory impairment. In *Aplysia,* where inhibitors can be applied directly to the isolated abdominal ganglion, the neural correlates of short-term retention of habituation were found not to require protein synthesis (Schwartz, Castellucci, and Kandel, 1971). It may now be possible to investigate whether or not new protein synthesis is required for long-term habituation. If it is required, one might also be able to specify when in the conversion from short- to long-term retention, protein synthesis becomes necessary.

However, before a meaningful biochemical study of these processes can be undertaken, it would be useful to have a more decisive analysis of the synaptic changes accompanying habituation and dishabituation. So far our studies have been quite superficial. Although we can localize the short-term change to specific synaptic sites, we have not yet specified whether the locus of the synaptic alterations is pre- or postsynaptic. Thus, we cannot rule out receptor desensitization as a possible mechanism for habituation, although the ease with which a decremented synapse can be facilitated makes a presynaptic explanation more likely. If one can determine that the change is presynaptic, it will be necessary to distinguish further between a change in the availability of transmitter, in the probability of release, or in the number of release sites. A quantal analysis of synaptic transmission at the synapses between sensory and motor neurons may help to distinguish between these possibilities. To probe further into the mechanism will prove more difficult because we know so little about the morphology of the synaptic neuropil. Indeed, the understanding of synaptic morphology in invertebrate is generally rather rudimentary. A more complete analysis of the neural basis of behavioral plasticity will ultimately require a better understanding of the synaptic fine structure underlying behavior.

ACKNOWLEDGMENTS

We thank Drs. Vincent Castellucci, Irving Kupfermann, John Koester, and William Alden Spencer for their comments on an earlier draft of this chapter. The original research reported in this paper was supported by grants NIMH 19795–02 and NS 09361–03. Dr. Kandel is also supported by a Career Scientist Award No. MH 18558–06 and Dr. Carew by a Special Fellowship from NIMH MH 5355 1–01.

REFERENCES

Agranoff, B. W., Davis, R. E., Casola, L., and Lim, R. (1967): Actinomycin D blocks formation of memory of shock-avoidance in goldfish. *Science*, 158:1600–1601.
Barondes, S. H., and Cohen, H. D. (1966): Puromycin effect on successive phases of memory storage. *Science*, 151:594–595.
Barondes, S. H., and Cohen, H. D. (1968): Memory impairment after subcutaneous injection of acetoxycyclohexamide. *Science*, 160:556–557.
Bennett, M. V. L. (1974): *This Volume*.
Bullock, T. H., and Horridge, G. A. (1965): *Structure and Function in the Nervous Systems of Invertebrates*. Freeman, San Francisco.

Carew, T. J., Castellucci, V. F., and Kandel. E. R. (1971): An analysis of dishabituation and sensitization of the gill-withdrawal reflex in *Aplysia. Intern. J. Neurosci.*, 2:79–98.

Carew, T. J., and Kandel, E. R. (1973): A cellular analysis of acquisition and retention of long-term habituation in *Aplysia. Science*, 182:1158–1160.

Carew, T. J., Pinsker, H. M., and Kandel, E. R. (1972): Long-term habituation of a defensive withdrawal reflex in *Aplysia. Science*, 175:451–454.

Castellucci, V. F., and Kandel, E. R. (1974): Properties of excitatory and inhibitory interneurons mediating the defensive withdrawal reflex of the mantle organ of *Aplysia. (in preparation)*

Castellucci, V., Pinsker, H., Kupfermann, I., and Kandel, E. R. (1970): Neuronal mechanisms of habituation and dishabituation of the gill-withdrawal reflex in *Aplysia. Science*, 167:1745–1748.

Chorover, S. L., and Schiller. P. H. (1965): Short-term retrograde amnesia in rats. *J. Comp. Physiol. Psychol.*, 59:73–78.

Davis, W. J., and Mpitsos, G. J. (1971): Behavioral choice and habituation in the marine mollusk *Pleurobranchaea californica*. MacFarland. (Gastropoda. Opisthobranchia) *Z. vergl. Physiol.*, 75:207–232.

Duncan, C. P. (1949): The retroactive effect of electroshock on learning. *J. Comp. Physiol. Psychol.*, 42:32–44.

Eccles, J. C. (1964): *The Physiology of Synapses.* Springer-Verlag, Berlin.

Farel, P. B. (1971): Long-lasting habituation in spinal frogs. *Brain Res.*, 33:405–417.

Flexner, J. B., Flexner, C. B., and Stellar. E. (1963): Memory in mice as affected by intra-cerebral puromycin. *Science*, 141:57–59.

Gerard, R. W. (1949): Physiology and psychiatry. *Am. J. Psychiat.*, 106:161–173.

Gerschenfeld, H. M. (1973): Chemical transmission in invertebrate central nervous systems and neuromuscular junctions. *Physiol. Rev.*, 53:1–119.

Glaser, E. M. (1966): *The Physiological Basis of Habituation.* Oxford University Press, London.

Groves, P. M., and Thompson. R. F. (1970): Habituation: A dual-process theory. *Psych. Rev.*, 77:419–450.

Hagbarth, K. E., and Kugelberg. E. (1958): Plasticity of the human abdominal skin reflex. *Brain*, 81:305–319.

Hebb, D. O. (1949): *The Organization of Behavior.* Wiley, New York.

Hilgard, E. R., and Bower. G. H. (1966): *Theories of Learning* (3rd edition). Appleton-Century-Crofts, New York.

Hinde, R. A. (1954): Factors governing the changes in strength of a partially inborn response, as shown by the mobbing behaviour of the chaffinch *(Fringilla coelebs)*. II: The waning of the response. *Proc. Roy. Soc. Lond. B*, 142:331–358.

James, W. (1890). *Principles of Psychology* (2 volumes). Holt, New York.

Kandel, E. R., and Gardner, D. (1972): The synaptic actions mediated by the different branches of a single neuron. In: *Neurotransmitters Res. Publ. A.R.N.M.D.*, 50:91–144.

Kandel, E. R., and Spencer, W. A. (1968): Cellular neurophysiological approaches in the study of learning. *Physiol. Rev.*, 48:65–134.

Kandel, E. R., and Tauc. L. (1965): Heterosynaptic facilitation in neurones of the abdominal ganglion of *Aplysia depilans. J. Physiol.*, 181:1–27.

Kling, J. W. (1971): Learning: Introductory Survey. In: *Woodworth and Schlosberg's Experimental Psychology* (3rd edition), edited by J. W. Kling and L. A. Riggs. pp. 551–613. Holt, Rinehart and Winston Inc., New York.

Koester, J., Mayeri, E., Liebeswar, G., and Kandel, E. R. (1974): Neuronal circuit controlling the circulation in *Aplysia*. II. Interneurons. *(in press)*

Konorski, J. (1948): *Conditioned Reflexes and Neuronal Organization.* Cambridge University Press, London.

Konorski, J. (1967): *Integrative Activity of the Brain: An Interdisciplinary Approach.* University of Chicago Press, Chicago.

Kopp, R., Bohdanecky, Z., and Jarvik, M. (1966): Long temporal gradient of retrograde amnesia for a well-discriminated stimulus. *Science*, 153:1547–1549.

Kupfermann, I., Carew, T. J., and Kandel, E. R. (1974): Local, reflex, and central commands controlling gill and siphon movements in *Aplysia. (in preparation)*

Kupfermann, I., Castellucci, V., Pinsker, H., and Kandel, E. R. (1970): Neuronal correlates of habituation and dishabituation of the gill-withdrawal reflex in *Aplysia. Science,* 167:1743–1745.

Kupfermann, I., and Kandel, E. R. (1969): Neuronal controls of a behavioral response mediated by the abdominal ganglion of *Aplysia. Science,* 164:847–850.

Kupfermann, I., Pinsker, H., Castellucci, V., and Kandel, E. R. (1971): Central and peripheral control of gill movements in *Aplysia. Science,* 174:1252–1256.

Lukowiak, K., and Jacklet, J. W. (1972): Habituation and dishabituation: Interactions between peripheral and central nervous systems in *Aplysia. Science,* 178:1306–1308.

Macpherson, S. J., Dees, V., and Grindley, G. C. (1949): The effect of knowledge of results on learning and performance. III. The influence of the time interval between trials. *Quart. J. Exp. Psychol.,* 1:167–174.

Mayeri, E., Koester, J., Liebeswar, G., Kupfermann, I., and Kandel, E. R. (1974): Neuronal circuit controlling the circulation in *Aplysia.* I. Motor neurons. *(in press)*

McDougall, W. (1901): Experimentelle beitrage zur lehre vom gedachtniss. edited by G. E. Müller and A. Pilzecker. *Mind,* 10:388–394.

McGaugh, J. L. (1966): Time-dependent processes in memory storage. *Science,* 153:1351–1358.

McGaugh, J. L., and Herz, M. J. (1972): *Memory Consolidation.* Albion Press. San Francisco.

McGeoch, J. A., and Irion, A. L. (1952): *The Psychology of Human Learning* (2nd edition). Longmans, Green and Co., New York.

Miller, N. E. (1967): Certain facts of learning relevant for its physical basis. In: *The Neurosciences,* edited by G. C. Quarton, T. Melnechuk, and F. O. Schmitt, pp. 643–652. Rockefeller University Press, New York.

Minami, H., and Dallenbach, K. M. (1946): The effect of activity upon learning and retention in the cockroach. *Amer. J. Psychol.,* 59:1–58.

Müller, G. E., and Pilzecker, A. (1900): Experimentelle beitrage zur lehre vom gedachtniss. *Journal de Psychologia. Erganzungband,* 1:1–300.

Nicholls, J. G., and Purves, D. (1970): Monosynaptic chemical and electrical connexions between sensory and motor cells in the central nervous system of the leech. *J. Physiol.,* 209:647–667.

Paine, T. J. (1963): Food recognition and predation on opisthobranchs by *Navanax inermis. Veliger,* 6:1–9.

Pavlov, I. P. (1927): *Conditioned Reflexes. An Investigation of the Physiological Activity of the Cerebral Cortex,* translated and edited by G. V. Anrep. Oxford University Press: Humphrey Milford, London.

Peretz, B. (1970): Habituation and dishabituation in the absence of a central nervous system. *Science,* 169:379–381.

Petrinovich, L. (1973): A species-meaningful analysis of habituation. In: *Habituation: Behavioral Studies and Physiological Substrates,* edited by H. V. S. Peeke and H. J. Herz. Academic Press, New York.

Pinsker, H., Hening, W., Carew, T., and Kandel, E. R. (1973): Long-term sensitization of a defensive withdrawal reflex in *Aplysia. Science,* 182:1039–1042.

Pinsker, H., Kupfermann, I., Castellucci, V., and Kandel, E. (1970): Habituation and dishabituation of the gill-withdrawal reflex in *Aplysia. Science,* 167:1740–1742.

Postman, L., and Alper, T. G. (1946): Retroactive inhibition as a function of the time of interpolation of the inhibitor between learning and recall. *Amer. J. Psychol.,* 59:439–449.

Quartermain, D., Paolino, R. M., and Miller, N. E. (1965): A brief temporal gradient of retrograde amnesia independent of situational change. *Science,* 149:1116–1118.

Russell, W. R. (1959): *Brain Memory Learning, A Neurologist's View.* Clarendon Press, Oxford.

Schwartz, J. H., Castellucci, V. F., and Kandel, E. R. (1971): Functioning of identified neurons and synapses in abdominal ganglion of *Aplysia* in absence of protein synthesis. *J. Neurophysiol.,* 34:939–953.

Sharpless, S., and Jasper, H. (1956): Habituation of the arousal reaction. *Brain,* 79:655–680.

Siegel, S. (1956): *Nonparametric Statistics (For the Behavioral Sciences).* McGraw-Hill, New York.

Sokolov, E. N. (1960): Neuronal models and the orienting reflex. In: *The Central Nervous System and Behavior,* edited by M. A. B. Brazier. Josiah Macy, Jr. Foundation, New York.

Sokolov, E. N. (1963): *Perception and the Conditioned Reflex,* translated by S. W. Waydenfeld, edited by R. Worters and A. Clarke. Pergamon Press, Oxford.

Spencer, W. A., and April, R. S. (1970): Plastic properties of monosynaptic pathways in mammals. In: *Short-term Changes in Neural Activity and Behavior*, edited by G. Horn and R. Hinde, pp. 433–474. Cambridge University Press, Cambridge.

Spencer, W. A., Thompson, R. F., and Neilson, D. R., Jr. (1966a): Response decrement of the flexion reflex in the acute spinal cat and transient restoration by strong stimuli. *J. Neurophysiol.*, 29:221–239.

Spencer, W. A., Thompson, R. F., and Neilson, D. R., Jr. (1966b): Decrement of ventral root electrotonus and intracellularly recorded PSPs produced by iterated cutaneous afferent volleys. *J. Neurophysiol.*, 29:253–274.

Tauc, L. (1967): Transmission in invertebrate and vertebrate ganglia. *Physiol. Rev.*, 47:521–593.

Thompson, R. F., and Spencer, W. A. (1966): Habituation: A model phenomenon for the study of neuronal substrates of behavior. *Psych. Rev.*, 173:16–43.

Thorpe, W. H. (1963): *Learning and Instinct in Animals* (2nd edition). Harvard University Press, Cambridge, Mass.

Wall, P. D. (1970): Habituation and post-tetanic potentiation in the spinal cord. In: *Short-term Changes in Neural Activity and Behavior*, edited by G. Horn and R. Hinde, pp. 181–210. Cambridge University Press, Cambridge.

Weiskrantz, L. (1966): Experimental studies of amnesia. In: *Amnesia*, edited by C. Whitty and O. Zangwill, pp. 1–35. Butterworth, London.

Weiskrantz, L. (1970): A long-term view of short-term memory in psychology. In: *Short-term Changes in Neural Activity and Behavior*, edited by G. Horn and R. Hinde, pp. 63–74. Cambridge University Press, Cambridge.

Wickelgren, B. G. (1967a): Habituation of spinal motoneurons. *J. Neurophysiol.*, 30:1404–1423.

Wickelgren, B. G. (1967b): Habituation of spinal interneurons. *J. Neurophysiol.*, 30:1424–1438.

Willows, A. O. D. (1968): Behavioral acts elicited by stimulation of single identifiable nerve cells. In: *Physiological and Biochemical Aspects of Nervous Integration*, edited by F. D. Carlson, pp. 217–243. Prentice-Hall, Englewood Cliffs, N.J.

Zucker, R. S. (1972): Crayfish escape behavior and central synapses. II. Physiological mechanisms underlying behavioral habituation. *J. Neurophysiol.*, 35:621–637.

SUBJECT INDEX

A

Acetylcholine
 axonal transport of, 248-251
 in cisternae, 75
 depolarizes *Aplysia* D cell, 10, 11
 distribution in zonal centrifugation
  of *Torpedo* electroplax, 221
 hyperpolarizes *Aplysia* H cell, 10, 11
 inhibitory action in snail neurons, 9
 ionic gates, activation of, 12
 kinetics of receptor interaction, 51
 rate of synthesis, 247
 release from synaptic vesicles upon
  stimulation of electroplax, 229-237
 release of labeled ACh from nerve
  upon stimulation, 253-256
 subcellular distribution, 251-253
 synthesis in cell body, 241-247
 uptake of choline limits synthesis
  rate, 241-245
Acetylcholinesterase, 46
 absence of activity in cultured neuromuscular preparations, 268
 distribution in zonal centrifugation of
  Torpedo electroplax, 221
 separation from receptor suspension,
  181-182
 and time course of end-plate currents,
  51
Acetylcholine receptor, nicotinic, 142,
  144, 179-189, 191-215
 assay for receptor, 180
 distribution of, on neuroblastoma
  cells, 320-322, 325-327
 ionic gates, 14-15
 localization by autoradiography,
  288-289, 292, 295
 metabolic inhibitors block incorporation of new receptors into
  membranes, 296-300
 morphogenesis, 291-300
 Naja naja venom binding, 179-180,
  184-185, 194-205, 328-331
 purification, 181-183, 191-194,
  205-213
 sites increased in denervation
  supersensitivity, 291

 synaptogenesis and receptor sensitivity, 316-318
Acetyl CoA, 247
Action potential presynaptic, 23
Adenosine triphosphate, 217, 229
 release from synaptic vesicles, 229-237
Amacrine cells, 88
γ-Aminobutyric acid, 11
 depolarizes *Aplysia* H cells, 12
 desensitization and, 13
 inhibits *Aplysia* D cells, 12
Ampullae of Lorenzini, skate, 120-134
 depolarizing post-synaptic potentials,
  124-129
 effect of altered ionic composition
  of medium, 126-130
 hyperpolarizing post-synaptic
  potentials, 122-124
 intracellular recordings, 121
Anion permselective channels, 8
Anodal bursts, 26
Aplysia
 behavioral modifications in, 339-380
 central mediation of long-term
  habituation, 352-354
 habituation and dishabituation,
  344-357
 methodological problems in studies
  of, 340-344, 357-359
 relation of short-term to long-term
  habituation, 373-378
 sensitization and dishabituation,
  363-373
 synaptic analysis of short-term
  habituation and dishabituation,
  359-363
Aspartate, 11
 effects on electroreceptors, 118-119
 as possible transmitter in photoreceptor synapse, 99-100
Axoplasmic flow
 acetylcholine transport, 248-251
 retrograde transport of horseradish
  peroxidase, 76

B

Barium, effect on synaptic electrogenesis, 16